MUSCULAR SYSTEM

Dr. Ahmed Taha

ALLIED HEALTH PRESS

Muscular System

Author: **Dr. Ahmed Taha**

Allied Health Press
4164 Lakeshore Road
Burlington ON L7L 1A4
Canada
www.alliedhealthpress.com
Email: orders@arclereducation.com

ISBN: 978-1-77956-227-2

ABOUT THE AUTHOR

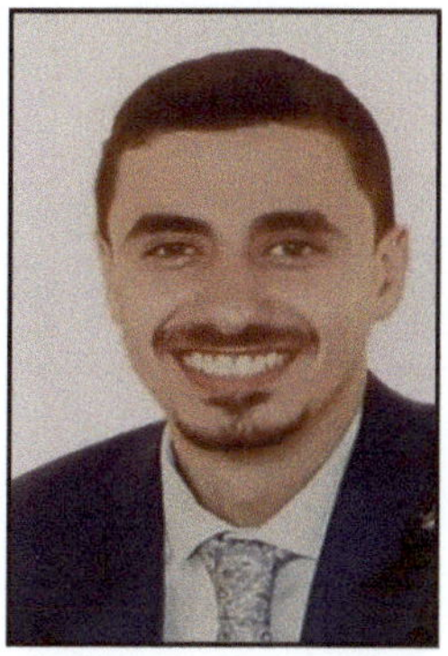

Dr. Ahmed Taha Abdel Sattar, MD, M.Sc. (c), MBChB, is a distinguished graduate of Fayoum University with a GPA of 4 (Summa Cum Laude). Currently a Teaching Assistant in Ophthalmology at Fayoum University Hospital, he has over 14 peer-reviewed publications with 100+ citations and five years of experience in international medical publications. Committed to advancing medical knowledge and patient care, he mentors future healthcare professionals while providing compassionate care to patients.

Word Roots, Prefixes, and Suffixes by Chapter

Chapter 1 Muscular System: An Overview

Duct/o: To draw
Leiomy/o: Smooth visceral muscle
Pronati/o: Facing down or backward
Rhabdomy/o: Skeletal or striated muscle
-desis: Surgical fixation
-ectomy: Surgical removal or excision
-graph: Instrument used to record

Chapter 2 Muscle Metabolism

Fasci/o: Fascia (band of tissue surrounding muscle)
Myocardi/o: Heart muscle
Sarc/o: Soft, fleshy, or connective tissue
-algia: Pain in fibrous tissue
-dynia: Pain
-gram: Record
-itis: Inflammation

Chapter 3 Skeletal Muscle Mechanics

Fibr/o: Fibers
Flex/o: Bend
Supinati/o: Facing up or forward
Tens/o: Stretch
-graphy: The process of recording
-ology: Study of, process of study
-oma: Tumor or mass

Chapter 4 Smooth Muscle

My/o: Muscle
Myos/o: Muscle
-otomy: To cut into
-pathy: Disease
-plasty: Surgical reconstruction, or shaping of
-rrhaphy: Suture repair

Chapter 5 Cardiac Muscle

transversus: abdominis (abdominal muscle)
aden-: glands
brachi-: the arm
capit-, cep-, ceph-: the head
cardi-, coron-: the heart

Chapter 6 Abdominal Muscle

adren-: the adrenal glands
bronch(i)-: the lungs
cerebr-, encephal-: the brain
cervic-: the neck
cholecyst-: the gallbladder
clav-, cleid-: collar bone

Chapter 7 Muscle Tissue

angi-: blood vessels
carp-: the wrist
enter-: the intestines
gastro-: the stomach
glut-: buttocks
gyno-, gyneco-: woman

Chapter 8 Muscle Adaptations

arthr-, articul-: joints
axill-: armpit region
cyst-: bladder
hepat-: the liver
kary-: nucleus
lumb-: loin, lower spine region
muscul-, myo-: muscle

Chapter 9 Spinal Muscular Atrophy

chondr-: cartilage
col-, colo-, colono-: the colon/large intestine
cost-, pleur-: the ribs
omo-: shoulder
pect-: chest

ped-: foot

plant-, sole-, tars-: sole of foot

Ot/o-: Ear

Ovar/i-, Ovario-, Ovi-, Ovo-: Ovary

Chapter 10 Muscle Disorders and Diseases

abdom-: the abdomen

adip-: fat/fatty tissue

arteri-: arteries

osse-, ossi-, ost(eo)-: bone

poll-: thumb

thromb-: blood clot

vas-, vasculo-: blood vessel

ven-, (phlebo): veins, venous blood

viscer-: the internal organs

Table of Contents

LIST OF FIGURES

kinase; mTOR = mammalian target of rapamycin; PI-3K = phosphatidylinositol-3 kinase; p70 S6K = 70 kDa ribosomal protein S6 kinase; 4E-BP1 = eukaryotic initiation factor 4 E

Figure 10.5. A schematic illustration of the main molecular mechanisms underlying muscle wasting and thereby to muscle fatigue (red lines/arrows indicate downregulation, blue lines/arrows indicate upregulation)

LIST OF TABLES

PREFACE

The musculoskeletal system is a crucial system in the human body that provides support, shape, and stability, allowing for joint movement. It is primarily composed of bones, skeletal muscles, tendons, ligaments, intervertebral discs, and articular cartilage tissue, along with associated nerves and blood vessels. These tissues are prone to injury due to their functions, making musculoskeletal disorders a prevalent health issue globally. Recent decades have seen significant advancements in understanding the pathophysiology of the musculoskeletal system, leading to the identification of new molecular targets for therapeutic interventions. Innovative approaches such as tissue engineering, regenerative medicine, gene therapies, drug delivery systems, microgravity studies, and nutritional interventions have expanded our knowledge of conditions like osteoarthritis, rheumatoid arthritis, sarcopenia, muscle wasting, osteoporosis, bone necrosis, and others.

The objective of "Muscular System: A Holistic Approach" is to provide a comprehensive understanding of the human musculoskeletal system and its interconnected nature. This book aims to bridge the gap between traditional reductionist views and holistic perspectives, offering insights into how different parts of the musculoskeletal system work together as a unified whole.

By exploring the intricate relationships between muscles, bones, joints, and connective tissues, this book seeks to enhance the reader's appreciation of the complexity and resilience of the human body. Through detailed anatomical descriptions, physiological explanations, and clinical insights, readers will gain a deeper understanding of how injuries or dysfunctions in one part of the body can affect seemingly unrelated areas.

The interconnected nature of the human body has been a subject of fascination and study for millennia. Ancient beliefs, such as the humors, sought to link specific organs with broader aspects of human experience, like courage and hope. Today, we recognize the gut-brain connection as a key example of how different parts of the body are intertwined, influencing each other in complex ways.

Despite this, there's often a conflict between this holistic view and the reductionist approach of modern science, which breaks the body down into its individual parts for study. While this reductionist approach has led to great advances, it can sometimes overlook the intricate relationships between different parts of the body.

The musculoskeletal system is a prime example of this interconnectedness. While medical practice often focuses on treating specific injuries or conditions in isolated parts of the body, such as the hand, foot, or ankle, clinicians understand that these injuries can have far-reaching effects. An ankle injury, for instance, can lead to changes in gait that result in chronic back pain, while a shoulder injury can affect posture and cause neck discomfort.

Understanding these complex interactions requires a holistic approach that considers the entire system, not just individual parts. In this book, we deal with this holistic perspective, exploring the fundamental relationships between different parts of the musculoskeletal system and how they can impact one another. The book is designed for a wide range of readers, including students and professionals in the fields of anatomy, physiology, physical therapy, sports medicine, and orthopedics. It is also valuable for anyone interested in learning more about their own musculoskeletal system and how to maintain its health and function.

Whether you are a healthcare professional seeking to enhance your clinical knowledge, a student exploring the complexities of the human body, or an individual curious about the inner workings of your own muscles and bones, this text provides a comprehensive and accessible resource. Through its detailed exploration of the musculoskeletal system, this book aims to inspire a greater appreciation for the interconnectedness of the human body and the importance of taking a holistic approach to health and well-being.

Chapter

MUSCULAR SYSTEM: AN OVERVIEW

1

Contents

Introduction

Muscle fibers are specialized cells that make up the muscular system. Their ability to contract is their main feature. Muscles attached to bones, internal organs, and blood vessels facilitate movement. Muscle contraction underlies nearly all bodily movements. Exceptions include the movement of cilia, the flagella of sperm cells, and the amoeboid movement of certain white blood cells. Movements as simple as walking and running are the result of the coordinated action of joints, bones, and skeletal muscles. More delicate skeletal muscle movements also result in different facial expressions, eye movements, and breathing patterns. Muscle contraction serves the body's needs for posture, joint stability, and heat production in addition to facilitating movement. Muscle contraction is responsible for maintaining posture, including sitting and standing. The skeletal muscles maintain the body's stationary postures by continuously making minute adjustments. Many muscles' tendons cover joints, which helps to maintain joint stability. Muscle tendons play a significant role in stabilizing the knee and shoulder joints, where this is especially noticeable. A crucial byproduct of muscle metabolism is the generation of heat, which is necessary to maintain body temperature. Muscle contraction generates almost 85% of the heat that the body produces.

Orientation and Directional Terms:

Term	Definition	Illustration
Blood vessel muscle	They handle a large amount of force and pressure from your blood flow but don't carry a large volume of blood. At any given time, only about 10% to 15% of your body's blood is in your arteries.	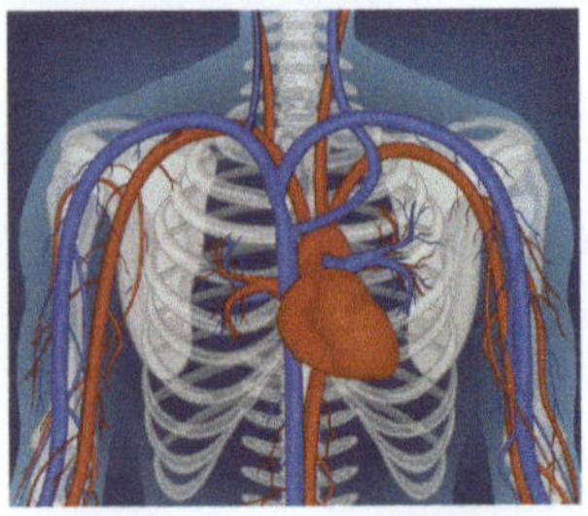
Cardiac muscle	One of three types of vertebrate muscle tissues, with the other two being skeletal muscle and smooth muscle. It is an involuntary, striated muscle that constitutes the main tissue of the wall of the heart.	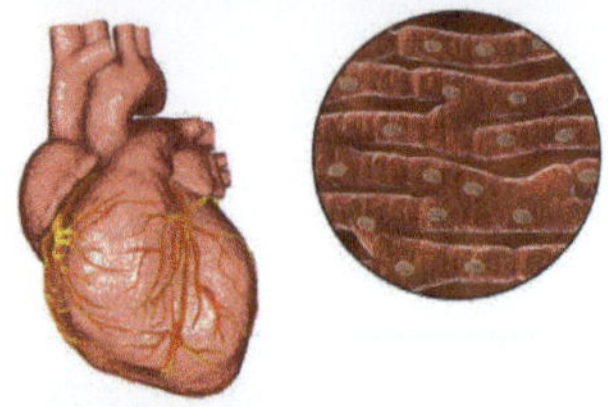
Fibromyalgia	Fibromyalgia is a disorder characterized by widespread musculoskeletal pain accompanied by fatigue, sleep, memory and mood issues. Researchers believe that fibromyalgia amplifies painful sensations by affecting the way your brain and spinal cord process painful and nonpainful signals.	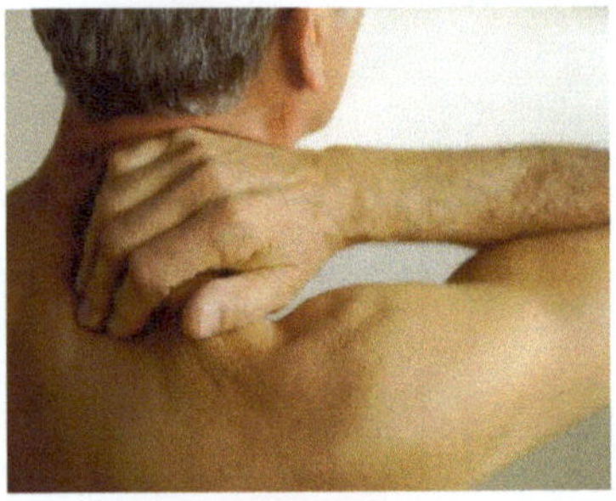
Muscle fiber	Muscle fibers are typically large cells, some 20–100 μm in diameter and many centimeters long, with the longest fibers being about 12 cm.	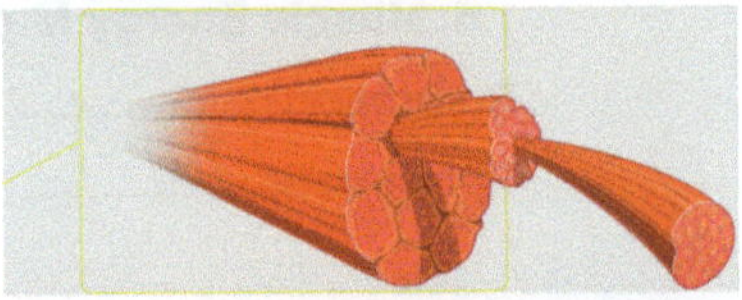
Muscle strain	An injury to a muscle or a tendon — the fibrous tissue that connects muscles to bones. Minor injuries may only overstretch a muscle or tendon, while more severe injuries may involve partial or complete tears in these tissues.	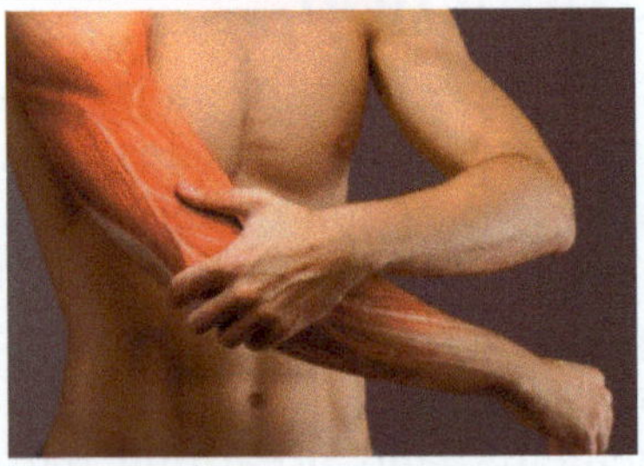

1.1. Human Muscle System

Human muscle system: the voluntary controllable muscles of the human body support the skeletal system and are involved in posture, movement, and balance. In general, skeletal muscles, smooth muscles, and cardiac muscles are the three types of muscle found in humans and all other vertebrates. Smooth muscle, which is found in the walls of blood vessels and organs like the stomach, intestines, and bladder, is controlled involuntarily. The heart's mass is made up of cardiac muscle, which is also controlled involuntarily and is in charge of the organ's regular contractions. The human heart and smooth muscle are arranged in exactly the same way as those of other vertebrate animals, with very few exceptions. The human body's skeletal muscles, with a focus on muscle function and the alterations brought about by the protracted evolutionary process that included the adoption of an erect posture. The article on muscle covers smooth muscle, cardiac muscle, and the physiology of muscle contraction in great detail.

1.1.1. Functions of Muscles

The main functions of the muscular system are as follows:

1. **Mobility**. The muscular system's main function is to allow movement. When muscles contract, they contribute to gross and fine movement.

   Gross movement refers to large, coordinated motions and includes:

   - walking
   - running
   - swimming

   Fine movement involves smaller movements, such as:

   - writing
   - speaking
   - facial expressions

   This kind of movement is usually the result of the smaller skeletal muscles. The majority of a person's muscle movement is controlled consciously. On the other hand, reflexive motions include pulling a hand away from a heat source.

2. **Stability.** Tendons of muscles wrap around joints and help maintain joint stability. Stabilization depends heavily on the shoulder and knee joints' tendon muscles. The muscles in the abdomen, back, and pelvis are known as the core muscles. They help with tasks like lifting weights and stabilizing the body.

3. **Posture**. Skeletal muscles support an individual's ability to maintain proper posture while sitting or standing. We call this posture. Strong, flexible muscles are essential for proper posture. Tight, weak, or stiff muscles can lead to bad posture and body misalignment. Long-term, bad posture leads to joint and muscle pain in the shoulders, back, neck, and elsewhere.

4. **Circulation**. One muscle that circulates blood throughout the body is the heart. The heart beats automatically in response to electrical signals; it is not conscious of its own movements. An additional factor in the movement of blood throughout the body is the smooth muscle found in the veins and arteries. In the event of blood loss or dehydration, these muscles keep the blood pressure and circulation stable. When engaging in vigorous

exercise, when the body needs more oxygen, muscles enlarge to improve blood flow.

5. **Respiration**. The diaphragm muscle is used during breathing. Beneath the lungs is a muscle dome called the diaphragm. The diaphragm pushes down when it contracts, expanding the chest cavity. Air then fills the lungs. The diaphragm muscle forces air out of the lungs when it relaxes. The muscles in the back, neck, and abdomen must cooperate for someone to breathe more deeply.

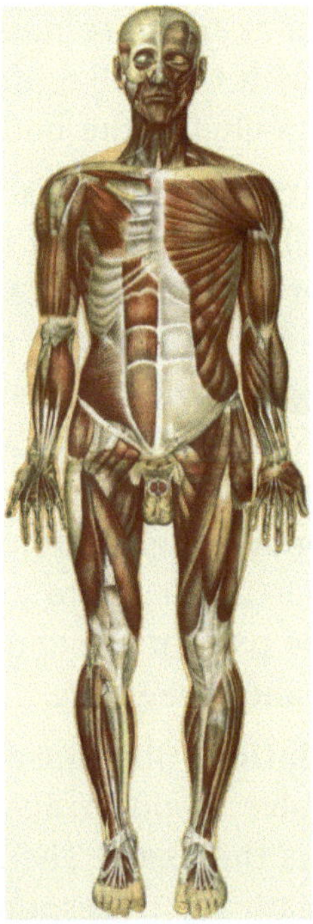

Figure 1.1. *The muscular system allows for movement within the body, for example, during digestion or urination.*

Source: By Bouglé, Julien. – https://www.nlm.nih.gov/exhibition/historicalanatomies/bougle_home.html, Public Domain, https://commons.wikimedia.org/w/index.php?curid=34979414.

6. **Digestion.** Digestion is regulated by smooth muscles in the gastrointestinal tract. The GIT extends from the mouth to the anus. The wave-like movement of food through the digestive system is known as peristalsis. Food is forced into the esophagus and stomach by the contraction and relaxation of muscles in the walls of these hollow organs (Figure 1.1).

Food particles are mixed with stomach acid and enzymes by the lower muscles of the stomach while the upper muscles relax to let food pass through. Peristalsis transports the food that has been digested from the stomach into the intestines. Further contractions of muscles result in the passage of food out of the body as stool.

7. **Urination**. The urinary system comprises both smooth and skeletal muscles, including those in the:
   - bladder
   - kidneys
   - penis or vagina
   - prostate
   - ureters
   - urethra

The muscles and nerves must work together to hold and release urine from the bladder.

Urinary problems, such as poor bladder control or retention of urine, are caused by damage to the nerves that carry signals to the muscles.

8. **Childbirth**. Smooth muscles in the uterus expand and contract during childbirth. These movements push the baby through the vagina. Also, the pelvic floor muscles help to guide the baby's head down the birth canal.

9. **Vision.** Six skeletal muscles around the eye control its movements. These muscles work quickly and precisely, and allow the eye to:
    - maintain a stable image
    - scan the surrounding area
    - track moving objects

If someone experiences damage to their eye muscles, it can impair their vision.

10. **Organ protection**. Muscles in the torso protect the internal organs at the front, sides, and back of the body. The bones of the spine and the ribs provide further protection. Muscles also protect the bones and organs by absorbing shock and reducing friction in the joints.
11. **Temperature regulation.** Keeping the body at a normal temperature is one of the muscles' major jobs. The human muscles contract to produce about 85% of the heat they produce in their bodies. Skeletal muscles contract more vigorously to generate heat when body temperature drops below ideal levels. One manifestation of this mechanism is shivering. To keep the body warm, blood vessel muscles also contract. It is possible to return body temperature to normal by relaxing the smooth muscle in the blood vessels. By doing so, more blood flows through the skin and extra heat is released.

1.1.2. Properties of Muscle

The ability of muscle cells to shorten when compelled to do so is known as contractility. Other traits shared by all muscle cells include excitability, extensibility, and elasticity. For example, to flex your elbow (reduce the angle of a joint), you must contract (shorten) the biceps brachii and other anterior arm elbow flexor muscles. The capacity to react to a stimulus, which can be sent by a hormone or a motor neuron, is known as excitability. Extensibility is the capacity of a muscle to be stretched. Think about the elbow flexing movement, for instance. Bending the elbow requires the extensor muscles to be stretched for flexion to occur. A lack of extensibility is referred to as spasticity. The capacity of a muscle to retract or return to its initial length following an extension beyond its maximum length is known as elasticity. The organs of the vertebrate muscular system, skeletal muscles are also referred to as muscles and are mainly joined to the skeleton by tendons. They are in charge of how the body moves. Some people refer to the muscle cells found in skeletal muscles as muscle fibers because they are significantly longer than the muscle cells found in other types of muscle tissue. The arrangement of the fibers in the muscle called sarcomeres gives skeletal muscle tissue its striped appearance.

To maintain proper posture and joint position, muscle spindles in skeletal muscles transmit information about the length and stretch of the muscle to the central nervous system. Proprioception is commonly associated with the sense of body awareness or the "unconscious" awareness of the different parts of the body at any given moment. Our ability to sense our position in space is known as proprioception. Based on the feedback data gathered from proprioception, multiple brain regions collaborate to coordinate movement and position. Particularly, the red nucleus and cerebellum continuously sample position against movement and make small adjustments to maintain smooth motion. Under a microscope, two contractile proteins called myosin and actin—two of the myofilaments present in the myofibrils of the muscle fibers—arrange themselves to produce the characteristic banding pattern seen in skeletal muscle. Myosin forms the thick filaments, while actin forms the thin filaments. Sarcomeres are repeating units made up of these filaments. The two proteins mentioned above interact to cause muscle contraction. The cytoskeleton's intermediate filaments, which link the sarcomere to other organelles like the mitochondria, aid in stabilizing the cell's structural integrity. The function of the costamere is to join the sarcomere and sarcolemma.

1.1.3. Disorders Affect Muscles

A wide range of disorders, diseases, drugs, and injuries can cause problems with how the muscles work. They include:

- **Cancer and other diseases:** Muscle disorders can result from various cancers, including sarcoma, and other illnesses. These comprise a variety of myopathies (muscle diseases), autoimmune illnesses like myasthenia gravis (MG), and neuromuscular conditions like amyotrophic lateral sclerosis (ALS). Muscle weakness results from inflammation in the muscles caused by a disease called polymyositis.
- **Cardiovascular disease:** Several kinds of venous disease and cardiovascular disease, including coronary artery disease, can cause problems with the heart and blood vessels. A heart attack can result when muscles in the blood vessels weaken.
- **Chronic pain disorders:** Fibromyalgia and other disorders cause chronic pain in the muscles all over the body.
- **Genetic disorders:** Muscular dystrophy is an inherited disorder (passed down through families). There are more than 30 types of muscular dystrophy. The disorder causes permanent muscle weakness.
- **Infections:** Bacterial and viral infections can damage muscle fibers. These infections include Lyme disease, malaria, and Rocky Mountain spotted fever.
- **Injuries:** Muscle strain is the result of muscles tearing or stretching too far due to a variety of injuries. Strains to the back are a very common injury. Clumps or spasms in the muscles can be brought on by trauma, accidents, and overuse injuries. In extreme situations, these wounds may result in paralysis.
- **Medications:** Certain drugs, such as chemotherapy medications, can cause muscle pain. Sore muscles can also result from medications that treat high blood pressure. Some people develop muscle weakness after having a severe allergic reaction to a medication or a toxic substance (Aiello & Dean, 1990; Agur & Dalley, 2009).

1.2. The Muscle Groups and Their Actions

The following sections provide a basic framework for the understanding gross human muscular anatomy, with descriptions of the large muscle groups and their actions. The various muscle groups work in a coordinated fashion to control the movements of the human body.

1.2.1. The Neck

The terms rotation, flexion, extension, and side bending are used to characterize the motion of the neck (i.e., the gesture that connects the ear to the shoulder). Actions can be carried out in either an ipsilateral (moving toward the side of the contracting muscle) or contralateral (moving away from the side of the contracting muscle) direction. One of the most crucial functions of the cervical (neck) spine is rotation. The sternocleidomastoid muscle, which bends the neck to the ipsilateral side and rotates it contralaterally, is principally responsible for rotation. The sternocleidomastoid muscles on either side of the neck work in tandem to help with forced inhalation by flexing the neck and raising the sternum. The first rib is raised, and the neck is rotated ipsilaterally by the anterior and middle scalene muscles, which are likewise found at the sides of the neck. Rotating the head is accomplished by the splenius capitis and splenius cervicis, which are muscles in the back of the neck (Figure 1.2).

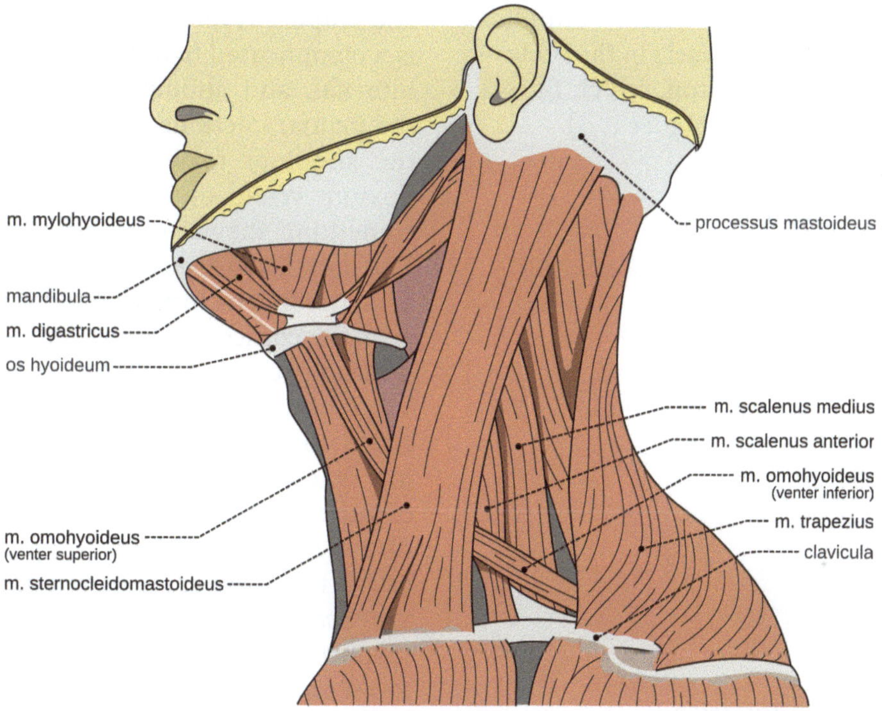

Figure 1.2. *Muscles of the neck.*

Source: By Olek Remesz (wiki-pl: orem, commons: orem) – own work, based on this picture from gray's anatomy., CC BY-SA 2.5, https://commons.wikimedia.org/w/index.php?curid=2339732.

Another crucial function of the cervical spine is side bending. Cervical side bending involves the sternocleidomastoid muscles. The neck is bent ipsilaterally to the side and the second rib is raised by the posterior scalene muscles, which are found on the lower sides of the neck. Neck side bending is also facilitated by the splenius capitis and splenius cervicis. Large, deep muscles that run the length of the back are called the erector spinae muscles, and they include the iliocostalis, longissimus, and spinalis. All three work to bend the neck to the side ipsilaterally. The action of touching the chin to the chest is referred to as neck flexion. The front of the neck muscles known as the longus colli and longus capitis help the sternocleidomastoid muscles in their primary function. Many of the same muscles that are used for other neck movements, such as the splenius cervicis, splenius capitis, iliocostalis, longissimus, and spinalis muscles, are also used for neck extension, which is the opposite of neck flexion.

1.2.2. The Back

A large number of the muscles used to move the neck and shoulders originate in the back. Furthermore, the spinal cord—which supplies innervation to nearly every muscle in the body—is shielded by the axial skeleton, which passes vertically through the back (Figure 1.3).

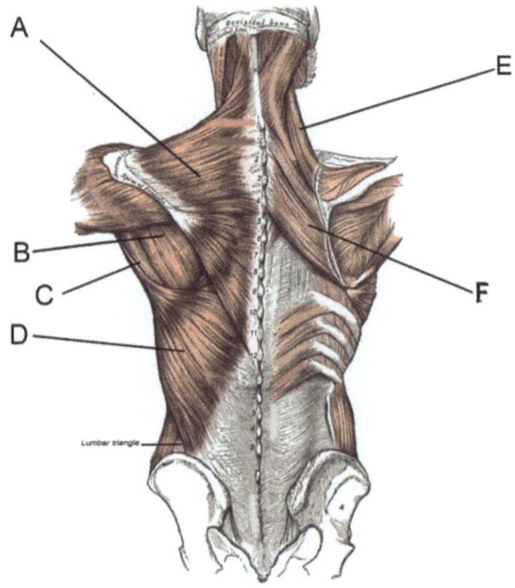

Figure 1.3. *Muscles of the back.*

Source: https://upload.wikimedia.org/wikipedia/commons/9/90/Back_Muscles.jpg.

Several back muscles are specifically used in back movements. For example, the erector spinae muscles extend (bend) the back, and they also side-bend it. The back is also extended by the semispinalis dorsi and semispinalis capitis muscles. The multifidi and rotators, two tiny muscles of the vertebrae, aid in side bending, extension, and rotation of the back. By stabilizing the lumbar spine at its insertion at the 12th rib (the last of the floating ribs), the quadratus lumborum muscle in the lower back helps with inspiration of air. The rhomboid major and minor muscles in the upper back, the levator scapulae muscle that runs along the side and back of the neck, and the trapezius muscle that extends from the back of the neck to the middle of the back all work together to elevate the scapula, or shoulder blade.

1.2.3. The Shoulder

With the humerus head, clavicle (collarbone), and scapula as its constituent parts, the shoulder is a complicated ball-and-socket joint. External, internal, and abduction rotations are among the primary actions of the shoulder. Motioning the shoulder forward is known as shoulder flexion. When one reaches forward to grasp something, they are exhibiting shoulder flexion. The muscles in the chest, the inside of the upper arm, the biceps brachii, the inside of the upper arm, the coracobrachialis, and the deltoid in the uppermost portion of the arm work together to accomplish that action. Shoulder flexion is equal to shoulder extension. In a relay race, for example, receiving a baton is an example of pure shoulder extension—moving the arm directly behind the body. The deltoid, latissimus dorsi, teres major, and triceps muscles, which are located in the back, armpit, and upper arm, respectively, are the muscles that work together to accomplish that movement. The term triceps refers to a muscle group that has three heads that come from different places and converge at the olecranon process of the ulna, a forearm bone. The combined action of the three heads extends the elbow. To lower the arm toward the body and raise it away from it, respectively, one uses shoulder adduction and abduction. Imagine someone doing jumping jacks to get an idea of what they look like. Primary muscles involved in adduction are the triceps, coracobrachialis, teres major, latissimus dorsi, and pectoralis major. The two major abductors of the shoulder are the deltoid and the supraspinatus, a muscle that runs along the back of the scapula (Figure 1.4).

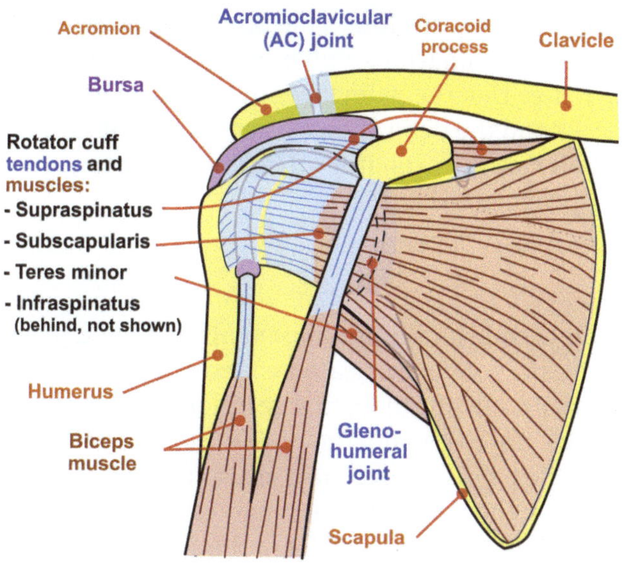

Figure 1.4. *Muscles of the shoulder.*

Source: By National institute of arthritis and musculoskeletal and skin diseases (NIAMS); SVG version by angelito7 – shoulderjoint.PNG, Public Domain, https://commons.wikimedia.org/w/index.php?curid=29907860.

An illustration of external rotation of the shoulder can be observed in a backhand tennis stroke. The deltoid, the teres minor in the armpit, and the infraspinatus muscle, which is located over the scapula, are the main muscles involved in external rotation. The opposite of external rotation in the shoulder is internal rotation. The motion of the shoulder when reaching into a back pocket serves as an illustration. The pectoralis major, latissimus dorsi, deltoid, teres major, and subscapularis muscles work in unison to accomplish that movement. On the anterior, or front-facing, surface of the scapula, there is a deep muscle called the subscapularis.

The rotator cuff, which is made up of the teres minor, subscapularis, supraspinatus, and infraspinatus muscles, stabilizes the humeral head, or ball part of the ball-and-socket shoulder joint. Adults frequently sustain injuries to their rotator cuff muscles, especially if they frequently perform overhead motions (e.g., hitting a ball or applying paint to a ceiling). Tendons from a number of the rotator cuff muscles pass beneath the acromion, a bony protrusion at the distal end of the scapula. The term "distal" refers to a relative position that is farther from the body's center; it is frequently used in contrast to the term "proximal," which refers to a relative position that is closer to the center. Shoulder impingement syndrome is a condition that can arise from the positioning of the tendons and the subacromial bursae, which are fluid-filled sacs situated beneath the acromion, making them susceptible to compression and pinching.

1.2.4. The Arm

The muscles in the upper arm not only facilitate movement of the shoulder but also generate different movements of the forearm.

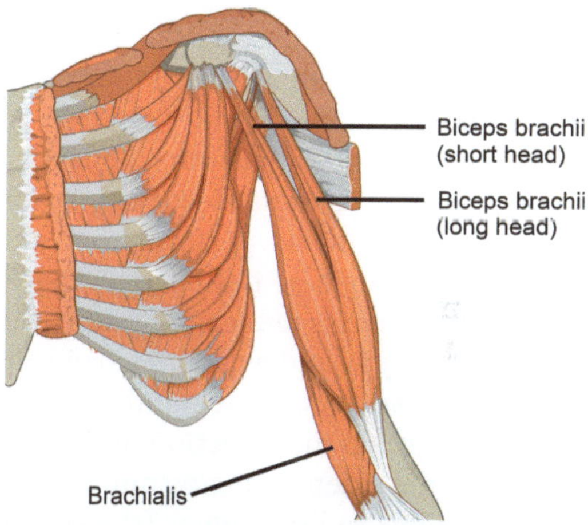

Figure 1.5. *Muscles of the upper arm.*

Source: By CFCF – Own work, CC BY-SA 4.0, https://commons.wikimedia.org/w/index.php?curid=44309314.

For instance, the main muscles used in forearm flexion, which reduces the angle formed at the elbow (i.e., the hand approaches the shoulder), are the brachialis (located in the upper arm beneath the brachii), the brachioradialis (whose origin is on the humerus), and the biceps brachii. The pronator teres, the flexor carpi radialis, the flexor digitorum superficialis, the palmaris longus, and the flexor carpi ulnaris are among the flexor muscles located in the anterior compartment of the forearm, also referred to as the palm side of the forearm, which contribute slightly to forearm flexion. The coracobrachialis also plays a role in this movement (Figure 1.5).

The hand is moved away from the shoulder when the forearm is extended, increasing the angle at the elbow. The triceps brachii are primarily responsible for that action. The extensor muscles of the posterior compartment of the forearm—also referred to as the extensor compartment—which include the extensor carpi radialis longus, extensor carpi radialis brevis, extensor digitorum, extensor carpi ulnaris, and the anconeus—are additional muscles that contribute slightly to forearm extension.

1.2.5. The Wrist

Wrist flexion is defined as a wrist motion that pulls the hand's palm downward. The flexor pollicis longus, flexor digitorum superficialis, flexor digitorum profundus, flexor carpi radialis, and flexor carpi ulnaris perform that action. In contrast, the angle at the back of the wrist shortens during wrist extension. The extensor carpi radialis longus and extensor carpi radialis brevis, which also abduct the hand at the wrist (moving the hand in the direction of the thumb, or first digit), the extensor digitorum, which also extends the index to little finger (the second to fifth digits), the extensor digiti minimi, which also extends the little finger and adducts the hand (moving the hand in the direction of the little finger), and the extensor carpi ulnaris, which also adducts the hand, are the muscles that cause that action. Wrist extension may also be slightly increased by other tiny muscles that cross the wrist joint. The wrist rotation known as wrist supination causes the palm to face upward. The posterior compartment's supinator muscle is responsible for supinating the forearm. Moreover, the biceps brachii increase supination. The opposite movement is called pronation, which involves rotating the wrist so that the palm faces downward. Pronator teres and the deep anterior compartment muscle known as the pronator quadratus work together to pronate the forearm.

1.2.6. The Hand

Comprising intricate components, the hand plays a crucial role in intricate task execution and fine motor control. Small, highly innervated muscles make up the majority of the body. The hand muscles must perform a multitude of precise movements even for seemingly simple tasks like typing on a keyboard. Only the primary action of each hand muscle is covered in the following paragraphs due to its complexity. Many muscles in the hand originate from the radius, the other forearm bone, or the posterior surface of the ulna. These include the thumb's abductor pollicis longus, which extends and abducts; the thumb's extensor pollicis brevis, which extends the thumb's metacarpophalangeal (MCP) joint; the thumb's extensor pollicis, which extends the thumb's distal phalanx, or finger bone; and the thumb's extensor indicis, which extends the index finger when it reaches the MCP joint. Between the phalanges, or tiny bones that make up the fingers, and the metacarpal bones, which are found in the hand, are MCP joints. While the forearm is the source of origin for many hand muscles, the hand itself is the site of origin and insertion for numerous small hand muscles. The hand's intrinsic muscles are known as such. Included in these are the palmaris brevis, which aids in grip; the umbrales, which flex the MCP joints and extend the finger phalangeal joints (IPs); the palmar interossei, which adduct the fingers toward the middle finger (the third digit); and the dorsal interossei, which abduct the fingers away from the middle finger. The MCP and IP joints are flexed and extended by all of the interossei. The median nerve innervates the abductor pollicis brevis, flexor pollicis brevis, and opponens pollicis, the three muscles that make up the thenar eminence, which is situated on the palm side of the base of the thumb. The flexor pollicis brevis flexes the thumb's MCP joint, the abductor pollicis brevis abducts the thumb, and the opponens pollicis acts to oppose the thumb in relation to the other fingers. The thumb is adducted by the adductor pollicis, which is not a component of the thenar eminence. On the hand's palm side, beneath the little finger, is the hypothenar eminence. It is composed of three muscles innervated by the ulnar nerve's deep branch. To abduct the little finger, use the abductor digiti minimi. To flex the little finger, use the flexor digiti minimi. Opponens digiti minimi is used to oppose the little finger against the thumb.

1.2.7. The Abdomen

The abdominal wall consists of three layers of muscle, plus a fourth layer in the middle anterior region. The rectus abdominis, which has vertically running muscle fibers that flex the trunk and stabilize the pelvis, makes up the fourth layer of the midregion. The remaining three layers of abdominal muscles are located on either side of the rectus abdominis. The transversus abdominis, the deepest of those layers, acts to compress and support the abdomen and provides static core stabilization. Its fibers run perpendicular to the rectus abdominis. The external oblique layers, which make up the outermost muscle layers of the abdomen, run downward and forward, while the internal oblique layers extend upward and forward from the sides of the abdomen. The trunk flexes and rotates toward the side of the contracting internal oblique (also known as the "same-side rotator") when the internal oblique layers work in tandem with the external oblique on the other side of the body (Figure 1.6).

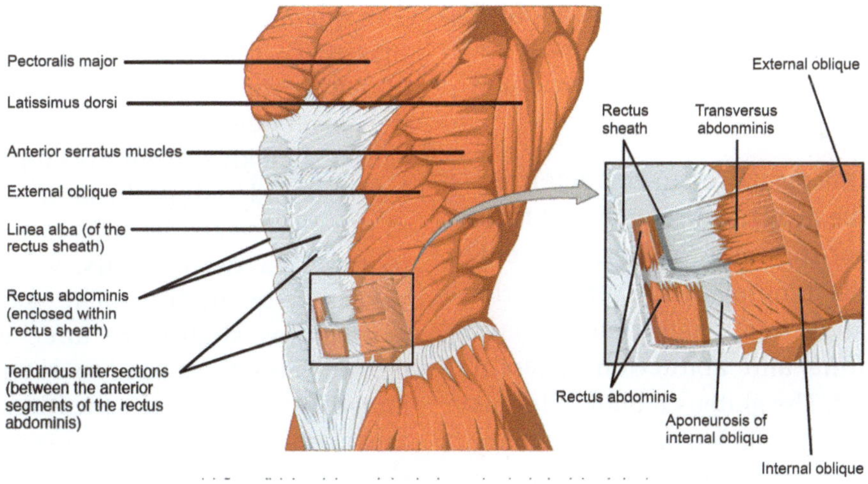

Figure 1.6. *Muscles of the abdominal wall.*

Source: By OpenStax College – https://cnx.org/contents/FPtK1zmh@8.108:y9_gDy74@5, CC BY 3.0, https://commons.wikimedia.org/w/index.php?curid=64291130.

1.2.8. The Hip

The hip joint is a complex weight-bearing ball and socket joint with significant load capacity. Because of the joint's relatively deep socket, stability is provided at the expense of some range of motion. Flexion, extension, abduction, and adduction are among the motions covered in this section. The action of the hip that moves the knee toward the chest is known as hip flexion. The iliacus, psoas major, and psoas minor together form the iliopsoas, one of the main muscles involved in hip flexion. When combined, those muscles primarily flex the hip, but they also aid in stabilizing the hip and flexion of the abdomen. The rectus femoris, pectineus, gracilis, and sartorius are additional hip flexors. Together with the rectus femoris, the sartorius is involved in external hip rotation, knee extension, and abduction. Additionally, internal rotation and hip adduction involve the pectineus. The majority of the muscles involved in hip extension are found in the posterior thigh and buttocks. These muscles contract to move the thigh from a flexed position toward the body's midline or the trunk from a bent position toward a more erect posture. The biceps femoris, which is separated into the long and short heads, the semitendinosus, the semimembranosus, and the gluteus maximus are the main muscles involved in hip extension. Other small pelvic muscles, such as the adductor magnus, also make a small contribution (Figure 1.7).

Adduction is the term used to characterize a limb's motion in the direction that moves it from a lateral alignment to a more axial alignment. For instance, in a jumping-jack exercise, the leg experiences adduction when it moves back toward the midline and abduction when it moves away from it. The gluteus medius, gluteus minimus, and tensor fascia lata are the primary abductors of the hip. Additionally, the thigh can be rotated externally in the flexed position and internally in the extended position using those three muscles. The piriformis is another small contributor. Three major adductors are found in the hip: the adductor longus, adductor brevis, and adductor magnus. The gracilis and pectineus make a small but significant contribution to hip adduction.

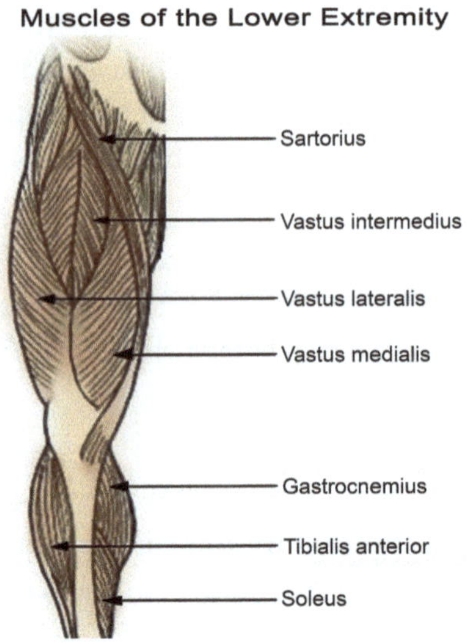

Figure 1.7. *Anterior view of the muscles of the human leg.*

Source: Public Domain, https://commons.wikimedia.org/w/index.php?curid=789660.

1.2.9. The Upper Leg and Knee

The quadriceps femoris is a group of muscles that work together to extend the knee. This increases the angle of the knee and straightens the lower leg. Knee extension is essential for actions like kicking and is employed during the forward and swing phase of the gait. Included in the quadriceps femoris group are the rectus femoris, vastus lateralis, vastus medius, and vastus intermedius. The sartorius muscle contributes slightly to knee extension. Knee flexion is the term used to describe bending the knee from its straight position. The hamstring muscles are the ones that carry out that action; they are usually thought of as the opposite of the knee extension muscles. The hamstring muscles, which comprise the semitendinosus, semimembranosus, and biceps femoris, are located in the rear of the thigh. A few minor muscles that cross the knee joint posteriorly and the gastrocnemius muscle in the rear of the calf both contribute slightly to knee flexion.

1.2.10. The Lower Leg and Foot

The foot and lower leg muscles are intricate and function on multiple planes. Their actions are dependent upon both the foot's position and whether the person is bearing weight or not. An overview of the movements of the lower leg and foot muscles is given in the paragraphs that follow. Ankle flexion toward the dorsum, or anterior surface of the foot, is referred to as dorsiflexion (the surface of the foot viewed from above). Many muscles, including the tibialis anterior, are involved in dorsiflexion. This muscle also performs inversion (tilting the foot toward the midline), stabilizes the foot when it strikes the ground, and locks the ankle during kicking. In addition to acting in dorsiflexion, the extensor digitorum longus (EDL) extends the last four toes. A muscle known as the peroneus tertius (fibularis tertius), which is present in some people in addition to the EDL, has a limited role in the dorsiflexion and eversion of the foot (tilting of the foot away from the midline). The extensor hallucis longus mainly facilitates dorsiflexion of the big toe (hallux), but it can also be used to dorsiflex the ankle and weakly invert it. The term "plantarflexion" describes an ankle's flexion toward the foot's sole. The easiest way to illustrate that is to have someone stand on their toes. The large calf muscles, such as the gastrocnemius and the soleus, which is located directly behind the gastrocnemius, are responsible for most of the plantarflexion of the ankle. Although the gastrocnemius and soleus are sometimes confused for two separate muscles, it is generally agreed upon that they are two separate muscles (Figure 1.8).

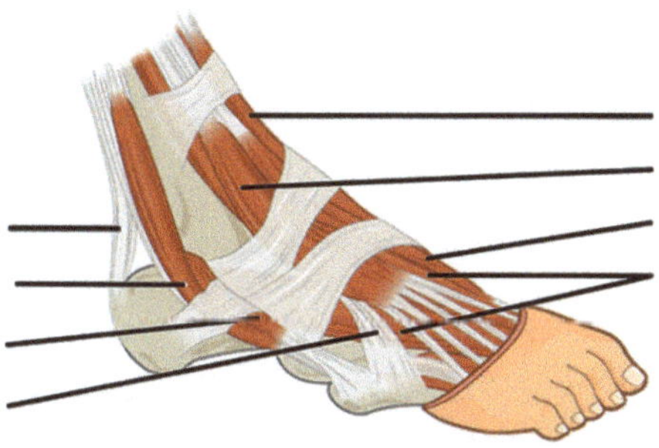

Figure 1.8. Dorsal view of the right foot, showing major muscles, tendons, and nerves.

Source: https://en.m.wikipedia.org/wiki/File:1124_Intrinsic_Muscles_of_the_Foot_a.png.

The plantaris, which runs obliquely between the gastrocnemius and the soleus, the flexor hallucis longus, which primarily functions in big toe flexion but also contributes to ankle flexion, the flexor digitorum longus, which flexes the second to fifth toes, the peroneus longus, which flexes the ankle and everts the foot, and the peroneus brevis, which performs plantarflexion and eversion of the foot, are some additional muscles of the lower leg and foot. The intrinsic muscles originate from the foot and do not pass over the ankle joint. As such, they can only move the foot. The lumbricals, which flex the metatarsophalangeal (MTP) joints and extend the distal IP and proximal IP joints of the toes, the flexor hallucis brevis, which flexes the big toe, the adductor hallucis, which flexes and contracts the big toe, and the quadratus plantae, which aids in toe flexion, are among the intrinsic muscles of the foot. There is a common insertion point for the two heads of the adductor hallucis, the oblique head and the transverse head, on the outside of the proximal phalanx of the big toe. The transverse head originates from the ligaments of the MTP joints of the third to fifth toes, while the oblique head originates from the base of the second to fourth metatarsal bones. The fifth toe is extended and adducted by the flexor digiti minimi brevis. The toes are abducted by the dorsal interossei and adducted by the plantar interossei (Aiello & Dean, 1990; Agur & Dalley, 2009).

1.3. Types of Muscles

The human body has roughly 600 muscles. From pumping blood and enabling movement to lifting large weights or giving birth, muscles serve a variety of purposes. Movement is produced by the contraction or relaxation of muscles. This movement could be involuntary—done without our conscious knowledge—or voluntary, meaning it is made consciously. In the body, there are three types of muscle: skeletal (striated); smooth; and cardiac.

1.3.1. Skeletal Muscle

The most prevalent of the three muscle types in vertebrates is skeletal muscle, also referred to as voluntary muscle. Tendons connect skeletal muscles to bones, and these muscles create all of the movements that occur between body parts. Skeletal muscle is controlled voluntarily, in contrast to cardiac and smooth muscle.

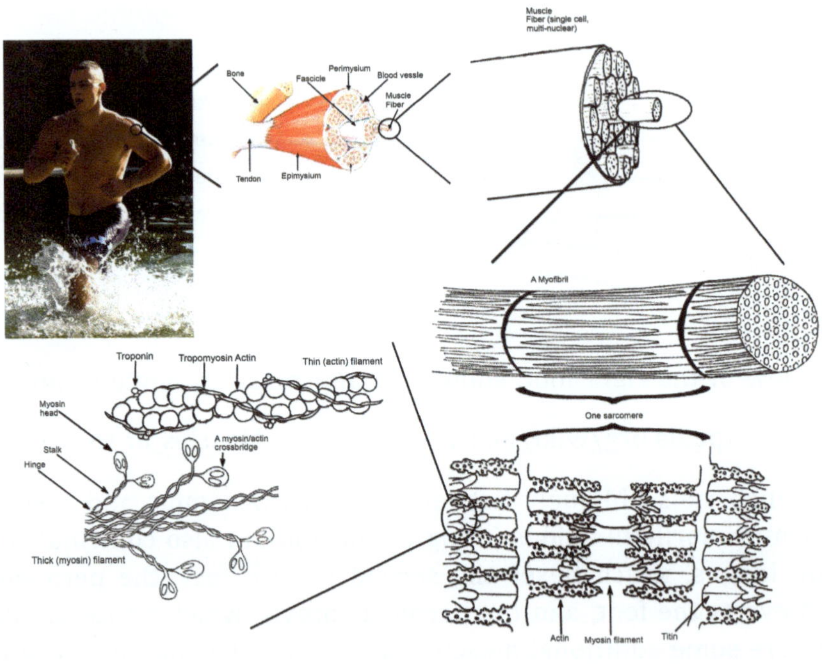

Figure 1.9. *Structure of Skeletal muscle.*

Source: CC BY-SA 3.0, https://commons.wikimedia.org/w/index.php?curid=73744.

But skeletal muscle is striated, too, just like cardiac muscle. Its long, thin, multinucleated fibers are crossed in a regular pattern of fine red and white lines, which gives the muscle its characteristic appearance. Connective tissue holds skeletal muscle fibers together while facilitating communication between them and blood vessels and nerves. One can regard a complete skeletal muscle as an organ of the muscular system. Each muscle or organ is made up of blood or vascular tissue, connective tissue, skeletal muscle tissue, and nerve tissue. The size, shape, and fiber arrangement of skeletal muscles vary widely. They vary in size from massive masses like the thigh muscles to minuscule strands like the middle ear's stapedius muscle. Certain skeletal muscles have a broad shape, while others are narrow. The muscle fibers can be oblique, converge to a narrow attachment, or run parallel to the muscle's long axis in certain muscles (Figure 1.9).

A single cylindrical muscle cell makes up each skeletal muscle fiber. A single skeletal muscle can consist of hundreds or even thousands of interconnected muscle fibers that are covered with connective tissue. The epimysium is a sheath of connective tissue that envelops every muscle. The connective tissue known as fascia, which lies outside the epimysium, envelops and divides the muscles. The epimysium projects inward in certain places, creating compartments within the muscle. There is a bundle of muscle fibers within each compartment. The fasciculus, a bundle of muscle fiber, is encircled by the perimysium, a layer of connective tissue. Every individual muscle cell, known as a muscle fiber, is encircled by connective tissue within the fasciculus, which is known as the endomysium. Like other body cells, skeletal muscle fibers are delicate and soft. The delicate cells are supported, shielded, and enabled to withstand the forces of contraction by the covering of connective tissue. Additionally, the coverings offer nerve and blood vessel passageways.

The epimysium, perimysium, and endomysium typically extend past the muscle's fleshy portion, the belly or gaster, to form an extensive, flat sheet-like aponeurosis or a thick rope-like tendon. Indirect attachments between muscles and the periosteum of bones or the connective tissue of other muscles are created by tendons and aponeurosis. The muscle usually extends across a joint and has tendons connecting its ends to the bones. When one end moves as a result of a muscle contraction, the other bone stays comparatively fixed or stable. There is an abundance of blood vessels and nerves in skeletal muscles. This has a direct bearing on contraction, the main job of skeletal muscle. Skeletal muscle fibers require an impulse from a nerve cell to contract. Every nerve that pierces a skeletal muscle's epimysium is usually accompanied by an artery and at least one vein. A nerve cell's muscle's connective tissue components are followed by branches of the nerve and blood vessels, which may have one or more tiny blood vessels known as capillaries.

1.3.1.1. Function

Every skeletal muscle is an organ made up of different tissues that are integrated together. These tissues include connective tissue, blood vessels, nerve fibers, and skeletal muscle fibers. The three layers of connective tissue, or fascia, that envelop and give structure to each skeletal muscle also serve to compartmentalize the muscle fibers within the muscle. The epimysium, a sheath of dense, asymmetric connective tissue, envelops every muscle and permits it to contract and move forcefully while preserving its structural integrity. Moreover, the epimysium permits muscle to move independently by dividing it from nearby tissues and organs. Muscle fibers within skeletal muscles are arranged into bundles called fascicles, which are encircled by the perimysium, a middle layer of connective tissue. This fascicular organization, which is typical of limb muscles, enables the nervous system to initiate a particular muscle movement by stimulating a subset of muscle fibers within a muscle fascicle. A thin layer of collagen and reticular fibers, known as the endomysium, encases each muscle fiber inside each fascicle. The endomysium, which envelops the cells' extracellular matrix, aids in the force transmission from the muscle fibers to the tendons.

The collagen in the three layers of connective tissue intertwines with the collagen of a tendon in skeletal muscles that pull on bones in concert with tendons. The tendon merges with the periosteum that covers the bone at the opposite end. To pull on the bone to allow the skeleton to move, the tension produced by the contraction of the muscle fibers is subsequently transmitted through the layers of connective tissue, to the tendon, and finally to the periosteum. In other locations, the mysia may unite with fascia, the connective tissue that lies between the skin and bones, or with an aponeurosis, a broad sheet resembling a tendon. An example of an aponeurosis is the broad sheet of connective tissue in the lower back into which the latissimus dorsi muscles, also known as the "lats," fuse. Additionally, blood vessels supply every skeletal muscle with an abundance of nutrients, oxygen, and waste-removal agents. Additionally, the axon branch of a somatic motor neuron supplies each muscle fiber in skeletal muscle, signaling the fiber to contract. Skeletal muscle can only contract functionally through nervous system signals, unlike cardiac and smooth muscle.

1.3.1.2. Skeletal Muscle Fibers

Skeletal muscle cells are often called muscle fibers (or myofibers) because they are long and cylindrical. In the Sartorius of the upper leg, skeletal muscle fibers can reach lengths of up to 30 cm (11.8 in) and diameters of up to 100 μm, making them relatively large compared to other cells. These big, protein-dense cells can produce the vast quantities of proteins and enzymes needed to sustain their regular functions because they have numerous nuclei. Skeletal muscle fibers contain cellular organelles like mitochondria and endoplasmic reticulum along with nuclei, which are found in other cells. However, some of these structures are unique to muscle fibers. The sarcoplasmic reticulum (SR), a specialized smooth endoplasmic reticulum, is responsible for storing, releasing, and retrieving calcium ions (Ca^{++}). The cytoplasm of muscle fibers is called sarcoplasm, and the plasma membrane is known as sarcolemma (from the Greek sarco, meaning "flesh"). Proteins are organized into organelles called myofibrils, which extend the length of the cell and contain sarcomeres connected in series. One muscle fiber can contain hundreds to thousands of myofibrils, each with thousands of sarcomeres, because myofibrils are only about 1.2 μm in diameter. The sarcomere is a highly ordered arrangement of contractile, regulatory, and structural proteins that make up the smallest functional unit of a skeletal muscle fiber. The contraction of an individual skeletal muscle fiber (and eventually the entire muscle) is caused by the shortening of these individual sarcomeres.

1.3.2. Smooth Muscle

Smooth muscles are distributed throughout the body and perform a multitude of tasks. They aid in digestion and nutrient absorption in the stomach and intestines. They are present throughout the urinary system and aid in the body's detoxification as well as electrolyte balance. They are present in all veins and arteries, where it is essential for controlling tissue oxygenation and blood pressure. The body could not sustain even the most basic functions in the absence of these essential functions. There are several ways in which smooth muscle differs from skeletal muscle, but its capacity for involuntary contraction and control may be the most significant. Without conscious effort by the human, the nervous system can use smooth muscle to tightly regulate many of the body's subsystems throughout life. When an individual engages in exercise, their blood pressure adjusts to the increased oxygen demands without their conscious awareness. Instead, the nervous system uses other receptors, hormones, and neurotransmitters to naturally regulate smooth muscle. A significant part of the disease process in the body is also played by smooth muscle.

For asthmatics, bronchodilators are a crucial and potentially life-saving treatment because they relax the smooth muscle of the airways. Metoclopramide is one example of a medication that increases smooth muscle signaling to stimulate and promote gastric emptying. When combined with ACEI, nitrates are used to treat ischemic heart disease, which is one of the most well-known uses of smooth muscle and medical therapy. This combination has been shown to reduce patient mortality. Understanding smooth muscle is crucial for medical professionals due to its unique influence on various parts of the body. Since the fundamental mechanism of many treatments is altering the signaling pathways that impact smooth muscle.

One kind of tissue that is present in the walls of hollow organs like the stomach, uterus, and intestines is called smooth muscle. Smooth muscle is also present in the walls of conduits, such as the veins and arteries that make up the circulatory system. The urinary, respiratory, and reproductive system tracts also contain this kind of involuntary non-striated muscle. Furthermore, smooth muscle is present in the eyes, where it functions to alter the pupil's size and the lens's shape. Additionally, smooth muscle in the skin enables hair to rise in reaction to fear or cold temperatures.

1.3.2.1. Structure

The length and thickness of a smooth muscle cell range from 20 to 200 μm. Most of the myofilaments make up the homogeneously eosinophilic cytoplasm. During contraction, the center-positioned nucleus assumes the shape of a cigar. Similar to the skeletal muscle's T-tubules, the cell membrane invades the cytoplasm to form tiny pouch-like structures called caveolae. A basal lamina connects the smooth muscle cells to the surrounding connective tissue (Figure 1.10).

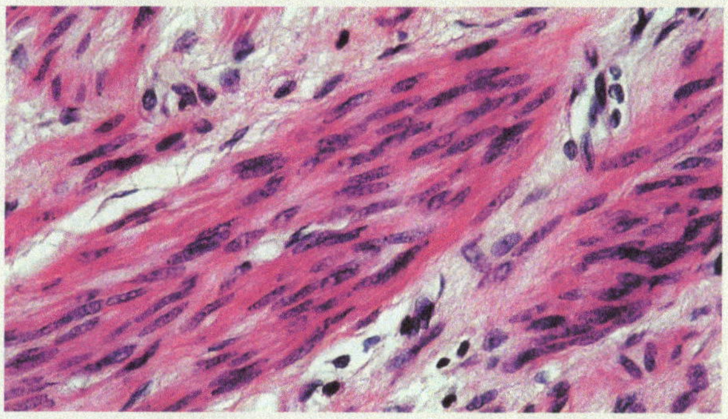

Figure 1.10. *Smooth muscle under magnification.*

Source: https://upload.wikimedia.org/wikipedia/commons/1/1a/Muscle_Tissue_Smooth_%2840087100000%29.jpg.

Branching bundles are the grouping of smooth muscle fibers. These bundles form a complex system rather than a strictly parallel and ordered structure like skeletal muscle fibers do. As a result, the cells have far greater contractile power than striated muscle. Stretched between dense bodies in the cytoplasm and attachment plaques at the cell membrane are the actin filaments. Actin filaments and myosin filaments are positioned between them. Furthermore, the cell structure is supported by intermediate filaments like vimentin and desmin.

1.3.2.2. Function

Smooth muscle has the same ability to contract as any other type of muscle tissue. The actin and myosin fibers shorten in the image above, causing the cell to effectively shrink. When compared to other muscle types, the smooth muscle contracts in a few significant ways differently. A signal travels from the somatic nervous system to the skeletal muscle, where it activates the muscle cell's organelles to release calcium. Actin's opening is rapidly occupied by myosin after a protein separates from it due to the action of calcium. The myosin uses the constant supply of ATP to rapidly contract the cell. In smooth muscle tissue, this is not the case. Nerve impulses, hormones, and other chemicals released by specialized organs are examples of signals from the autonomic nervous system that control smooth muscle contraction instead of the somatic nervous system. Unlike skeletal muscle, which must contract and relax rapidly, smooth muscle is designed to contract continuously. Smooth muscle functions more like a car's throttle than a calcium trigger that initiates a contraction reaction. The cell receives a signal from an external stimulus or nerve impulse telling it to release calcium. Actin does not have a unique protein on smooth muscle cells that stops myosin from binding. Actin and myosin, on the other hand, bind continuously. However, myosin can only cling to and advance in response to energy. A sophisticated mechanism found inside smooth muscle cells enables calcium levels to regulate the quantity of ATP that myosin can use. Therefore, the cells do not immediately relax after the stimulus is removed. Myosin keeps attaching to actin and moving along the filaments until the calcium level drops.

1.3.2.3. Location

Smooth muscle has been adapted to many different parts of the body because of its unique ability to contract for extended periods of time and maintain that force. In addition to lining many sections of the digestive and circulatory systems, smooth muscle is also in charge of raising the hairs on your arms. Smooth muscle is essential to the circulatory system because it regulates and maintains blood pressure and oxygen flow throughout the body. All veins and arteries are lined with smooth muscle, even though the heart exerts the majority of the pressure. These tiny muscles can contract to put pressure on the system or to relax and let blood flow more freely. Experiments have demonstrated that these smooth muscles respond to oxygen availability or deficiency by contracting the veins to deliver sufficient oxygen. For similar reasons, smooth muscle lines most of the digestive tract. The stimuli that affect the cells in the digestive system differ from those in the circulatory system, though. For example, when you swallow, your gut's smooth muscle sheets contract. Tension is put on one side of the sheet when you swallow. In response, the cells on that side contract, causing a wave to start moving down your digestive tract. Food is moved through the numerous twists and turns of the stomach by a process called peristalsis. Smooth muscle has a wide range of functions throughout the body due to its capacity to contract and hold. In addition to the functions mentioned above, smooth muscle is also in charge of contracting your irises, lifting the tiny hairs on your arm, sphincter contraction, and even the movement of fluids through your organs through pressure. Smooth muscle is much better at producing steady, elastic tension even though it doesn't contract or relax as quickly as skeletal or cardiac muscle.

1.3.3. Cardiac Muscle

One of the three main muscle types exclusively present in the heart of vertebrates is cardiac muscle, also known as the myocardium. The fact that cardiac muscle has sarcomeres, which are contractile units, sets it apart from smooth muscle, the third major muscle type, but it also makes cardiac muscle similar to skeletal muscle, another major muscle type. Cardiac muscle, unlike skeletal muscle, isn't controlled voluntarily and shows rhythmic contractions. The sinoatrial node, acting as the heart's pacemaker, regulates the rhythmic contraction of cardiac muscle. The majority of the heart is composed of myocardium, or cardiac muscle cells. The heart's pumping action, driven by its contractility, and the rhythmicity of its contractions, contribute to its remarkable function. To fulfill the metabolic needs of various tissues like skeletal muscles, kidneys, brain, skin, liver, heart, and gastrointestinal tract, the cardiac output, or the amount of blood pumped by the heart per minute, fluctuates. The cardiac output is determined by the contractile force of cardiac muscle cells and their rhythmic activation. The heart's ability to pump blood effectively and adjust to changes in demand relies heavily on factors influencing the frequency and force of heart muscle contraction (Figure 1.11).

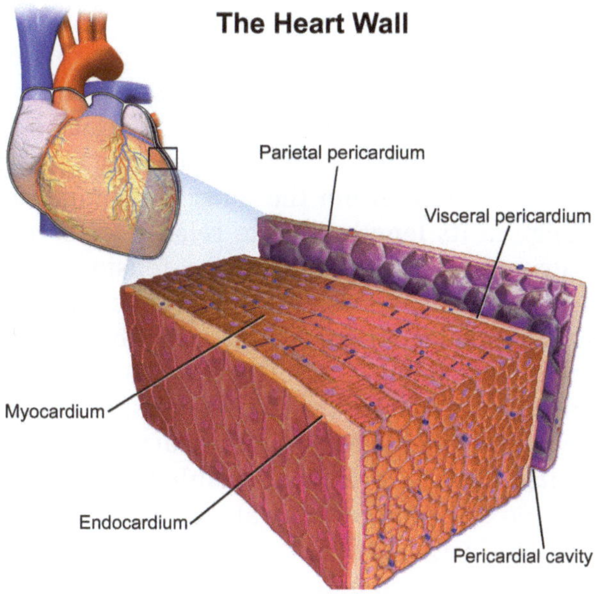

Figure 1.11. *Structure of cardiac muscle.*

Source: By BruceBlaus. When using this image in external sources it can be cited as:Blausen.com staff (2014). "Medical gallery of Blausen Medical 2014." WikiJournal of Medicine 1 (2). DOI:10.15347/wjm/2014.010. ISSN 2002-4436. - Own work, CC BY 3.0, https://commons.wikimedia.org/w/index.php?curid=28761820.

It is a specific type of muscle that has evolved to contract repeatedly and continuously, allowing blood to circulate throughout the body. The heart is an organ that is quite basic. There are only three layers that are visible despite all of the kinks and turns and different chambers. The cardiac muscle is encircled on the outside by the epicardium, also referred to as the visceral pericardium. This keeps it safe from harm from other organs. By adhering to this outer layer, the parietal pericardium forms a fluid-filled layer that aids in lubricating the heart. The muscle and the blood it pumps through the heart's chambers are separated by the inner layer, or endocardium. The heart muscle lies between these two sheets. Myocardium is another term for cardiac muscle. Heart muscle is made up of layers of cells that are connected like a lattice when we take a closer look at it. An intercalated disc is a type of specialized junction that locks two cells together at their meeting point. Under a microscope, this area appears as a dark disc, but it is actually the interlocking of hundreds of projections that resemble fingers from individual cells. Gap junctions, which are tiny holes in these projections, allow connected cells to receive the impulse to contract. Neural and vascular networks are entwined within and surrounding these cells, transmitting signals and oxygen to the heart muscle. The structure of cardiac muscle is similar to that of skeletal muscle at the microscopic level. Both muscle tissues are striated, which means that, when examined under a microscope, they display bands of light and dark. The incredibly well-organized sarcomeres are what form these bands. A sarcomere is a collection of protein fibers that contracts in response to a signal. These sarcomeres are supported by the same proteins and consist of actin and myosin in both cardiac and skeletal muscle. Actin is wrapped by a protein called tropomyosin, which prevents myosin from attaching to it. Tropomyosin is held in place by the protein troponin until a signal to contract is received. The skeletal and cardiac muscles share the same proteins.

1.3.3.1. Function

An action potential is used as the contracting signal, just like in skeletal muscle. But in the case of skeletal muscle, the somatic, or voluntary, nervous system is typically the source of this signal. The autonomic nervous system regulates cardiac muscle. Your brain and heart cells work together to release precisely timed nerve impulses that instruct your heart's cells to contract in the proper sequence. The signal's source may differ, but the signal's reception and the remainder of the contraction are remarkably similar. A specialized organelle is stimulated by the action potential, also known as the nerve impulse, on the cell surface to release calcium ions (Ca^{2+}). Derived from the endoplasmic reticulum present in a general cell, this organelle is known as the sarcoplasmic reticulum. Troponin is a protein that is affected by the release of Ca^{2+} ions into the cytoplasm, which causes it to release tropomyosin. Myosin is permitted to attach to actin when tropomyosin changes positions. Subsequently, myosin reduces the length of each sarcomere by walking along the actin filaments using the energy contained in ATP molecules. The $Ca^{2+}$is swiftly reabsorbed into the sarcoplasmic reticulum after the impulse has passed. When troponin and tropomyosin reattach, the heart muscle cells relax. Your heart goes through this general process each time it beats. A force can be applied to the heart's chambers as a result of the muscle cells' coordinated action. The cardiac muscle sheets are arranged such that they are perpendicular to one another. This has the effect of causing the heart to contract in various directions. The contraction of these multiple layers of muscle fibers causes the ventricles and atria of the heart to contract from top to bottom and from side to side. This causes the ventricles to pump and twist vigorously, pushing blood throughout the body (Aiello & Dean, 1990; Agur & Dalley, 2009).

1.4. Muscle Contraction

The tightening, shortening, or lengthening of muscles during an activity is known as muscle contraction. It can occur during weightlifting, stretching, or holding or picking up objects. Muscle relaxation, or the return of contracted muscles to their normal state, frequently occurs after muscle contraction. The fibers in your muscles are known as myosin. Myosin fibers either tighten and shorten or loosen and stretch out depending on how your muscles must be used. Muscle contractions that occur at regular intervals, such as your heartbeats, are also caused by myosin. Two factors are the foundation of the physiological theory of muscle contraction: length and tension. Muscle contraction and muscle shortening are not interchangeable terms in physiology. As in the case of holding a sleeping child in your arms or gripping a dumbbell in the same position, tension can be created within the muscle without any change in its length. Muscle relaxation, or the return of muscle fibers to a low-tension state, happens when muscle contraction ends. Skeletal, cardiac, and smooth muscles are the three types found in mammals. The body's strength and structure come from the skeletal muscles, which are joined to the bones. The heart's walls, or cardiac muscle, are what enable blood to be pumped through the vasculature. All throughout the blood vessels, GI tract, bronchioles, uterus, and bladder is smooth muscle.

The human body's muscle contraction can be categorized according to the specialization of the individual muscle subtypes. Muscle fibers can be broadly divided into two groups: smooth muscle fibers and striated muscle fibers. The actin and myosin filaments found in striated muscle fibers, which are arranged into repeating arrays known as sarcomeres and have a striated microscopic appearance, are what drive contraction. The body's autonomic nervous system (ANS) controls the striated muscle fibers that make up cardiac muscle tissue in an involuntary manner. A voluntarily controlled striated muscle fiber makes up skeletal muscle tissue. Sarcomeres are absent from smooth muscle fibers, which contract using actin and myosin to narrow blood vessels and shift the contents of hollow organs within the body. The body's nervous system (ANS) and reflexes control these fibers involuntarily.

1.4.1. Cellular Level

1.4.1.1. Striated Muscle

It is crucial to comprehend the structure of striated muscle before attempting to comprehend its mechanism of contraction. Our body's striated muscles are made up of numerous separate muscle fibers. Myofibrils, which are smaller units composed of parallel thin and thick filaments, are found inside these muscle fibers. Sarcomeres are the tiny longitudinally arranged units of filaments that, when viewed under a microscope, give the muscle its striated appearance. The protein myosin, which has one pair of heavy chains and two pairs of light chains—different from the thin and thick filaments of myofibrils—is what makes up the thick filaments. The two heavy chains are entangled in a helical formation at the thick filament's tail. Each heavy chain is paired with two light chains at the opposite end of the thick filament to create two heads. An actin-binding site on the myosin heads facilitates their attachment to the thin filaments. The actin, tropomyosin, and troponin make up the thin filaments. Actin is a globular protein that forms two entwined strands with positive and negative ends when it joins with other actin globules. Tropomyosin coats the double-stranded actin filaments, preventing myosin and actin from interacting when the muscle is not contracting. The trio of troponins, I, T, and C, make up the troponin group, which is situated next to tropomyosin along actin filaments.

Excitation-contraction coupling, a complicated process that results in muscle contraction, starts when an action potential depolarizes the myocyte membrane. Transverse (T) tubules, which are extensions of the muscle cell membrane, aid in the depolarization process by dispersing depolarization signals throughout the muscle fiber. The sarcoplasmic reticulum (SR), the site where calcium is stored in muscle cells, has adjacent ryanodine receptors that open as a result of the T tubules depolarising and changing their conformation. Calcium binds to troponin C upon release from the SR. As a result, tropomyosin undergoes a conformational shift that causes the myosin heads to attach to the actin filaments, forming a cross-bridge. When ATP attaches to an ATP-binding domain on the myosin head, cross-bridge cycling starts. Actin and myosin separate, rupturing the cross-bridge. After that, ATP is hydrolyzed into ADP and P, which causes the myosin heads to cock—move toward the positive end of the actin strand—by changing their conformation. Myosin bound to ADP releases its phosphate and binds to a new spot on the actin filament. After that, ADP is released, causing the myosin to revert to its initial position. This pulls on the actin filament, causing the sarcomere to contract, which in turn causes the muscle fiber to contract. These cycles continue until the myocyte's calcium levels drop, at which point tropomyosin covers the myosin-binding sites on actin filaments.

1.4.1.2. Smooth Muscle

Smooth muscles contain the same thin and thick filaments that were mentioned in striated muscles. Nevertheless, these filaments are not arranged into sarcomeres in smooth muscle tissue. Smooth muscle has a different mechanism of controlling contraction because it lacks the troponin complex necessary for skeletal muscle contraction. The three ways that calcium (Ca) enters the cell to increase intracellular concentration define this difference:

1. Voltage-gated Ca channels are activated by membrane depolarization, allowing Ca to enter the cell.
2. Hormones or neurotransmitters can open ligand-gated channels on the cell membrane.
3. Hormones and neurotransmitters

such as norepinephrine and angiotensin II can, via the phospholipase-C (PLC) pathway, cause an increase in intracellular inositol triphosphate (IP3).

Ca can be released when IP3 binds to receptors on the SR. Upon release, calcium binds to a protein called calmodulin rather than to troponin C, as it does in striated muscle. Myosin light chain kinase (MLCK), as its name implies, phosphorylates the myosin light chain when calmodulin activates it. Because of its ATPase activity, the phosphorylated myosin light chain increases the affinity of ATP for actin. Actin can then be easily bound by myosin. Cross-bridge cycling is the same as in striated muscle from this point on. As long as calcium is bound to calmodulin and the MLCK is phosphorylated, the smooth muscle will stay contracted. This permits blood vessel vasoconstriction for extended periods.

1.4.2. Development

Mesoderm is the source of smooth, cardiac, and skeletal muscles. More precisely, the lateral splanchnic mesoderm gives rise to cardiac muscle, the paraxial mesoderm gives rise to skeletal muscle, and the splanchnic mesoderm gives rise to smooth muscle fibers. The sphincter and dilator pupillae of the iris, as well as the myoepithelial cells of the mammary and sweat glands, are examples of smooth muscles that are not derived from the mesoderm. Instead, they are derived from mesenchymal cells that originate from the ectoderm.

1.4.3. Reasons for Muscle Contraction

Muscles serve several purposes in your body. Your muscles contract for any number of reasons, but they primarily do the following:

- Offer stability to your joints and connective tissues – Your muscles lengthen and shorten, sometimes involuntarily, as your body needs them.
- Produce heat to maintain your body temperature – Around 40% of your body's temperature converts into muscle work. Shivering is your body's response to feeling cold, and your skeletal muscles activate to warm your body.
- Maintain posture – Muscles help you maintain a position like sitting or standing.

1.4.4. Types of Muscle Contraction

There are three types of Muscle Contraction are:

1. *Concentric Contractions.* Your muscles contract in this way when they are actively shortened. Tension is created when you activate your muscles to lift something heavier than usual, causing them to tighten. Remember that this kind of muscle contraction occurs when the load is less than the maximal strength of your muscles. Without physically shortening the fibers to move the object, your muscles are unable to lift the load. Taking up a heavy box is an example of a concentric muscle contraction. Your leg muscles tighten as you stand up with the extra weight after squatting down to lift a box, even though your arm muscles may have contracted to support the weight.
2. *Eccentric Contractions.* Eccentric contractions occur when a muscle lengthens while under tension. Unlike concentric contractions, where the muscle shortens as it

contracts, eccentric contractions involve the muscle lengthening while still generating force. These contractions play a crucial role in various activities, such as controlling movement and decelerating the body's motion. During eccentric contractions, muscle fibers are actively stretched, leading to microscopic damage that triggers muscle growth and adaptation. This process contributes to muscle strength, flexibility, and overall function. Examples of eccentric contractions include lowering weights during resistance training and controlling movements during downhill running or walking downhill.

3. *Isometric Contraction*. This type of muscle contraction happens when your muscle is actively held at a set length. Instead of lengthening and shortening as it would during some activities, you hold it in a position that requires a specific length once activated. An example of this type of contraction is carrying something in your arms in front of you. You aren't trying to raise or lower the object but keep it at a steady position.

1.4.5. Uses of Muscle Contraction

1.4.5.1. Isometric Muscle Contractions

When your muscle remains in one position and the joint to which it is attached remains motionless, you use this kind of contraction. It doesn't give the muscle group general strengthening. Rather, it fortifies your muscle for that one particular motion. It is beneficial to practice using a muscle in a specific way after an injury by performing an isometric muscle contraction.

1.4.5.2. Concentric and Eccentric Muscle Contractions

Combinations of these two contraction types are common. When lifting something heavy, a concentric muscle contraction comes in handy. Positive work is the term used to describe it most frequently. Negative work is the contraction of an eccentric muscle. To assist you in lowering something heavy, your muscle contracts eccentrically. During an exercise routine, lifting a dumbbell is an example of these two contractions. Your biceps muscles contract and tighten as you pick up the dumbbell in order to lift the weight.

1.4.5.3. Passive Stretching

This type of muscle contraction is helpful for gently lengthening your muscles. You can contract your muscles passively by stretching them as far as they can physically go. This lengthens your muscles in a way that activates them without using force.

1.4.6. Function

Skeletal muscle contraction is primarily responsible for enabling the execution of particular movements. In addition, skeletal muscle stores amino acids, maintains posture, offers structural support, and shivers to regulate body temperature. Heart muscle cells come in two varieties: contractile and autorhythmic. Instead of contracting, autorhythmic cardiac cells set the pace at which other cardiac muscle cells contract, a function that the ANS can control. Most of the heart muscle is made up of contractile cardiac cells, or cardiomyocytes. Smooth muscle cells come in two varieties: single-unit and multi-unit. The gastrointestinal tract and blood vessels contain single-unit smooth muscle cells. They can contract as a functional syncytium because gap junctions connect them. They can also be modulated by the ANS and contract myogenically. The base of hair follicles and the muscles of the eye both contain multiunit smooth muscle cells. Fine control and gradual response are made possible by their contraction, which is triggered independently by ANS nerves.

1.4.7. Mechanism

1.4.7.1. Types of Striated Muscle Contraction

Muscle contractions can be classified as isometric, isotonic, concentric, or eccentric. Muscle tension changes without corresponding changes in muscle length during an isometric striated contraction. Isometric contractions occur when one tries to lift a weight that is too heavy or pushes against an immovable object. Constant muscle tension without a change in muscle length is the hallmark of isotonic striated muscle contraction. When the force used to contract a muscle equals the total load on it, this kind of contraction takes place. Exercises like running, squatting, and walking cause isotonic contractions. When there is enough muscle tension to overcome the load, the muscle contracts and shortens, resulting in a concentrated striated contraction. The sliding filament theory states that a muscle is stimulated to contract during this kind of contraction. Concentric contractions occur when performing exercises like a biceps curl or getting up from a squat. When a muscle works to slow down a joint after a movement rather than pulling it in the direction of the contraction, this is known as eccentric striated muscle contraction. This kind of contraction can happen unintentionally (e.g., while making an effort to lift a weight that is too heavy for the muscle to support, or freely (e.g., when the muscle is defying gravity or "smoothing out" a movement (like when walking downhill). To prevent damage to joints, eccentric contractions function as a braking force in opposition to concentric contractions.

1.4.7.2. General Mechanism of Skeletal Muscle Contraction

Skeletal muscle contraction initiation and execution occur in the following steps.

1. An action potential (AP) travels along a motor nerve to its endings on muscle fibers.
2. At each motor nerve ending, the nerve secretes acetylcholine (ACh).
3. ACh acts locally on the muscle fiber membrane to open ACh-gated cation channels.
4. The opening of ACh-gated channels allows large quantities of sodium (Na) ions to diffuse into the interior of the muscle fiber membrane.
5. This action causes a local depolarization, leading to the opening of voltage-gated sodium (Na) channels, which initiates an AP at the membrane.
6. The AP depolarizes the muscle membrane, causing the sarcoplasmic reticulum (SR) to release large quantities of Ca ions stored within the reticulum.
7. The Ca ions produce attractive forces to act between actin and myosin filaments, causing them to slide alongside each other, leading to the contractile process.
8. After a fraction of a second, the Ca ions are pumped back into the SR by a Ca-membrane pump and remain stored in the SR until a new muscle AP occurs.
9. The removal of Ca ions from the

myofibrils causes muscle contraction to cease.

1.4.7.3. General Mechanism of Cardiac Muscle Contraction

The process of excitation-contraction coupling (ECC), which uses a mechanism known as calcium-induced calcium release (CICR), is how cardiac muscle contracts. ECC is the procedure that transforms an electrical stimulus (AP) into a contraction of a muscle mechanism. In CICR, calcium ions are conducted into the cardiomyocyte, which causes additional ion release into the cytoplasm. Ca increases the amount of time that cardiac muscle cells are depolarized before they repolarize. The mechanical force of contraction in cardiac muscle is produced by the binding of the myosin head to ATP, which pulls actin filaments to the center of the sarcomere.

Cardiac muscle contraction initiation and execution occur in the following steps.

1. An action potential (AP), induced by the pacemaker cells in the sinoatrial (SA) and atrioventricular (AV) nodes, is conducted to contractile cardiomyocytes through gap junctions.
2. As the AP travels between sarcomeres, it activates the Ca channels in the T tubules, leading to an influx of Ca ions into the cardiomyocyte.
3. Ca in the cytoplasm then binds to cardiac troponin C, which moves the troponin complex away from the actin-binding site. Removal of the troponin complex frees actin, which becomes bound by myosin and initiates contraction.
4. Intracellular Ca is then removed by the SR, dropping the concentration of intracellular Ca. This decrease in intracellular Ca concentration returns the troponin complex to its inhibiting position on the active site of actin, ending contraction as the actin filaments return to their initial position, relaxing the muscle.

1.4.7.4. General Mechanism of Smooth Muscle Contraction

The contraction of smooth muscle is not regulated by the binding of Ca to the troponin complex, as is seen in cardiac and skeletal muscle contraction. Smooth muscle instead utilizes calmodulin, an intracellular second messenger that binds calcium.

Smooth muscle contraction initiation and execution occur in the following steps.

1. Intracellular Ca concentration increases when calcium enters the cell and is released from the SR.
2. Calcium binds to calmodulin.
3. Ca-calmodulin activates myosin light chain kinase (MLCK).
4. MLCK phosphorylates myosin head light chains and increases myosin ATPase activity.
5. Active myosin cross-bridges slide along actin and create muscle tension.
6. Smooth muscle relaxation occurs as free Ca in the cytosol decreases when Ca is pumped out of the cell or back into the SR.
7. Ca unbinds from calmodulin.
8. Myosin phosphatase removes phosphate from myosin, decreasing myosin ATPase activity and muscle tension.

1.4.8. Testing

1.4.8.1. Manual Muscle Testing (MMT)

MMT is used in the physical examination of patients to assess muscle strength. It may be used to evaluate weakness and can effectively differentiate true weakness from imbalance or poor endurance. The Oxford scale is the most widely and commonly accepted method of assessing muscle strength, as it does not require special equipment and demonstrates reliability among independent evaluators. The Oxford scale involves testing key muscles from the upper and lower extremities against an examiner's resistance and grading the patient's strength on a scale of 0 to 5, documented as x/5 (e.g., 1/5, 2/5 muscle strength).

- 0: no contraction
- 1: visible/palpable muscle contraction but no movement
- 2: movement with gravity eliminated
- 3: movement against gravity only
- 4: movement against gravity with some resistance
- 5: movement against gravity with full resistance

1.4.8.2. Electromyography (EMG)

The main application of electromyography (EMG) is to differentiate between myopathic and neurogenic muscle weakness and wasting. EMG is the recording of electrical activity that occurs within a muscle. By identifying the distribution of neurogenic abnormalities, EMGs can distinguish focal nerve, plexus, or radicular pathology and detect fasciculations or chronic denervation in muscles that appear clinically normal. The pathophysiology of a peripheral myopathy can be supported by EMGs, which are a necessary investigation in motor neuron disease to show the widespread fasciculation and denervation needed to establish a diagnosis. A needle electrode is inserted into the muscle to record electromyography readings. A typical EMG needle records a radius of about 1 mm, and there can be up to 100 muscle fibers in this volume. Diagnostic data can be obtained by examining the waveforms and firing rates of single- or multiple-motor units.

1.4.9. Pathophysiology

Since muscles are present all over the body, there are many different pathologies linked to abnormal muscle contraction. As such, although this list outlines high-yield pathophysiological conditions associated with the contraction of muscles, it is not all-inclusive.

1.4.9.1. Skeletal Muscle Contraction Pathology

- Duchenne muscular dystrophy
- Becker muscular dystrophy
- Myotonic dystrophy
- Lambert-Eaton syndrome
- Myasthenia gravis
- Myositis
- Bell's palsy

1.4.9.2. Smooth Muscle Contraction Pathology

- Asthma
- Gastroparesis
- Nephrolithiasis
- Chronic kidney disease
- Neurogenic bladder
- Infertility
- Pulmonary hypertension

1.4.9.3. Cardiac Muscle Contraction Pathology

- Congestive heart failure
- Cardiomyopathy (e.g., dilated, hypertrophic, restrictive)

1.4.10. Clinical Significance

1.4.10.1. Troponin Assays

Subtypes of troponin I and T have the potential to act as indicators of damage to the heart muscle. Since unstable angina and myocardial infarction (MI) can have similar symptoms, blood levels of troponin are used to distinguish between the two conditions. Elevated troponin levels in MI would not be present in unstable angina. Troponin levels can stay high for up to two weeks after an injury and peak a few hours later. Since troponin release only signifies the presence of cardiac muscle damage, it is not unique to MI. For this reason, diseases like amyloidosis, pericarditis, and heart failure may also have increased troponin levels. Moreover, conditions other than heart failure, like sepsis or renal failure, can also raise troponin levels.

1.4.10.2. Muscle Spasm

Muscle spasms, sometimes referred to as cramps, are painful, localized, and involuntary contractions of a single muscle, a group of muscles, or specific muscle fibers. The duration of a muscle spasm varies, ranging from a few seconds to several weeks, contingent upon the impacted muscle and the underlying mechanism. Muscle spasms related to exercise are the most common conditions in sports that need medical attention. The precise cause of the spasms is unknown, and potential explanations vary depending on the physiological or pathological context in which they manifest. It is crucial to understand that a painful contraction that is localized does not always indicate that the cramp's origin is nearby. In some clinical situations, chronic spastic muscle contractions that have a major impact on bodily functions may be the underlying etiology. One common site of manifestation for this condition is the sternocleidomastoid muscle. Clinically, this is known as either spasmodic or congenital torticollis. Other pertinent conditions in this field include piriformis syndrome and cramping in the muscles brought on by exercise and heat.

1.4.10.3. Manual Muscle Testing (MMT)

MMT is rated on a scale of 0 to 5, and as was previously mentioned, it is used as a clinical tool to evaluate muscle strength. Assessing deficiencies and impairments in muscle performance, such as strength, power, and endurance, is another use of MMT in rehabilitation and recovery procedures. The rehabilitation process, which may involve specific therapy exercises, bracing, or functional movement training, depends on the identification of impairment in particular muscles or groups of muscles.

1.4.10.4. Pharmacology

Clinically, it is essential to recognize that many medications today will affect muscle contraction at some level. Therefore, whether it is the main effect of the drug or a side effect, it is crucial to understand the uses and consequences of administering medications to patients. Pharmacological agents that directly affect muscle contraction include, but are not limited to:

- Skeletal muscle relaxants (e.g., botulinum toxin, cyclobenzaprine, methocarbamol)
- Vasodilating medications (e.g., hydralazine, nitrates, milrinone)
- Volatile anesthetics or succinylcholine can lead to malignant hyperthermia

(Aiello and Dean, 1990; Agur & Dalley,2009)

1.5. Muscle Energy Metabolism

Body tissue known as muscle is distinguished by its ability to contract, typically in reaction to a nervous system stimulus. Skeletal and cardiac muscles are the highest energy consumers among the three main types of muscle. The circulatory system pumps blood through the heart, a muscular pump. Heart muscle is relatively small in relation to other muscle types, but it has a remarkable blood supply share and a vibrant energy metabolism. The respiratory, urinary, and gastrointestinal tracts, as well as the reproductive system and blood vessels, are the primary locations for smooth muscle. The contraction and tone of smooth muscle in these tissues and organs regulate many essential processes, including blood pressure and flow regulation, respiratory tract air flow direction, and the transmission of contents in the intestines and urinary tract. Smooth muscle has a high workload, but it consumes very little energy. Approximately two-thirds of the body's mass is made up of the skeletal muscle that makes up the locomotor system. Its portion of the cardiac output at rest is one-sixth of the total, matching the brain's share. Muscle consumes the most oxygen during maximal activation in aerobic work, and its blood circulation accounts for four-fifths of the cardiac output.

The metabolism of energy is distinct in skeletal muscle. Its adaptation for brief anaerobic exercise, in addition to its aerobic capacity, enables both prolonged lower-intensity endurance exercise and brief high-energy output. For skeletal muscle, the dynamic range of the change in the rate of ATP utilization is greater than a hundredfold. Circulatory, cardiac, and respiratory functions must be adjusted to compensate for changes in ATP utilization. Skeletal muscle in humans at rest receives approximately 5 milliliters of blood per 100 grams of tissue. The percentage of muscle tissue's cardiac output that comes from heavy exercise can reach up to four-fifths or higher in trained subjects. The extraction of oxygen also increases during heavy exercise, as shown by the rising arteriovenous difference, which goes from 25% at rest to 80% or higher during maximal exercise. As a result, when human muscle is worked, the amount of oxygen used can increase by approximately 100 times. This is actually quite a small increase when compared to some animals, where the increase can reach a thousand times.

Muscle metabolism can be understood from a set of basic statements about the biochemical energy balance:

- Chemical energy is stored in muscle cells as ATP and creatine phosphate, which are biochemical capacitors.
- ATP provides the energy for all forms of muscle work.
- ATPases, the enzymes that break down ATP and release the energy for muscle work and metabolism, are the demand side of the balance and define energetic states; and
- This demand is supplied mainly by continuous aerobic metabolism.

The fundamental component of every muscle is the myofibril, a tiny, thread-like structure made up of intricate protein structures. Numerous myofibrils, which are made up of thin and thick myofilaments arranged in a regular pattern, are found inside each muscle cell, or fiber. When skeletal muscle contracts, the plasma membrane typically depolarizes, causing the sarcoplasmic reticulum's intracellular calcium ion stores to release calcium ions. A protein's conformation changes when calcium ions attach to troponin C, a regulatory protein connected to thin filaments. The actin subunits of the thin filaments can interact with the nearby myosin molecules, which are made up of thick filaments, as a result of this shape change that is transferred to the other thin filament components (troponin T, troponin I, tropomyosin, and actin). When calcium ions are absorbed by the sarcoplasmic reticulum via the action of an ATP-driven pump, also referred to as Ca2+ ATPase, the contraction stops.

1.5.1. Anaerobic Energy Metabolism

The cytosolic pathway for the catabolism of glucose is called glycolysis. Glycolysis is distinct in that it can operate without oxygen (pyruvate → lactate) or with oxygen if it is available (pyruvate → acetyl-CoA). Different tissues use glycolysis differently as a source of energy; the heart uses it less than other tissues, while the brain and red blood cells use it more. Glycolysis allows skeletal muscle to function at a high level when aerobic metabolism is insufficient. Glycolysis produces almost half of the acetyl-CoA required for the citric acid cycle in skeletal muscle at rest. Six-carbon glucose is catabolized into three-carbon pyruvate and then acetyl-CoA during this process, producing two NADH and two ATP net. With a net yield of two ATP per NADH, NADH produced by glycolysis is moved into the mitochondria by the malate shuttle and oxidized in the respiratory chain. So, during the aerobic full oxidation of one mole of glucose, the citric acid cycle produces thirty ATP and glycolysis produces eight ATP. Anaerobiosis can also easily occur in skeletal muscle. This characteristic enables short-term performance that is significantly higher than what is possible to sustain aerobically. Two of the three ways that ATP is synthesized involve anaerobic metabolism or metabolism that does not require oxygen. Anaerobic energy metabolism, also referred to as anaerobic glycolysis, is the process by which carbohydrates are partially broken down into lactic acid through anaerobic metabolic pathways. When aerobic metabolism is insufficient to meet the energy needs of muscle activity, which can occur in as little as a few minutes, anaerobic glycolysis is triggered. Even though ATP is produced quickly during this cytoplasmic process, anaerobic glycolysis is not as efficient as aerobic glycolysis.

The amount and duration of exercise are directly correlated with the lactic acid end-product of anaerobic energy metabolism. Lactic acid buildup lowers intracellular pH, which stops phosphofructokinase—the enzyme that limits the rate of glycolysis—from working. Additionally, during low-intensity exercise, muscle NADH decreases, but during high-intensity exercise, it increases above resting values. Limited O2 availability in the contracting muscle may be the cause of the increase in muscle NADH. Intense exercise causes an increase in cytosolic NADH, which inhibits pyruvate dehydrogenase and increases the extraction of hydrogen atoms from NADH to reduce pyruvate to lactate. To facilitate the process of glycolysis and supply energy for the reconstitution of the energy-rich phosphates, oxidized NAD can function as a hydrogen acceptor. However, the cost of producing ATP anaerobically is high. Just two moles of ATP are produced net when one mole of glucose is oxidized. Increased lactic acid production can impair the function of vessels, neuromuscular junctions, muscle fibers, and connective tissue cells. However, it can also trigger adaptive changes in metabolism, which are crucial for training, particularly in sports. Excessive oxygen consumption also leads to the profound production of various forms of oxygen, such as reactive oxygen species (ROS) in fibroblasts, endothelium, neutrophils, and erythrocytes in skeletal muscle fiber and endothelium. ROS induces tissue damage and muscular exhaustion. Several aqueous and lipid phase antioxidant defense systems exist in muscle tissue, protecting the tissue from the harmful effects of excessively produced ROS. The synthesis of glutathione (GSH), which is essential for maintaining the antioxidant defense, is a function of skeletal muscle. It helps maintain the reduced forms of vitamin C (in the soluble phase) and vitamin E (in the lipid phase) as an oxidisable substrate itself.

In the metabolism of peroxides, enzymes of the glutathione system such as glutathione-S-transferases and glutathione peroxidase work together with catalase.

1.5.2. Aerobic Metabolism

The respiratory cascade delivers oxygen to the site of oxidation in living tissues. Since over 90% of energy is used by muscle cells during intense exercise, the aerobic demand is primarily determined by active skeletal muscle cells. Substances are transported in plasma, while oxygen is carried in the bloodstream bound to erythrocyte hemoglobin. Because most mammalian species have very small oxygen reserves in their bodies and large amounts of substrates stored in tissue substrate stores as well as within muscle cells, a constant oxygen supply is necessary.

1.5.2.1. Mitochondrial Oxidative Phosphorylation

The mitochondria are the site of aerobic energy metabolism, which releases the most energy. However, as the name suggests, it needs oxygen. For the production of energy, aerobic glycolysis is the most efficient process. In the absence of oxygen, a single mole of glycogen can produce only two moles of ATP anaerobically, but in the presence of oxygen, the same amount of glycogen can produce 38 moles of ATP. After deducting the 2 moles of ATP consumption, the net yield amounts to 36 moles of ATP (with 38 molecules in the heart muscle, liver, and kidney). Oxidative phosphorylation is the process by which hydrogen atoms are taken out of the reducing equivalents created during the citric acid cycle in the mitochondria of muscle cells. As a result, unique electron transport proteins take electrons from hydrogen atoms and ultimately move them to molecules of oxygen. ATP is a form of energy conservation that is produced during the transfer of electrons to oxygen. In the respiratory chain, electrons move from more electronegative to more electropositive oxygen molecules in an order that increases redox potential. The rate of mitochondrial respiration in cells under high oxygen pressure is determined by energy demand, while the cellular energy level at which that rate is reached is determined by substrate supply. When compared to the energy needed by contracting muscle cells, the pool of ATP and CP is considerably smaller. For very brief intervals of time, the rate of ATP utilization can be higher or lower than the rate of ATP synthesis due to the small size of the high-energy phosphate pool. Therefore, the rate at which ATP is synthesized needs to be, on average, equal to the rate at which it is hydrolyzed by cellular processes. As a result, mitochondrial oxidative phosphorylation is closely linked to numerous metabolic processes and reacts fast to variations in the ATP requirements of tissues. But the respiratory chain's coupling isn't flawless. Superoxide is thought to escape from the respiratory chain at rest in an amount of 1–3%. Reactive oxygen species production like this could have effects during exercise and while at rest.

1.5.2.2. Citric Acid Cycle

The majority of oxygen in skeletal muscle is used by the mitochondria, which also provide the main metabolic energy source for prolonged activity. The citric acid cycle, sometimes referred to as the Krebs or tricarboxylic acid cycle, is a set of events that occur in the mitochondria that catabolize acetyl-CoA and release hydrogen equivalents, which are then utilized in oxidative phosphorylation to produce ATP from ADP. An essential component of aerobic metabolism is the citric acid cycle. The common final pathway for the catabolism of proteins, lipids (fatty acid beta-oxidation), and glucose (glycolysis) is the citric acid cycle. Fatty acid beta-oxidation and glycolysis contribute more than 95% of the acetyl-CoA that enters the citric acid cycle, both at rest and during exercise. Acetyl-CoA condenses with oxaloacetate to form citrate in the citric acid cycle. Oxaloacetate is once more created in the reactions that follow. Three NADH, one FADH2, one GTP, and two CO2 are produced during the process. After that, the hydrogen equivalents go through oxidative phosphorylation. In the process, 11 ATP are produced by the 3 NADH and 1 FADH2. Consequently, 12 ATP are produced by one citric acid cycle turn.

1.5.3. Metabolism of Glucose and Glycogen in Muscle Fibers

Glycogen is obtained by skeletal muscle through either transport from the blood or glycogenolysis. Glycogen can be stored in muscle tissue up to a maximum of 4–5% of the tissue's wet weight. The primary source of glucose during moderate to intense exercise is glycogen, which also poses a constraint on endurance events like marathons. The best way to characterize the glycogen and glucose catabolic rates is as exponential functions of exercise intensity, with the glycogen response having a higher gain in slope than the glucose response. Using insulin-dependent processes, muscle takes up glucose from the blood. Insulin sensitivity in skeletal muscle is increased by exercise. Muscle increases its uptake of glucose during exercise by an increased metabolic rate and an increase in membrane permeability to glucose brought on by contraction. It has been demonstrated that glucose uptake is inhibited by additional regulatory mechanisms, such as elevated glycogenolysis or higher resting glycogen concentration. Increased concentrations of free fatty acids may also reduce the uptake of glucose during exercise, though this is a contentious claim. Exercise training causes an increase in muscle glucose transporter levels, including GLUT4, an essential limiting factor of glucose utilization, and glycogen synthase activity. However, elevated GLUT4 levels may not always correlate with increased uptake of glucose. Furthermore, the balance of substrate utilization during intense muscle work is influenced by both phenotypic adaptations to short- and long-term physical activity and genotypic adaptation for aerobic capacity (Aiello & Dean, 1990; Agur & Dalley, 2009).

A Closer Look

Muscle Regeneration and Repair

Muscle regeneration after injury is a complex and highly orchestrated process involving a variety of cellular and molecular mechanisms. At the forefront of this regeneration are satellite cells, a specialized population of stem cells located within the muscle tissue. These satellite cells are normally quiescent but become activated in response to injury or exercise-induced stress. Upon activation, satellite cells undergo proliferation and differentiation, giving rise to myoblasts, which are the precursor cells for muscle fibers. Myoblasts then fuse together or with existing muscle fibers to repair and regenerate damaged muscle tissue.

The role of satellite cells in muscle regeneration is pivotal, as they not only contribute directly to muscle fiber formation but also play a crucial role in maintaining the pool of stem cells for future repair. Additionally, satellite cells are capable of self-renewal, ensuring the sustainability of the regenerative process over time. Moreover, satellite cells are regulated by a complex interplay of signaling molecules, growth factors, and transcription factors, which orchestrate their activation, proliferation, and differentiation in response to injury.

Despite the remarkable regenerative capacity of skeletal muscle, severe injuries or chronic conditions can sometimes overwhelm the regenerative capacity of satellite cells, leading to impaired muscle repair and fibrosis. In such cases, therapeutic interventions aimed at enhancing muscle regeneration may be necessary. One promising approach involves the transplantation or activation of exogenous stem cells, such as mesenchymal stem cells or induced pluripotent stem cells, to supplement or augment the regenerative capacity of endogenous satellite cells. These exogenous stem cells can differentiate into myogenic cells and contribute to muscle repair, thereby accelerating the regeneration process.

In addition to stem cell-based therapies, various other strategies have been explored to promote muscle regeneration and repair. These include the administration of growth factors, such as insulin-like growth factor 1 (IGF-1) and hepatocyte growth factor (HGF), which stimulate satellite cell activation and proliferation. Furthermore, advances in tissue engineering and biomaterials have enabled the development of scaffolds and matrices that mimic the native muscle microenvironment and facilitate the recruitment, proliferation, and differentiation of satellite cells.

Summary

- The muscular system is composed of specialized cells called muscle fibers. Their predominant function is contractility. Muscles, attached to bones or internal organs and blood vessels, are responsible for movement.
- The human muscle system is the muscles of the human body that work with the skeletal system, are under voluntary control, and are concerned with movement, posture, and balance.
- Elasticity is defined as the ability of a muscle to recoil or bounce back to its original length after being stretched beyond its maximum length.
- The motion of the neck is described in terms of rotation, flexion, extension, and side bending (i.e., the motion used to touch the ear to the shoulder). The direction of the action can be ipsilateral, which refers to movement in the direction of the contracting muscle, or contralateral, which refers to movement away from the side of the contracting muscle.
- The shoulder is a complex ball-and-socket joint comprising the head of the humerus, the clavicle (collarbone), and the scapula. The shoulder's main motions are flexion, extension, abduction, adduction, internal rotation, and external rotation.
- Wrist flexion refers to the movement of the wrist that draws the palm of the hand downward. That action is carried out by the flexor carpi radialis, the flexor carpi ulnaris, the flexor digitorum superficialis, the flexor digitorum profundus, and the flexor pollicis longus.
- The hip joint is a complex weight-bearing ball-and-socket joint that can sustain considerable load. The socket of the joint is relatively deep, allowing for stability but sacrificing some degree of range of motion. The movements described in this section include flexion, extension, abduction, and adduction.
- Skeletal muscle, also called voluntary muscle, in vertebrates, is the most common of the three types of muscle in the body. Skeletal muscles are attached to bones by tendons, and they produce all the movements of body parts in relation to each other.
- Smooth muscle is found throughout the body where it serves a variety of functions. It is in the stomach and intestines where it helps with digestion and nutrient collection. It is found throughout the urinary system where it functions to help rid the body of toxins and works in electrolyte balance.
- Cardiac muscle, also called myocardium, in vertebrates, is one of three major muscle types, found only in the heart. Cardiac muscle is similar to skeletal muscle, another major muscle type, in that it possesses contractile units known as sarcomeres; this feature, however, also distinguishes it from smooth muscle, the third muscle type.
- Muscle contraction is the tightening, shortening, or lengthening of muscles when you do some activity. It can happen when you hold or pick up something, or when you stretch or exercise with weights. Muscle contraction is often followed by muscle relaxation when contracted muscles return to their normal state.

References

1. Agresta, C., Kessler, S., Southern, E., Goulet, G. C., Zernicke, R., & Zendler, J. D. (2018). Immediate and short-term adaptations to maximalist and minimalist running shoes. *Footwear Science, 10*(3), 151–166.
2. Agur, A. M. R., & Dalley, A. F. (2009). Knee Joint. In A. M. R. Agur & A. F. Dalley (Eds.), *Grant's Atlas of Anatomy* (12th ed., p. 414). Lippincott Williams & Wilkins.
3. Aiello, L., & Dean, C. (1990). *An Introduction to Human Evolutionary Anatomy*. Oxford: Elsevier Academic Press.
4. Alam, M., Choudhury, I. A., & Mamat, A. B. (2013). Mechanism and design analysis of articulated ankle foot orthoses for drop-foot. *The Scientific World Journal, 2014*, Article 258096. https://doi.org/10.1155/2014/258096.
5. Alves, F., Towers, J. R., Baird, R. W., Bearzi, G., Bonizzoni, S., Ferreira, R., Halicka, Z., Alessandrini, A., Kopelman, A. H., Yzoard, C., Rasmussen, M. H., Bertulli, C. G., Jourdain, E., Gullan, A., Rocha, D., Hupman, K., Mrusczok, M.-T., Samarra, F. I. P., Magalhaes, S., Weir, C. R., Ford, J. K. B., & Dinis, A. (2017). The incidence of bent dorsal fins in free-ranging cetaceans. *Journal of Anatomy, 231*(6), 885–893. https://doi.org/10.1111/joa.12702.

Chapter

MUSCLE METABOLISM

2

Contents

Introduction

The complex biochemical reactions that take place inside muscle cells to produce energy, aid in muscular contraction, and preserve cellular processes are referred to as muscle metabolism. The range of activities from the lightest movements to high levels of physical exertion requires these processes. The process of converting nutrients into adenosine triphosphate (ATP), the main energy unit of cells, is the basis of muscle metabolism. The energy required for different cellular functions and muscle contraction is provided by ATP. The breakdown of creatine phosphate (CP) and aerobic metabolism are the three primary metabolic pathways that muscle cells use to produce ATP. In aerobic metabolism, which takes place in the presence of oxygen, ATP is produced by the citric acid cycle and oxidative phosphorylation in the mitochondria through the breakdown of carbohydrates, fats, and occasionally proteins. The main source of ATP during extended, low-to-moderate intensity exercise is this highly efficient pathway.

Anaerobic metabolism, on the other hand, uses oxygen as a fuel and consists of two primary pathways: the phosphagen system and glycolysis. A tiny quantity of ATP is produced in the cytoplasm during glycolysis, which converts glucose from blood glucose or muscle glycogen stores into pyruvate. When oxygen availability is reduced during vigorous exercise, pyruvate is changed into lactate, which permits glycolysis to proceed. A quick-acting but transient source of ATP is produced by the phosphagen system, which breaks down CP, during high-intensity, brief activities. When CP is broken down by creatine kinase, energy is released, allowing adenosine diphosphate (ADP) to be converted back into ATP. Exercise intensity, duration, and personal fitness levels are some of the variables that affect how much each of these pathways contributes to the synthesis of ATP. For instance, the phosphagen system and anaerobic glycolysis predominate during brief bursts of high-intensity exercise, such as sprinting or weightlifting, providing quick energy but causing lactate to build up and fatigue. On the other hand, aerobic metabolism takes over as the main source of ATP during extended endurance exercises like distance running or cycling, using fats and stored glycogen as fuel. Muscle metabolism includes many metabolic activities, including protein turnover, lipid metabolism, and the synthesis and breakdown of glycogen, in addition to the synthesis of ATP. These procedures guarantee that the muscle cells can adjust to shifting metabolic demands and have a sufficient supply of substrates for energy production.

Orientation and Directional Terms

Term	Definition	Illustration
Aerobic respiration	A chemical process in which oxygen is used to make energy from carbohydrates (sugars).	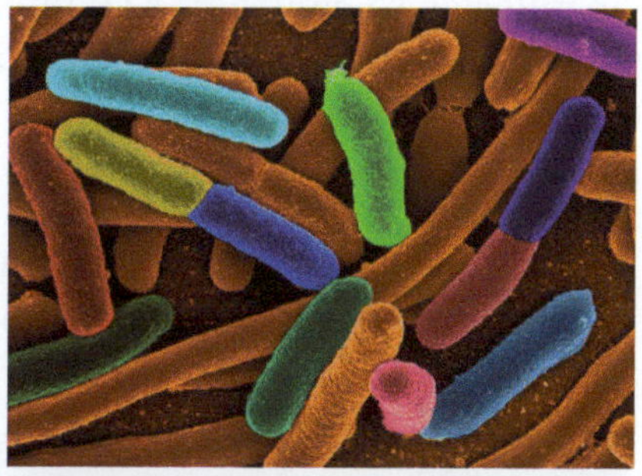
Cerebral metabolism	The brain is metabolically one of the most active of all organs in the body. The brain does not store excess energy and derives almost all of its energy needs from aerobic oxidation of glucose. Therefore, it requires a continuous supply of glucose and oxygen to meet its energy requirements.	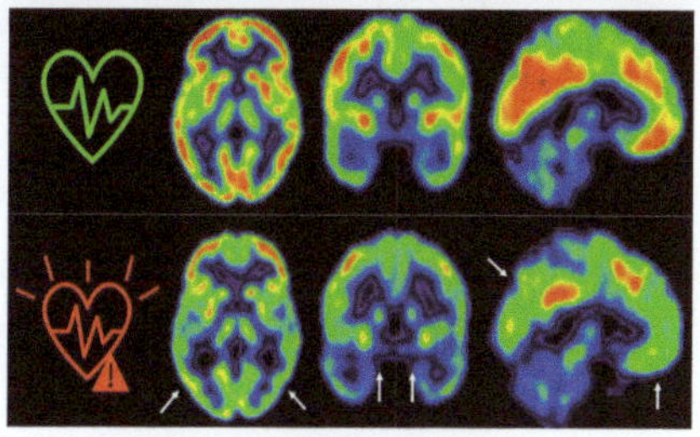
Glycogen synthesis	The first committed step in glycogen synthesis is the formation of UDP glucose by UDP glucose pyrophosphorylase.	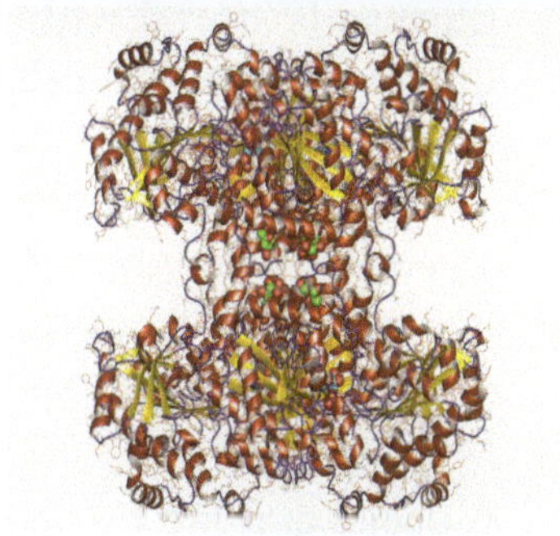
Hyperthyroidism	Hyperthyroidism happens when the thyroid gland makes too much thyroid hormone. This condition also is called overactive thyroid. Hyperthyroidism speeds up the body's metabolism. That can cause many symptoms, such as weight loss, hand tremors, and rapid or irregular heartbeat.	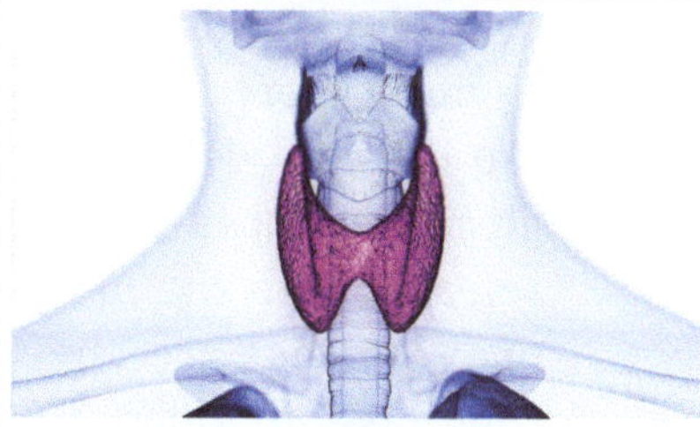
Serum hypokalemi	Hypokalemia is generally defined as a serum potassium level of less than 3.5 mEq/L (3.5 mmol/L). Moderate hypokalemia is a serum level of 2.5-3.0 mEq/L, and severe hypokalemia is a level of less than 2.5 mEq/L.	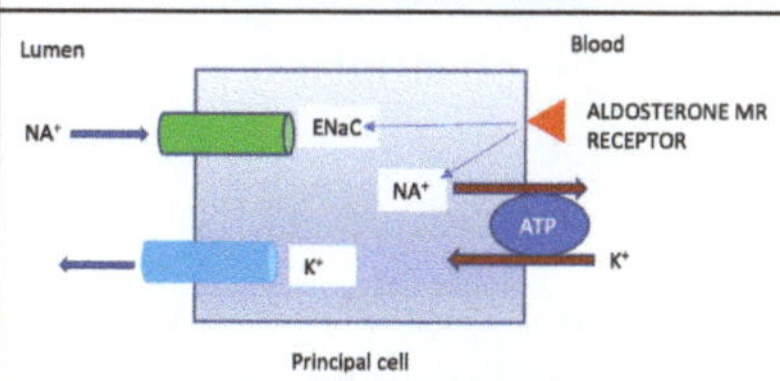

2.1. Fundamentals of Muscle Metabolism

For muscles to contract, ATP must be available in the muscle fiber. ATP is available from the following sources:

- Within the muscle fiber. ATP available within the muscle fiber can maintain muscle contraction for several seconds.
- Creatine phosphate. Creatine phosphate, a high-energy molecule stored in muscle cells, transfers its high-energy phosphate group to ADP to form ATP. The creatine phosphate in muscle cells can generate enough ATP to maintain muscle contraction for about 15 seconds.
- Glucose is stored within the cell. Glucose within the cell is stored in the carbohydrate glycogen. Through the metabolic process of glycogenolysis, glycogen is broken down to release glucose. ATP is then generated from glucose by cellular respiration.
- Glucose and fatty acids are obtained from the bloodstream. Fatty acids from fat stored in adipose cells and the liver, as well as glucose from glycogen stored in the liver, are released into the bloodstream when energy needs are high. Muscle cells then take up glucose and fats from the circulation. Cellular respiration uses these energy-dense molecules to produce ATP.

Cellular respiration is the process by which ATP is obtained from energy-rich molecules. Several major metabolic pathways are involved, some of which require the presence of oxygen. Here's a summary of the important pathways:

- Even though there is no oxygen present during glycolysis, glucose is converted to pyruvic acid and two ATP molecules are produced. Anaerobic respiration is the process of producing ATP without the use of oxygen. Anaerobic glycolysis is the process of producing ATP without the use of oxygen during any of the pathway's metabolic steps.
- During anaerobic respiration, pyruvic acid is converted to lactic acid. Lactic acid (via liver enzymes) can be converted back to pyruvic acid and, with the presence of oxygen, pyruvic acid can enter the mitochondria.

Anaerobic respiration has advantages and disadvantages:

- Advantages: Anaerobic respiration is relatively rapid, and it does not require oxygen.
- Disadvantages: Only two ATPs are produced by anaerobic respiration, along with lactic acid. The majority of lactic acid diffuses into the bloodstream after leaving the cell, where it is then absorbed by the liver. Muscle fatigue is a result of some of the lactic acid that is still present in the muscle fibers. Much ATP must be produced during intense exercise. The anaerobic pathway is how the body attempts to produce ATP when an individual exercises more quickly than they are taking in oxygen. Lots of lactic acid and ATP are produced as a result. The muscles and liver must change the lactic acid back into pyruvic acid after exercise. Much of the oxygen the body is now consuming is used in the conversion process rather

than being used in other ways to accomplish that. The phrase "oxygen debt" refers to this process of "repaying the debt."

- In aerobic respiration, pyruvic acid (from glycolysis) and fatty acids (from the bloodstream) are broken down, producing H_2O and CO_2 (carbon dioxide) and regenerating the coenzymes for glycolysis. A total of 36 ATP molecules are produced (including the two from glycolysis). However, oxygen is required for this pathway.

Aerobic respiration also has advantages and disadvantages:

- Advantages: Aerobic respiration generates a large amount of ATP.
- Disadvantages: Aerobic respiration is relatively slow and requires oxygen.

Anaerobic respiration starts when the ATP produced from creatine phosphate is exhausted due to the immediate need to contract muscle fibers. ATP can be produced by anaerobic respiration for roughly 30 seconds. The slower ATP-producing pathway, aerobic respiration, starts if muscle contraction doesn't stop and produces a lot of ATP as long as oxygen is available. When oxygen levels drop, aerobic respiration comes to an end. Anaerobic respiration's ability to produce ATP, however, might still be able to sustain some additional muscle contraction. In the end, muscle fatigue and the cessation of muscular contraction are caused by the buildup of lactic acid from anaerobic respiration and the depletion of resources (ATP, oxygen, and glycogen).

2.1.1. Muscle Metabolism During Contraction

The need to generate energy to sustain muscular contractions is what propels muscle metabolism. Adenosine diphosphate (ADP) is created when ATP cleaves its third phosphate group, releasing energy in the process. Muscle fibers also contain creatine phosphate, another molecule with high-energy bonds. A muscle fiber's intrinsic ATP supply can only sustain a contraction for a brief period of time. During contraction, the phosphate group transfers from creatine phosphate to the ADP molecule, providing energy. This gives you enough energy to contract for an additional fifteen seconds. Subsequently, the body needs to break down fats and carbohydrates to produce energy, initially from within the muscle fiber and subsequently from other sources.

Glycogen, a carbohydrate polymer that, when broken down enzymatically into individual subunits, yields the simple sugar glucose, is the primary intrinsic source of metabolic energy in a muscle fiber. Anaerobic glycolysis is the breakdown of a glucose molecule into lactic acid without the presence of oxygen. Two ATP molecules are produced in this process. This process can only support mild physical activity for approximately sixty seconds and is inefficient in terms of energy. However, the immediate energy produced by anaerobic glycolysis is approximately 100 times greater than that of the rapid breakdown of ATP and creatine phosphate. Beyond that, a process known as oxidative metabolism or aerobic respiration requires the injection of O_2 into the body to permit prolonged muscular activity. A glucose molecule is broken down into CO_2 and H_2O in the presence of O_2 and by the actions of mitochondria, producing 36 molecules of ATP as opposed to the two that are produced by anaerobic glycolysis (Figure 2.1).

From intrinsic muscle sources of metabolites, aerobic respiration can maintain muscle activity until intramuscular glycogen and certain lipid supplies are depleted.

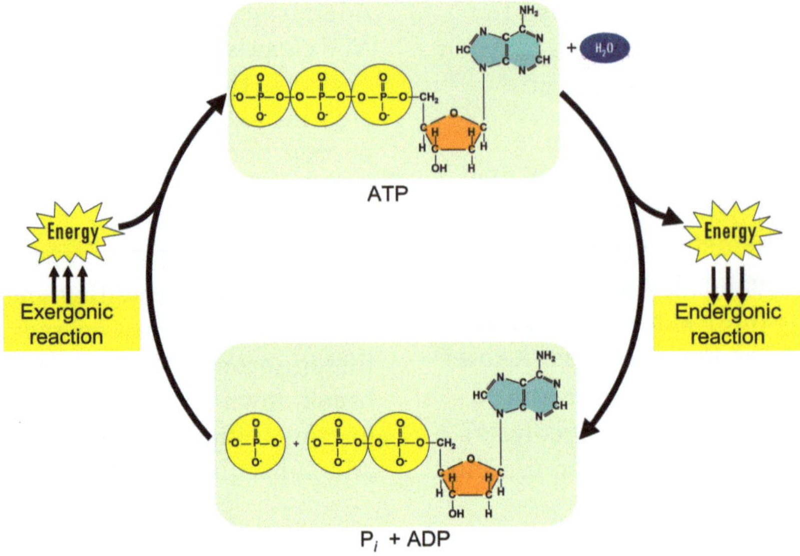

Figure 2.1. *Abbreviated scheme of ATP production in muscle through aerobic and anaerobic pathways.*

Source: https://commons.wikimedia.org/wiki/File:ATP_cycle.png.

At that point, the blood must carry energy sources for the muscles from other parts of the body, particularly the liver. The body's oxygen supply is insufficient during rest to support intense muscular activity, and it takes the heart and lungs one to two minutes to boost oxygen delivery and glucose supply to the muscles. Three mechanisms are involved in the body's reaction to the increased oxygen needed for exercise: (1) increased lung intake of oxygen (O_2), (2) quicker circulatory system delivery of O_2 to the muscles, and (3) increased extraction of O_2 from red blood cells into the mitochondria of the muscle fiber. Muscle fibers can obtain energy in a variety of ways, each with pros and cons. Anaerobic glycolysis builds up lactic acid in the muscle and happens quickly without the need for oxygen. However, it produces comparatively little ATP. Although it starts slowly and needs oxygen to function, aerobic respiration generates a lot of ATP. Muscles can use each of these energy production methods most efficiently because of adaptations in their muscle fibers. However, muscle functions at only about 20% efficiency when measured as an aggregate (mechanical work/metabolic cost).

Although cerebral and muscle metabolism are typically separate processes, certain illnesses cause both cerebral and muscle impairments. For example, proximal muscle weakness and wasting (steroid myopathy) are often the result of prolonged steroid treatment for conditions such as organ transplantation, brain tumors, vasculitis, or asthma. A round face, acne, and an obese body with spindly limbs—a "cushingoid" appearance—are other side effects of steroid treatment. When taken in excess, steroids can lead to mood swings, agitation, and irrational behavior, which is sometimes referred to as "steroid psychosis." Patients with brain tumors, cerebral vasculitis, and other central nervous system disorders are more likely to experience these mental abnormalities. When combined with exercise, testosterone and other steroids can enhance the size and strength of muscles. This regimen is used by bodybuilders and athletes to improve their strength and appearance. Steroid myopathy and steroid psychosis are conditions that are also experienced by those who abuse steroids. The fact that profound weakness, hypokalemic myopathy, and cardiac arrhythmias can result from low serum potassium concentrations (hypokalemia) demonstrates the delicate nature of muscle metabolism, which can occasionally be noticeably independent of cerebral metabolism. Hypokalemic myopathy is frequently an iatrogenic condition resulting from the use of potassium supplements in conjunction with diuretics or steroids, which are often self-administered covertly. Psychiatrists often treat hypokalemia resulting from laxative abuse and chronic alcoholism that progresses to cirrhosis.

Confusion, agitation, stupor, and seizures are the results of hyponatremia (sodium deficiency), as opposed to hypokalemia, which does not affect mental status. Psychiatrists may treat patients who have hyponatremia and its side effects because it can be brought on by excessive water consumption, the use of lithium, carbamazepine (Tegretol), oxcarbazepine (Trileptal), and selective serotonin reuptake inhibitors (SSRIs), among other medications. Hypokalemic periodic paralysis is a different disorder involving the metabolism of potassium. Patients experience dramatic episodes of areflexic quadriparesis that can last anywhere from a few hours to two days. Patients experience widespread paralysis during attacks, but they are awake and fully conscious, breathing normally, moving their eyes purposefully, and their blood tests reveal serum hypokalemia. The timing of the attacks is irregular rather than "periodic," despite the name of the illness. Every few weeks, they usually happen on their own, but they can also be triggered by heavy carbohydrate meals, exercise, or sleep. The attacks are distinct from cataplexy and sleep paralysis due to their prolonged duration and hypokalemia. These conditions, which include catatonia, are all distinguished from psychogenic episodes by hypokalemia and areflexia.

Adolescent boys who have hypokalemic periodic paralysis typically show signs of autosomal dominant patterning. It is caused by a mutation in the calcium ion channel gene and is indicative of another channelopathy in most cases. A variety with an adult onset is linked to hyperthyroidism. Changes in mental status can occasionally be indirectly related to other common metabolic myopathies. For instance, alcoholism causes alcohol cardiomyopathy, which is the wasting of cardiac and limb muscles. Weakness appears as a complication of hyperthyroidism in hyperthyroid myopathy. While heat intolerance and hyperactivity are the typical symptoms of hyperthyroidism, older people may have apathetic hyperthyroidism, which is markedly absent of overactivity symptoms. Metabolic myopathies typically go away when regular metabolism is resumed. Certain drugs, like clozapine, rarely result in a myopathy that is clinically discernible, but they can raise the serum CK concentration. There are times when other drugs, like the lipid-lowering "statins," can lead to muscle damage that can range from minor inflammation to potentially fatal rhabdomyolysis.

2.1.2. Nutrient Utilization in Muscle Metabolism

The process by which muscle cells use the energy contained in different nutrients to power contraction, sustain cellular processes, and enhance exercise performance is known as nutrient utilization in muscle metabolism. Proteins, lipids, and carbohydrates are the main building blocks for the synthesis of ATP, the cell's energy currency. Muscle cells experience increased metabolic demands during exercise, which causes a change in how nutrients are used to meet energy needs. Because they can be quickly converted into ATP through the process of glycolysis, carbohydrates—which are stored as glycogen in muscle tissue and the liver—are the favored fuel source for intense physical activity. In the process of glycolysis, glucose molecules are broken down to produce pyruvate and ATP in the cytoplasm. Pyruvate can be changed into lactate in low-oxygen environments, such as during strenuous exercise, enabling anaerobic glycolysis to occur. This process produces ATP quickly but insufficiently, which increases tiredness during extended high-intensity exercises. On the other hand, during endurance exercises and low-to-moderate intensity exercise, fats provide a rich source of energy. Adipose tissue-stored triglycerides are converted into glycerol and fatty acids, which are subsequently delivered to muscle cells where they undergo beta-oxidation in the mitochondria. In beta-oxidation, fatty acid chains are broken down one after another to produce acetyl-CoA molecules, which then enter the citric acid cycle and undergo oxidative phosphorylation to produce ATP. Although fatty acid oxidation uses more oxygen and is therefore more prevalent during aerobic exercise, it offers a more sustained energy supply than glycolysis.

Additionally, proteins are involved in muscle metabolism; mainly, they serve as a substrate of last choice after stores of fat and carbohydrates are exhausted. Muscle proteins may be broken down into amino acids for direct oxidation to produce ATP or for conversion into glucose (gluconeogenesis) during extended endurance exercise or in energy-deficient conditions. However, hormonal control and metabolic adjustments meant to maintain muscle mass and function usually minimize protein catabolism during exercise. Exercise intensity, duration, nutritional status, and personal metabolic traits are some of the factors that tightly control the interaction between the metabolism of carbohydrates, fats, and proteins. Performance and recovery can be impacted by optimal nutrient availability and timing. For example, loading on carbohydrates before endurance events or consuming protein right after exercise to replenish glycogen stores and encourage muscle growth and repair are two strategies that can help. To maximize training adaptations, refueling tactics, and overall athletic performance, athletes, coaches, and practitioners must comprehend the dynamics of nutrient utilization in muscle metabolism.

2.1.3. Muscle Metabolism and Exercise Performance

The regulation of energy production, substrate utilization, and metabolic adaptations in response to physical activity is a crucial aspect of muscle metabolism, which in turn influences exercise performance. Strength, power output, and endurance during exercise are all influenced by the effectiveness and adaptability of a person's muscle metabolism. To maintain extended endurance activities like long-distance running or cycling, an aerobic metabolism that is primarily powered by carbohydrates and fats is necessary. Muscle cells need oxygen to effectively metabolize substrates and produce energy during aerobic exercise, and this is achieved through the process of oxidative phosphorylation. To improve aerobic energy production and endurance performance, endurance training induces changes in muscle cells, such as increased mitochondrial density and enzyme activity. With brief bursts of high-intensity exercise, like sprinting or weightlifting, on the other hand, anaerobic metabolism takes over. Through the oxygen-free breakdown of carbohydrates, especially muscle glycogen, anaerobic glycolysis offers a quick but constrained source of ATP. But lactate and other metabolic waste products can build up and limit your ability to exercise. Maximal power output and explosive strength are the results of strength and power training, which increases anaerobic metabolism through increased muscle fiber recruitment, glycolytic enzyme activity, and buffering capacity.

Furthermore, during various forms of exercise, muscle metabolism demonstrates metabolic flexibility, which enables cells to adjust to changing energy requirements and substrate availability. To optimize performance outcomes, metabolic adaptations can be influenced by environmental factors, nutritional strategies, and training interventions. For instance, loading up on carbohydrates before endurance events restores glycogen stores and postpones fatigue, whereas ketogenic diets may improve the rate at which fat is burned during extended periods of exercise. Hormone control is also essential for controlling muscle metabolism and exercise capacity. Hormones that control substrate mobilization, glycogen breakdown, and protein synthesis, including insulin, glucagon, cortisol, and catecholamines, orchestrate metabolic responses to exercise stimuli. While resistance training raises growth hormone and testosterone levels, which aid in muscle protein synthesis and hypertrophy, endurance training improves insulin sensitivity and encourages lipid oxidation. Exercise performance is also impacted by individual variability in muscle metabolism, which is influenced by genetics, training status, age, and sex. While some people may have higher anaerobic or aerobic metabolism capacities, others may show metabolic changes that improve performance in particular sports. Comprehending these individual variations can help develop individualized exercise regimens and dietary plans based on a person's metabolic type.

2.1.4. Regulation of Muscle Metabolism

A complex web of mechanisms controls how energy is produced, how substrates are used, and how metabolism adjusts to different physiological and environmental stimuli in muscle tissue. Through the preservation of metabolic homeostasis, these regulatory mechanisms guarantee that muscle cells can effectively meet energy demands during exercise. Hormonal signaling, cellular energy status, and exercise stimuli are some of the major components that control muscle metabolism. The coordination of metabolic responses in muscle cells is largely dependent on hormone regulation. Substance mobilization, glucose uptake, glycogen synthesis and breakdown, and protein metabolism are all significantly impacted by hormones like insulin, glucagon, cortisol, and catecholamines. Insulin facilitates the synthesis of glycogen and increases the absorption of glucose by muscle cells, which helps with anabolic and energy storage processes. In contrast, catecholamines like norepinephrine and epinephrine, as well as hormones like glucagon, promote lipolysis and glycogenolysis to increase the availability of substrate during times when energy is needed. Released in response to stress or exercise, cortisol promotes gluconeogenesis and protein breakdown, which modulates protein metabolism, especially during prolonged endurance activities or catabolic states.

Muscle metabolism is also regulated by intracellular metabolites and signaling molecules, which sense the cellular energy status. One important energy sensor is adenosine monophosphate-activated protein kinase (AMPK), which is activated in response to low ATP or high AMP levels, as in the case of exercise or energy depletion. AMPK activation inhibits ATP-consuming activities like protein synthesis while promoting ATP-producing metabolic pathways like fatty acid oxidation and glycolysis. On the other hand, in response to exercise-induced muscle damage or hypertrophic stimuli, the mammalian target of rapamycin (mTOR) pathway integrates nutrient and growth factor signals to regulate protein synthesis and cellular growth, promoting anabolic processes. Muscle metabolism and metabolic adaptations are strongly impacted by exercise stimuli, which include activity type, intensity, and duration. Exercises with high intensities, like running or resistance training, cause the anaerobic pathways to activate quickly to meet the body's immediate energy needs. This increases the amount of lactate produced and the amount of glycolytic flux. Long-term, low-to-moderate intensity exercise increases aerobic metabolism and fatty acid oxidation by promoting mitochondrial biogenesis and oxidative enzyme activity. Resistance training also promotes muscle protein synthesis and glycogen storage by inducing muscular hypertrophy and metabolic adaptations through mechanical tension and metabolic stress. Moreover, environmental elements that affect muscle metabolism and exercise-induced metabolic changes include altitude, temperature, and nutritional status. Nutritional interventions, like loading on carbohydrates or supplementing with protein, maximize the availability and recovery of substrates, thereby enhancing performance and facilitating adaptation to training stimuli. Exercise performance and metabolic adaptations are impacted by environmental stressors like heat or hypoxia, which change metabolic demands and metabolic pathways (Acín-Pérez et al., 2004; Acín-Pérez et al., 2008).

2.2. Molecular and Biochemical Regulation of Skeletal Muscle Metabolism

Since catabolic and anabolic processes are integrated into major metabolic pathways and result in skeletal muscle hypertrophy, skeletal muscle metabolism regulation may have an impact on the efficiency of animal growth. The diverse population of muscle fibers that make up muscle can be categorized according to their contractile speed (fast or slow) and type of metabolism (oxidative or glycolytic). While type I slow fibers primarily rely on oxidative metabolism to support extended or continuous work, type IIa, IIx, and IIb fast fibers have varying metabolic capacities, ranging from high glycolytic to high oxidative. Because muscle is malleable, it can continuously adapt to changing extrinsic and intrinsic stimuli, changing the classification of muscle fibers and affecting protein turnover rate, fiber size, and nutrient utilization.

Beyond its primary roles in locomotion and thermogenesis, skeletal muscle is crucial for maintaining the metabolic balance of the entire body. Skeletal muscle makes up roughly 40% of body mass in healthy people, plays a major role in basal energy expenditure, and facilitates 70–90% of insulin-mediated glucose disposal. Therefore, it has been demonstrated that regulating insulin sensitivity and skeletal muscle metabolism can effectively treat metabolic diseases in people. The diverse population of muscle cells that make up skeletal muscles each have unique metabolic traits. These cells exhibit great plasticity in responding to a wide range of external stimuli, such as changes in activity level, load, nutrition, and environmental circumstances. For instance, resistance training and endurance training raise metabolic demand, which in turn raises the mitochondrial content and oxidative capacity of skeletal muscle. On the other hand, factors that contribute to the development of obesity, such as consuming too many calories coupled with a decrease in workload, and lower oxidative capacity, which is linked to metabolic syndrome and inadequate insulin sensitivity.

When compared to healthy individuals, the insulin sensitivity of diabetic and obese patients who undergo exercise training regimens has improved, but it has still been significantly blunted. Increased muscle oxidative capacity has the potential to mitigate age-related muscle atrophy, protect against metabolic disorders, and alleviate metabolic defects linked to certain myopathies. While the fight against metabolic disorders in humans has focused much of its attention on skeletal muscle metabolism, little is known about how to modulate skeletal muscle metabolism in meat-producing animals to increase production efficiency.

While it is evident that the glycolytic metabolism of skeletal muscle is linked to more effective lean growth, the regulatory mechanisms underlying these metabolic alterations remain unclear. For instance, high feed efficiency (FE) pigs have a higher inclination towards glycolytic metabolism, while low FE pigs show higher expression of oxidative enzymes. Additionally, ractopamine, a pharmacological agent that enhances FE and encourages lean accretion, causes a change in the composition of muscle fibers to boost glycolytic capacity. The adaptive mechanism that makes these changes possible, though, is still unknown. In the next section, we go over the fundamentals of skeletal muscle metabolism before delving into the state of our knowledge regarding skeletal muscle metabolic regulation.

2.2.1. The Biochemistry of Skeletal Muscle Metabolism

The amazing capacity of skeletal muscle to modify its energy consumption in response to energy requirements. Muscle can go from a resting to an active state by expelling 100 times as much energy in milliseconds. Adenosine triphosphate (ATP) concentrations stay largely constant despite these significant variations in energy demands, indicating the remarkable accuracy of cellular energy production systems in matching demand. Complex signaling and feedback loops that relay the cellular energy status to change the metabolic pathways within the cell are in charge of this metabolic control.

2.2.1.1. ATP homeostasis

Adenosine triphosphate (ATP) is the chemical energy produced by several intricate biochemical reactions that make up skeletal muscle metabolism (Figure 2.2). Muscle cells contain a variety of metabolic pathways with differing subcellular locations, substrate utilization, and duration. The phosphagen system, a reversible reaction that catalyzes the breakdown of phosphocreatine (PCr) by creatine kinase to produce creatine (Cr) and brief supplies of ATP from adenosine diphosphate (ADP) (PCr + ADP → Cr + ATP), is used for the quick, rapid mobilization of ATP. Furthermore, the adenylate kinase enzyme works in tandem with the phosphagen system to facilitate short-term energy buffering by converting 2 ADP into 1 ATP and 1 adenosine monophosphate (AMP) (2 ADP → 1 ATP + 1 AMP). Adenylate kinase plays a significant role in reporting the energy status of cells by converting relatively small changes in the ATP:ADP ratio into significant changes in the concentrations of AMP. Several metabolic enzymes are potent allosteric activators that increase the production of ATP when there is a slight increase in the concentration of cellular AMP, making it a sensitive indicator of the state of cellular energy. For instance, 5'-adenosine monophosphate-activated protein kinase (AMPK) enhances glucose uptake by increasing glucose transporter type 4 (GLUT4) expression and translocation and increases glycogenolysis by activating glycogen phosphorylase. Indeed, long-term AMPK activation changes the metabolic properties of skeletal muscle. Additionally, by activating hexokinase, the initial step in glycolysis, AMPK activation raises glucose conversion to glucose-6-phosphate. Until other energy-producing systems are fully operational, these transient energy buffering systems keep ATP levels stable.

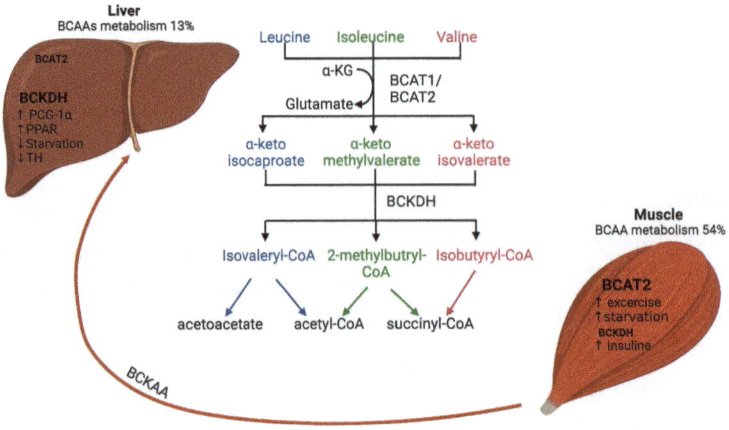

Figure 2.2. *Major metabolic pathways in skeletal muscle.*

Glucose or glycogen can be metabolized through glycolysis to yield pyruvate, which can be converted to acetyl-CoA by PDH or converted to lactate by LDH. Alternatively, the glycolytic intermediates G6P or F6P can be redirected to the PPP for biosynthetic processes, or to the HBP for metabolic signaling. If pyruvate is converted to acetyl-CoA, it can feed into the TCA cycle to be fully oxidized, producing the reducing equivalents NADH and $FADH_2$, or exit the cycle to contribute to biosynthetic processes such as fatty acid or amino acid synthesis.

Source: Trillos-Almanza MC, Martinez-Aguilar M, Arroyave-Ospina JC, van Vilsteren F, Blokzijl H, Moshage H. Clinical and therapeutic implications of bcaas metabolism during chronic liver disease in humans: crosstalk between skeletal muscle and liver. Muscles. 2024; 3(1):71–87. https://doi.org/10.3390/muscles3010008.

2.2.1.2. Glycolysis

A sequence of enzymatic reactions known as glycolysis turns glucose into pyruvate, and it can produce ATP 100 times more quickly than oxidative phosphorylation (OxPhos). Glycogen phosphorylase in the muscle can quickly mobilize muscle glycogen stores to fuel glycolysis, the primary energy source during high-intensity exercise. This process produces glucose-1-phosphate. On the other hand, the uptake of plasma glucose is allowed by GLUT4, but the rate of uptake is restricted by GLUT4's transportation to the cell surface. When blood glucose levels are high after a meal, insulin can trigger the translocation of GLUT4 vesicles; however, insulin resistance and/or diabetes can impair this translocation. Conversely, GLUT4 translocation can be stimulated by acute exercise-induced contractile activity without insulin. To prevent glucose from diffusing outward and to maintain the concentration gradient necessary for continuous glucose inflow, glucose is quickly phosphorylated by hexokinase once it has entered the cells. This results in glucose-6-phosphate (G6P). Depending on what the cell requires, G6P can then branch into the anabolic (pentose phosphate pathway), catabolic (glycolysis), or metabolic signaling (hexosamine biosynthetic pathway) pathways in either scenario of glycogen breakdown or glucose absorption.

2.2.1.3. Pentose Phosphate Pathway

The pentose phosphate pathway (PPP) derives from the glycolytic molecules G6P and F6P to produce necessary metabolites for skeletal muscle growth, such as ribulose-5-phosphate for nucleic acid synthesis, erythrose-4-phosphate for aromatic amino acid synthesis, and NADPH for reductive biosynthesis reactions. The enzymes G6PDH and 6PGDH are key in assessing PPP activity, with G6PDH catalyzing the initial step and 6PGDH the final step. While PPP activity is typically low in skeletal muscle due to its specialized nature, it significantly increases during muscle regeneration and in cases of muscle hypertrophy induced by AKT1 overexpression. These findings suggest that enhancing PPP flux can lead to greater skeletal muscle growth.

2.2.1.4. Hexosamine Biosynthetic Pathway

A metabolic signaling pathway called the hexosamine biosynthetic pathway (HBP) steals between two and three percent of the glucose produced by cells from glycolysis. It starts with the glycolytic intermediate F6P and is catalyzed by fructose 6-phosphate amidotransferase (GFAT), which changes glutamine and F6P into glucosamine-6-phosphate and glutamate. GFAT is the enzyme that limits the rate of this reaction. UDP-GlcNAc, or uridine diphosphate N-acetylglucosamine, is produced by the HBP's later stages. Altogether, UDP-GlcNAc integrates protein, lipid, carbohydrate, and nucleotide metabolism to represent the cellular nutrient flux. Because it reflects the conditions of nutrient excess or scarcity, the level of UDP-GlcNAc is therefore a useful indicator of the nutritional status of cells. In the end, O-linked-N-acetylglucosaminylation, or O-GlcNAcylation, is a post-translational modification that uses UDP-GlcNAc as a donor substrate to change the way cells behave in response to changing nutritional circumstances.

2.2.1.5. The TCA Cycle and Oxidative Phosphorylation

However, F6P is committed to glycolysis after being converted to fructose-1,6-bisphosphate by phosphofructokinase (PFK), and then goes through a multi-step, sequential conversion to pyruvate. Next, pyruvate can be transformed by lactate dehydrogenase (LDH) or pyruvate dehydrogenase (PDH) into lactate or acetyl CoA. In times of high glycolytic flux, or in anaerobic environments, pyruvate is transformed into lactate, which can be transported from the cell to the liver via monocarboxylate transporters (MCT) for hepatic gluconeogenesis, replenishing glycogen reserves. Alternatively, pyruvate can be moved into the mitochondrial matrix for oxidation, passing through the mitochondrial pyruvate carrier located in the inner membrane and the porin channel in the outer membrane. Once within the matrix, pyruvate is converted by PDH into acetyl-CoA, allowing it to enter the tricarboxylic acid cycle (TCA), or, less frequently, pyruvate carboxylase, converting pyruvate into oxaloacetate, which helps maintain anaplerosis. Being the primary connection between the TCA cycle and glycolysis, PDH is a crucial molecular switch that manages the changeover between the two metabolic pathways and is strictly controlled by phosphorylation. In response to nutritional status, the pyruvate dehydrogenase complex (PDC) is regulated by a balance between pyruvate dehydrogenase kinases (PDK) and pyruvate dehydrogenase phosphatases (PDP). Since pyruvate dehydrogenase kinase 4 (PDK4) is mostly located in skeletal muscle and is more active during times of fasting or high-fat feeding, diet likely plays a significant role in controlling the rate at which carbohydrates are oxidized.

Additionally, fatty acids catalyze the TCA cycle employing β-oxidation, which cleaves two carbons in each cycle of fatty acid chains to produce acetyl-CoA. Acetyl-CoA dehydrogenase, enoyl-CoA hydratase, hydroxyacyl-CoA dehydrogenase, and ketoacyl-CoA thiolase are the four primary enzymes that participate in the β-oxidation cycle. Nicotinamide adenine dinucleotide (NADH), flavin adenine dinucleotide (FADH2), and acetyl-CoA—a fatty acid chain that is two carbons shorter—are the products of one cycle. The reducing equivalents are oxidized in the electron transport chain (ETC) to produce ATP after acetyl-CoA enters the TCA cycle. Allosteric regulators of β-oxidation enzymes, along with their intermediate product, the NADH/NAD+ ratio, and acetyl-CoA levels are the end products of these reactions. The primary transcriptional regulators of β-oxidation are coactivator peroxisome proliferator-activated receptor-gamma coactivator 1α (PGC1α) and peroxisome proliferator-activated receptors (PPARs). Actually, skeletal muscle PPARβ deletion causes a metabolic shift that lowers muscle oxidative capacity, and skeletal muscle PGC1α ablation increases the number of glycolytic fibers, which may affect feed efficiency. In fact, pigs with higher feed efficiency values have lower levels of mitochondrial energy metabolism enzymes.

In the TCA cycle, acetyl-CoA can either be completely oxidized to yield the reducing equivalents FADH2 and NADH for ATP synthesis, or its intermediates can be released from the cycle through biosynthetic processes. Despite the multiple entry and exit points of the TCA cycle that permit both catabolic and anabolic processes in response to various cellular demands, the term "cycle" often refers to it as if it were a unidirectional and well-defined series of reactions. For the synthesis of fatty acids, amino acids, and nucleotides under anabolic conditions, TCA intermediates can be transported from the mitochondrial matrix into the cytosol. High energy demands, on the other hand, trigger catabolic processes. To resupply ATP stores through OxPhos, intermediates go through several oxidation steps to provide the electron transport chain (ETC) with reducing equivalents (NADH and FADH2). It should come as no surprise that the TCA cycle is intimately linked to energy consumption via intricate feedback loops. The TCA cycle, for instance, is affected by malfunctions in the ETC because the accumulation of NADH is a strong inhibitor of all TCA cycle regulatory enzymes. The inhibition of multiple TCA enzymes is also caused by elevated ATP concentrations or the build-up of TCA cycle intermediates. However, AMP, an allosteric activator of the regulatory TCA cycle enzymes, is elevated in response to high energy demands. While allosteric regulation offers a dynamic feedback loop to control the TCA cycle, additional signaling pathways regulate it as an additional layer of control. Because mitochondria are mostly found attached to the sarcoplasmic reticulum (SR) in skeletal muscle, there is a bidirectional signaling pathway between the two organellar systems. More specifically, the mitochondria can sequester the calcium released from the SR during muscle contraction, which in turn activates the F1F0-ATPase, pyruvate dehydrogenase, α-ketoglutarate dehydrogenase, and isocitrate dehydrogenase, stimulating the TCA cycle and mitochondrial ATP production. Muscle contraction and ATP synthesis are simultaneously initiated by the parallel activation of mitochondrial metabolism and muscle contraction, which efficiently balances energy supply and demand.

2.2.2. Mitochondria Bioenergetics and Dynamics

2.2.2.1. Multifaceted Functions of Mitochondria

While ATP synthesis is the primary function of mitochondria, they are also essential for metabolic signaling, scavenging and production of reactive oxygen species (ROS), cell death, ion and metabolite transport, iron-sulfur protein biogenesis, and calcium homeostasis. The internal membrane space (IMS) and mitochondrial matrix are produced by the porous outer mitochondrial membrane (OMM) and the selective inner mitochondrial membrane (IMM) found in mitochondria. Electron transport chain complexes reside in the IMM and create an electrochemical gradient by transferring electrons from reducing equivalents to electron acceptors through a series of redox reactions coupled with protons being transferred from the matrix to the IMS (Figures 2.2 and figure 2.3). In addition to being used for ATP synthesis, the mitochondrial membrane potential, or electrochemical gradient, is what powers the other key metabolic functions of the organelle.

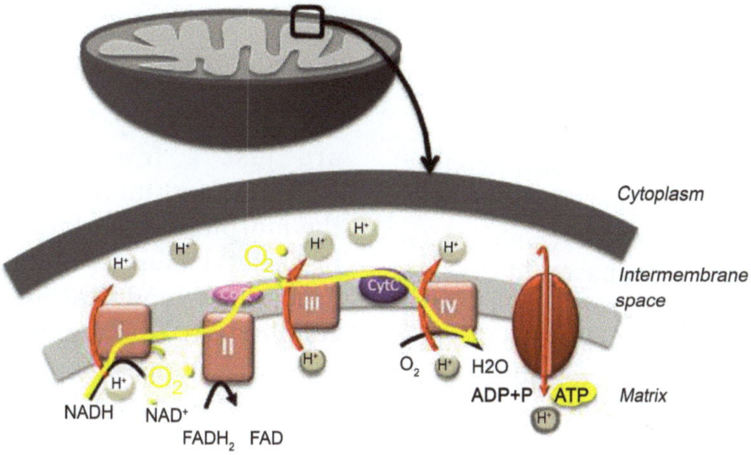

Figure 2.3. *The electron transport chain and generation of the electrochemical gradient.*

Source: May-Panloup P, Bognet M, El Hachem H, Bouet P-E, Reynier P. Embryo and its mitochondria. antioxidants. *2021; 10(2):139. https://doi.org/10.3390/antiox10020139.*

Two electron transfer carriers, ubiquinone and cytochrome c, and four protein complexes (CI-CIV) make up the electron transfer chain (ETC). The first electron carrier, ubiquinone, is reduced to ubiquinol by CI or CII oxidizing the electron donors, $FADH_2$ and NADH, respectively. While CI and CII both move electrons through the IMS, CI additionally moves four protons there, while CII does not move protons. In addition to pumping four protons into the IMS, CIII catalyzes the transfer of electrons from the first to the second electron carrier (ubiquinol to cytochrome c). To create water and pump protons, Complex IV catalyzes the transfer of electrons from cytochrome c to the terminal electron carrier oxygen. In the cristae, complexes are organized into super complexes, frequently consisting of dimers of ATP synthase (CV), III2 + IV, and I + III2 + IV arrangements. Proton re-entry into the matrix under normal physiological conditions is primarily mediated by ATP synthase (CV), which links ATP production to the electrochemical gradient. Nonetheless, there exist alternative re-entry points that are not linked to the production of ATP, like the production of heat by uncoupling proteins (UCPs) and the replenishment of NADPH pools for biosynthetic processes and ROS scavenging by nicotinamide nucleotide transhydrogenase (NNT).

Additionally, the roles that mitochondria play in the physiology of skeletal muscle vary depending on their subcellular location. Muscle contraction is supported by the rapid distribution of ATP to myofibrillar ATPases, which is facilitated by the presence of intrafibrillar mitochondria

(IFM), which are positioned between myofibrils that wrap around the I-band of the sarcomere and form extensive networks. More matrix and cristae volume are produced by peripherally located mitochondria (PM), which are larger and less branched than IMF. PM localize to capillaries (paravascular mitochondria; PVM) or nuclei (paranuclear; PNM). What differentiates PVM and PNM bioenergetically, however, is still unknown.

2.2.2.2. Electron Transport Chain

The mitochondrial membrane potential is produced by two electron carriers and four transmembrane protein complexes (Figure 2.3). Protons are pumped from the matrix to the IMS while electrons are moved from complex to complex through a sequence of redox reactions. To decrease the electron carrier ubiquinol, complex I (CI) and complex II (CII) oxidize the electron carriers FADH2 or NADH, respectively. Protons are pumped across the IMM by CI during this process, but not by CII. Then, to produce water and pump protons, complex III (CIII) and complex IV (CIV) catalyze the electron transfer from ubiquinol to cytochrome c and from cytochrome c to oxygen, respectively. The F1F0 ATPase, also referred to as complex V (CV), allows protons in the IMS to re-enter the matrix. Here, the energy produced by protons moving along a concentration gradient is used to phosphorylate ADP and create ATP, or OxPhos. While ATP synthesis accounts for most proton re-entry, other pathways avoid CV, such as heat-producing uncoupling of proteins or nicotinamide nucleotide transhydrogenase's ability to restore the NADPH pool for biosynthetic activities (Figure 2.3). Although ETC complexes are frequently reduced to linear complexes in numerical order with a 1:1 complex ratio, their stoichiometry varies widely. Complexes can be found freely floating or in superassembled structures called supercomplexes within the IMM folds, also known as cristae. Supercomplexes in mammalian cells are primarily made up of CI, CIII, and CIV, while it is still unclear how much CII and CV contribute to the formation of supercomplexes. Though their exact formation is unknown, it has been proposed that they are involved in complex stability, electron transport efficiency, and ROS production control. It's interesting to note that supercomplex formation rises with exercise, suggesting that supercomplexes are an adaptive response to higher energy requirements.

2.2.2.3. Mitochondrial Dynamics

Exercise, dietary factors, aging, and disease are just a few of the intermittent and continuous stimuli that can significantly alter the morphology and functions of mitochondria in skeletal muscle. Mitochondrial adaptations encompass modifications to their abundance, coupling, structure, and ETC activity (oxidative capacity). Of these, the structural alteration that enables dynamic mitochondrial remodeling to adjust to the cellular environment is the fastest and most flexible response. Because they allow damaged mitochondria to be removed (a process known as mitophagy; Figure 2.4), mitochondrial dynamics are a coalition of fusion and fission events that are crucial for mitochondrial biogenesis, stress mitigation, and quality control. The inner and outer mitochondrial membranes are fused via the action of mitofusion proteins (Mfn1 and Mfn2) and optic atrophy protein 1 (Opa1). In skeletal muscle, deletion of Mfn1 and Mfn2 results in a reduction in muscle mass, oxidative capacity, mitochondrial DNA (mtDNA) abundance, and eventually lethality. However, for fission events to wrap around and cleave the outer membrane, dynamin-related protein 1 (Drp1) must translocate from the cytosol. While other proteins are also involved in fission, Drp1 loss prevents fission and causes an increase in mitochondrial hyperfusion. Muscle atrophy, deformed mitochondrial morphology, and compromised mitochondrial respiration are the outcomes of skeletal muscle-specific Drp1 ablation. While overloaded muscle showed a decrease in Drp1, an increase in fusion proteins, and a larger mitochondrial area, it is possible that a physiological decrease in Drp1 could promote hypertrophy. Muscle hypertrophy may be influenced by the equilibrium of appropriate mitochondrial fusion and fission, which is necessary for maintaining the homeostasis of skeletal muscle.

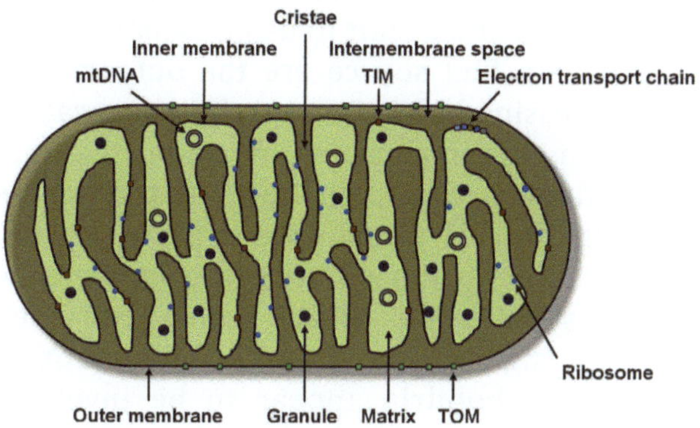

Figure 2.4. *An overview of mitochondrial structures.*

Skeletal muscle mitochondria form a dynamic network that is constantly adapting to changing external and internal stimuli. Punctate mitochondria can fuse together to form an interconnected network permitting an increase in oxidative capacity, dispersal of mitochondrial damage to promote survival, or an exchange of mitochondrial content (mtDNA and metabolites). Contrarily, mitochondria can undergo fission to remove damaged mitochondria through mitophagy, facilitate mitochondrial trafficking, or adapt to metabolic changes.

Source: Schniertshauer D, Wespel S, Bergemann J. Natural mitochondria targeting substances and their effect on cellular antioxidant system as a potential benefit in mitochondrial medicine for prevention and remediation of mitochondrial dysfunctions. Current issues in molecular biology. 2023; 45(5):3911–3932. https://doi.org/10.3390/cimb45050250.

Additionally, mitochondrial dynamics enable a flexible reaction to shifting dietary parameters. For instance, muscle cells isolated from the extensor digitorum longus (EDL) treated with glucose for the same length of time had less extensive (fused) mitochondrial networks than those incubated in media containing acetoacetate, an oxidative substrate, for 24 hours. While punctate mitochondria are more common in glycolytic fibers, fused mitochondrial networks are more common in oxidative fibers and have high rates of fusion. Mitochondrial networks share matrix content, allowing for quick distribution of cellular energy and mobility of metabolites, ions, proteins, and mtDNA. Thus, while glycolytic fibers have less extensive networks that support brief bursts of work through glycolysis, oxidative fibers with extensive mitochondrial networks facilitate energy homeostasis. Conversely, in the absence of nutrients, mitochondria lengthen by suppressing fission events to guard against mitophagy and optimize energy generation. These results show that mitochondria can easily adjust to a variety of nutrient environments to maintain muscle physiology.

2.2.3. Molecular Regulators of Skeletal Muscle Growth and Metabolism

A hierarchy of intricate anabolic and catabolic biological processes that control the rate of protein accretion governs the growth of skeletal muscle. The diverse population of muscle cells, or myofibers, that make up skeletal muscle varies in the rate at which myofibrillar, mitochondrial, and sarcoplasmic protein turnover occurs. Therefore, the rate of protein accretion depends on many myofiber properties. Myofibers can be categorized based on their contraction speed (fast or slow) and predominant energy metabolism (oxidative or glycolytic). Because mitochondrial proteins have higher fractional synthesis rates than myofibrillar proteins, slow-twitch muscle fibers have a higher rate of protein synthesis than fast-twitch fibers. This difference in protein synthesis can be attributed to the length of contraction and mitochondrial abundance. However, slow fibers also have high rates of protein degradation, which leads to low rates of protein accretion and relatively small fiber sizes. This is likely because slow fibers have a high mitochondrial content that is vulnerable to damage from reactive oxygen species. As a result, metabolism influences the rate at which muscles accumulate and can be used to control the rate at which muscles grow and the effectiveness with which they use substrates.

2.2.3.1. IGF-Akt Signaling

In muscle, the two main regulatory pathways that control protein accretion are the myostatin pathway, which is a positive regulator of protein synthesis, and the insulin-like growth factor 1 (IGF-1)/phosphoinositide-3-kinase-Akt (PI3K-Akt)/protein kinase B (PKB)/mammalian target of rapamycin (mTOR) pathway. PIP2 is phosphorylated by PI3K, which in turn generates PIP3, serving as a docking site for PIP3-dependent kinase 1 (PDPK1) that activates Akt when IGF-1 binds to its receptor. By stimulating protein synthesis through mTOR and glycogen synthase kinase 3β (GSK3β) activation, Akt prevents protein degradation by repressing transcription factors belonging to the forkhead box protein (FOXO) family. IGF-1 overexpression promotes hypertrophy, while IGF-1 receptor loss leads to muscular atrophy in skeletal muscle. Similarly, skeletal muscle experiences significant hypertrophy when its downstream target Akt is activated, but postnatal growth is hindered and severe myopathy develops when the downstream target mTOR is deleted. Further evidence supporting mTOR1's regulation of the metabolic properties of skeletal muscle comes from the reduced oxidative capacity in the soleus and EDL muscles due to mTOR1 loss. Reduced oxidative capacity may contribute to the development of myopathies in mTOR1-deficient muscle since it is linked to the onset of many metabolic disorders and muscle atrophy. The goal of scientists working in animal agriculture is very different from that of treating age-related illnesses: they want to enable effective lean accretion, even though it is clear that oxidative metabolism is essential for human longevity and disease prevention. Still, the field of animal agriculture benefits from these discoveries. For instance, increased muscle mass and a shift to using carbohydrates as the main fuel source are the outcomes of overexpressing IGF-1. Conversely, there was no change in oxygen consumption, indicating that the oxidation of carbohydrates is the source of energy for IGF-1-mediated hypertrophy. All in all, these results point to the importance of glucose as a fuel source being prioritized by IGF-1 signaling to promote hypertrophy. While mitochondria appear to be involved, more research on this junction is required to translate these findings into creative ways to promote effective muscle hypertrophy.

2.2.3.2. Myostatin Signaling

A negative regulator of muscle growth is myostatin. Myostatin gene mutations that occur naturally in sheep, cattle, dogs, and humans have been found to disrupt the gene and cause an increase in muscle mass. Myostatin overexpression causes a decrease in muscle mass in mice, while myostatin deletion causes a two-fold increase in muscle mass and a decrease in adipose tissue deposition. A lack of myostatin also enhances the metabolism of glucose and reduces mitochondrial respiration. Myostatin and IGF-1 dynamically interact to control the two pathways that lead to muscle accretion. Both pathways share the PI3K/Akt axis, which allows for crosstalk and is necessary for healthy muscle growth and physiology. For instance, myostatin overexpression reduces protein synthesis by downregulating Akt/mTOR signaling. On the other hand, myostatin deletion raises PKB and mTOR activity, even though effective hypertrophy requires the IGF-1 receptor to be present. When combined, these pathways influence metabolism and are important for controlling muscle hypertrophy.

2.2.3.3. AMPK Signaling

It is evident that maintaining metabolic homeostasis is as important for muscle physiology and growth as proper myostatin and IGF-1 crosstalk. Highly integrated signaling pathways that are closely related to cellular energy status and nutrient availability regulate the metabolism of skeletal muscle. One such pathway is the dynamic intracellular energy sensor AMPK, which relays signals of energetic stress to control muscle metabolism. When AMP levels rise in response to ATP hydrolysis, the ATP:AMP ratio drops, activating AMPK, which then stimulates catabolic processes while suppressing anabolic processes to restore ATP stores. Therefore, AMPK activation reduces the anabolic process of protein synthesis, as shown by a forty-five percent decrease in the fractional rate of protein synthesis in skeletal muscle one hour after the injection of 5-aminoimidazole-4-carboxamide ribonucleotide (AICAR), a drug that activates AMPK. By inhibiting mTOR activity and triggering FOXO and uncoordinated 51-like kinase 1 (ULK1), two autophagy pathway regulators, AMPK activation reduces the rates at which proteins accumulate. To produce ATP and meet the increased energy demand, there is also greater catabolism in response to the downregulation of anabolic pathways from AMPK activation. For instance, constitutive activation of AMPK is caused by mutation of the AMPKγ3 subunit in mice and pigs, which boosts glycolytic muscle's oxidative capacity and mitochondrial biogenesis. It may be due to a compensatory or adaptive mechanism that can override the negative regulation of AMPK on protein synthesis that its chronic activation surprisingly does not affect muscle growth. The AMPKγ3^{R200Q} mutant pigs exhibited normal growth, possibly due to increased expression of Akt, a positive regulator of muscle growth. Because increased oxidative capacity improves the muscle's ability to avoid energetic stress and provides protection against muscle wasting and metabolic diseases, the AMPK pathway has become a target to combat metabolic disorders without adversely affecting muscle mass. In fact, hypertrophy and an increase in oxidative capacity can happen at the same time, indicating the possibility of an unidentified compensatory pathway that can force hypertrophy regardless of metabolic characteristics. In conclusion, there are downstream effects on lean accretion efficiency due to the intricate and complex signaling pathways that modulate muscle hypertrophy and skeletal muscle metabolism (Acín-Pérez et al., 2004; Acín-Pérez et al., 2008).

2.2.4. Nutrient Sensing and Skeletal Muscle Adaptation

2.2.4.1. O-GlcNAcylation

Muscle is a malleable tissue that allows metabolic adaptations to environmental changes because muscle cells can sense the state of cellular energy and the availability of substrates. Muscles can "sense" the availability of substrates and increase protein accretion when there is a nutritional surplus, such as right after feeding. In contrast, times of nutrient scarcity cause nutrients to be redistributed away from anabolic activities. By cycling on and off O-GlcNAc moieties to serine and threonine residues of nuclear, cytosolic, and mitochondrial proteins, the dynamic post-translational modification O-linked-β-D-N-acetylglucosamine (O-GlcNAc) functions as a ubiquitous nutrient gauge. UDP-GlcNAc, the donor substrate, is a byproduct of the HBP. By integrating the metabolism of nucleotides, carbohydrates, lipids, and proteins, its levels represent the overall cellular nutrient flux. To change the function of target proteins and adapt to the abundance of cellular nutrients, two enzymes, O-GlcNAc transferase (OGT) and O-GlcNAcase (OGA), add and remove O-GlcNAc from them, respectively (Figure 2.5). Because levels of O-GlcNAcylation and UDP-GlcNAc are indicative of cellular nutrient status, this post-translational modification collectively functions as a nutrient-sensing pathway.

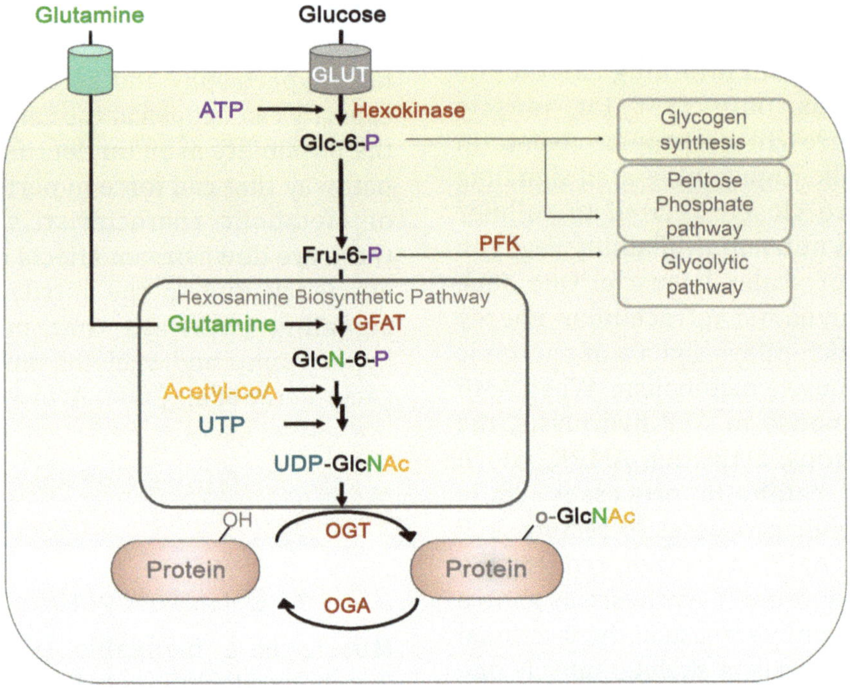

Figure 2.5. *O-GlcNAc signaling pathway.*

Source: Kim E, Kang JG, Jho E-h, Yang WH, Cho JW. O-GlcNAcylation: An Emerging Protein Modification Regulating the Hippo Pathway. Cancers. 2022; 14(12):3013. https://doi.org/10.3390/cancers14123013.

Step 1: UDP-GlcNAc is produced by the hexosamine biosynthesis pathway, which combines metabolites from the metabolism of proteins, carbohydrates, fats, energy, and nucleotides. The amount of this compound varies depending on the nutritional status of the cell. *Step 2:* To modify protein function, OGA extracts the O-GlcNAc moiety, also referred to as O-GlcNAcylation, and OGT transfers UDP-GlcNAc to any of its thousands of target proteins. O-GlcNAcylation is mediated exclusively by the enzymes OGT and OGA, and it happens similarly to phosphorylation in terms of how widely it occurs. However, O-GlcNAcylation patterns are correlated with the nutritional status of cells. The glycolytic muscle in skeletal muscle has more O-GlcNAcylated proteins in it. Since OGT targets several glycolytic enzymes and mitochondrial proteins, O-GlcNAcylation can actually alter skeletal muscle metabolism in response to dietary changes.

2.2.4.2. O-Glcnac Transferase

OGT is encoded by a single gene; however, alternative splicing produces three isoforms. Nucleocytoplasmic OGT (ncOGT) and mitochondrial OGT (mOGT), which has an N-terminal mitochondrion targeting sequence, are the two main isoforms. There is a brief version of OGT, but not much is known about it. Up until recently, ncOGT was primarily responsible for the global

O-GlcNAcylation observed in cells. Nevertheless, the pyrimidine nucleotide carrier is responsible for transporting UDP-GlcNAc into the matrix and inhibiting this transporter reduces the O-GlcNAcylation found in mitochondria, indicating that strong O-GlcNAc cycling takes place inside the mitochondria. These findings imply that there is crosstalk between the two isoforms of OGT to mediate mitochondrial integrity and function, but it is still unclear how this crosstalk relates to nutritional status.

2.2.4.3. OGT Substrates

O-GlcNAcylation is directed towards several metabolic enzymes. The rate-limiting glycolytic enzyme phosphofructokinase-1 is inhibited by O-GlcNAcylation, which causes glucose to be redirected to the PPP in cancer cells. The PPP's rate-limiting enzyme, G6PDH, is O-GlcNAcylated, which raises the PPP's activity and glucose flux through lung cancer cells. Extended exposure to glucose raises the amount of O-GlcNAcylation in cells, which in turn raises the rate of glycolytic flux. It's interesting to note that removing O-GlcNAcylation in high glucose environments returns mitochondrial function to levels seen in cells exposed to regular glucose. These findings demonstrate that increased O-GlcNAcylation of important regulatory proteins to modulate metabolism is signaled by elevated glucose availability.

2.2.4.4. HBP Pathway

Since both glucose and glutamine are thought to be rate-limiting in the HBP, they are strong inducers of O-GlcNAcylation and UDP-GlcNAc synthesis. In rat skeletal muscle, excess free fatty acids also raise UDP-GlcNAc levels; however, the subsequent glucose uptake and handling differ significantly from that induced by excess glucose. High-fat exposure raised UDP-GlcNAc levels in cultured pancreatic beta-cells and produced dysregulated metabolites that were different from those exposed to high glucose. This shows that while UDP-GlcNAc levels rise in response to various nutrients, their downstream metabolic adaptations are specific to each nutrient.

2.2.4.5. Implications of Skeletal Muscle O-GlcNAcylation in Farm Animals

O-GlcNAcylation in skeletal muscle has a long history and has been shown to be crucial for maintaining healthy skeletal muscle insulin sensitivity and glucose handling. Skeletal muscle O-GlcNAcylation is important for global metabolism because skeletal muscle is the body's largest metabolically active tissue and handles most insulin-mediated glucose disposal. An association between nutrient abundance and insulin resistance in rodents was observed in early muscle research. In fact, chronic glucose exposure to skeletal muscle caused by GLUT4 overexpression leads to increased UDP-GlcNAc levels and the development of insulin resistance in mice. Moreover, extended exposure to uridine and fatty acids raises UDP-GlcNAc levels and lowers insulin sensitivity in skeletal muscle. On the other hand, obesity and insulin resistance caused by high-fat diets are prevented in mice by ablation of OGT and consequently O-GlcNAcylation in skeletal muscle. These results show that whole-body metabolism is affected by O-GlcNAcylation in muscle. (Banerjee et al., 2015)

2.2.5. Metabolic and Nutritional Regulation of Satellite Cells

Satellite cells (SC), a diverse population of stem cells found in adult skeletal muscle, support the development, upkeep, and repair of postnatal muscle. The majority of adult stem cells are in a quiescent state, but they can become active to support multiple rounds of proliferation before going through terminal differentiation or self-renewal. The coordinated execution of these actions is closely timed by interconnected signaling chains that transmit developing internal and external stimuli.

2.2.5.1. Metabolic Regulation of Satellite Cells

Essentially, metabolism functions as a powerful regulator of SC behavior, causing metabolic changes to adapt to the needs of various growth phases (Figure 2.6). Despite having a comparatively low metabolic rate, quiescent SC can be divided into two different metabolic groups. A lower metabolic rate is associated with a population that enters the cell cycle later, mitoses more slowly, and is less transcriptionally primed for myogenic commitment. On the other hand, people who have higher metabolic activity respond better to activation. When SC are activated, they start to multiply and increase their rates of glycolysis and glutaminolysis to meet their energy needs and to support the biosynthesis of macromolecules, which is necessary for the proliferation of cells. After 48 hours of differentiation, there is a shift to a more oxidative metabolism with an increase in mitochondrial content and oxidative capacity. If this transition is disturbed by inhibiting mitochondrial DNA replication, mitochondrial fission, mitochondrial protein synthesis, or OxPhos, myoblasts are restricted to a proliferative single-cell state and are unable to differentiate. Although differentiation requires an oxidative shift, glucose remains a vital nutrient, indicating that glucose oxidation promotes myogenesis. In fact, differentiation is hampered when glucose entry into the TCA cycle is blocked by PDH deletion. These results characterize the metabolic alterations that promote myogenesis.

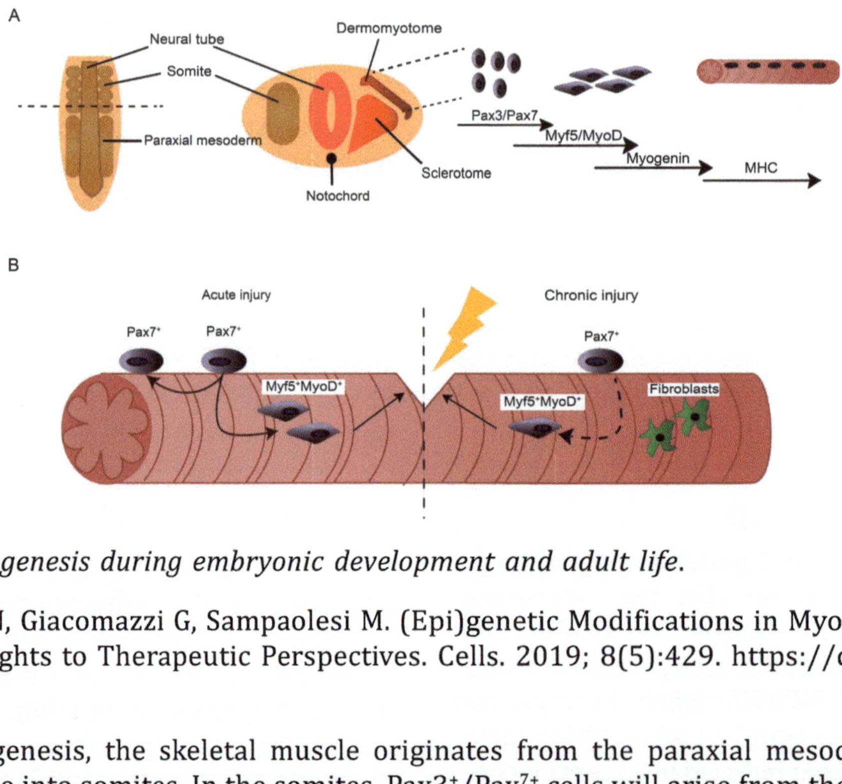

Figure 2.6. *Myogenesis during embryonic development and adult life.*

Source: Breuls N, Giacomazzi G, Sampaolesi M. (Epi)genetic Modifications in Myogenic Stem Cells: From Novel Insights to Therapeutic Perspectives. Cells. 2019; 8(5):429. https://doi.org/10.3390/cells8050429

During embryogenesis, the skeletal muscle originates from the paraxial mesoderm, which will further subdivide into somites. In the somites, $Pax3^{+}/Pax^{7+}$ cells will arise from the dermomyotome and will form muscle fibers through the sequential upregulation of Myf5, MyoD, and myosin heavy chain (MHC) (A). During adult life, Pax^{7+} satellite cells are the main cell type responsible for muscle regeneration upon injury. However, when the injury is of chronic nature, this stem cell pool becomes exhausted and fibroblasts are recruited to form scar tissue (B).

2.2.5.2. AMPK Signaling

Myogenesis is also affected by changes in the energy status of cells. AMPK is a metabolic stress sensor that signals times of energy stress to enable adaptations to shifting internal conditions. It is activated by variations in the ratios of AMP to ATP. The medication AICAR inhibits G1/S cell cycle progression and decreases myotube formation when it activates AMPK. However, the loss of AMPKα1 in SC hinders adult regenerative myogenesis, and transplanting SC without AMPKα1 into control muscles results in a reduced capacity for myogenic growth. These findings imply that the loss of AMPKα1 in SC cannot be restored by outside factors. These cells divide more slowly in culture in addition to having poorer regeneration, which is explained by the absence of AMPK, which prevents Warburg-like glycolysis. While non-proliferating cells have a higher ratio of ATP to ADP along with greater mitochondrial function, proliferating cells use AMPK to stimulate an increase in Warburg-like glycolysis through a decrease in ATP to ADP ratios to support proliferation. All of these results emphasize how crucial it is for AMPK to translate the state of cellular energy to control myoblast metabolism and promote effective myogenic advancement.

2.2.5.3. Nutrient Conditions on Satellite Cell Fate

Extrinsic nutrient abundance or scarcity is also sensed by SC, and they adapt their behavior accordingly. The common nutrient sensing pathway in SC, O-GlcNAcylation, is necessary for normal SC behavior. Both adult regenerative myogenesis and SC proliferation are hampered by OGT loss, which also affects O-GlcNAcylation. More precisely, through the mTOR pathway—a cellular nutrient sensor that controls the rates of protein synthesis—high circulating levels of amino acids facilitate the progression of the SC lineage. For instance, adding lysine, the first amino acid that limits blood sugar levels, to a diet raises mTOR activity, which in turn inhibits proteolysis by the autophagic-lysosomal system and promotes the growth of stem cells. Moreover, leucine restriction inhibits differentiation while leucine supplementation stimulates proliferation, differentiation, and skeletal muscle regeneration via the mTORC1 pathway. In fact, myoblasts cultured in high leucine concentrations exhibit decreased proliferative capacity and protein synthesis upon mTOR inhibition. According to the same findings, adult SC's conditional deletion of mTOR hinders muscle regeneration, differentiation, and proliferation. All of these results point to the necessity of the mTOR pathway in converting variations in nutrient availability into altered myoblast function. Myf5 and MyoD, which are involved in SC activation and transient proliferation, as well as myogenin, which is necessary for terminal myoblast differentiation, are examples of the myogenic regulatory factors whose expression mTOR regulates in addition to encouraging protein synthesis to support myogenesis. All of these results point to the necessity of sufficient nutrient availability and downstream signaling for cellular nutrient status for SCs to function properly.

Conversely, excessive substrate availability or overfeeding has a deleterious effect on SC function. For instance, high glucose causes C_2C1_2 myotubes to become insulin-resistant and inhibits myogenic differentiation, which is followed by a reduction in Akt phosphorylation. Actually, differentiation is inhibited and the high glucose phenotype is recapitulated by inhibition of Akt or PI3-kinase. Thus, for effective glucose absorption, the PI3-kinase/Akt pathway must be activated. In fact, myogenic differentiation is salvaged when Akt is pharmacologically activated under conditions of elevated glucose. These results show that SC behavior can be changed by the PI3-kinase/Akt pathway by "sensing" changes in nutrient concentrations. On the other hand, brief caloric restriction enhances oxidative metabolism and strengthens

SC. Nonetheless, differences in the response to and efficacy of calorie restriction have been discussed for age, sex, and length of restriction.

2.3. Energy Metabolism Design of the Striated Muscle Cell

One important area of research that needs to be addressed is the architecture of the striated muscle energy metabolism system. A physiological function evaluation of the entire process is necessary to comprehend the architecture of energy conversion and distribution in the muscle cell. The cellular energy conversion process, which mainly consists of glycolysis and oxidative phosphorylation (OxPhos), is comprised of the vascular supply of basic substrates, carbon sources, and oxygen. Lastly, there are structural and biochemical techniques to regulate and distribute the potential energy produced by the energy conversion processes throughout the cell. We have made an effort to concentrate our attention on the muscle's ability to perform at near maximum workloads under typical physiological conditions despite the wide scope. A crucial component of muscle design is its maximum workload, which dictates how much blood flow, intermediate metabolism, and mechanical strength the muscle can produce to support its maximum workload. Weibel et al. have also proposed the idea of symmorphosis, in which every component linked to a specific physiological function is adjusted to just satisfy the tissue's maximum demand for work output with minimal to no surplus. Simply expressed, symmorphosis suggests that biology makes optimal use of both space and protein to complete the task at hand without the need for a significant amount of extra protein to be used as a "reserve" or as a component of the regulatory system. When it comes to the heart, the answer is clear-cut: given that the heart functions primarily in a sustainable way, providing a steady workload over an extended time supported in the steady state by coronary blood flow and OxPhos, what are the maximum workload conditions for these two physiological systems? The maximum sustained cardiac output under physiological conditions is therefore defined as the maximum work of the heart. Given its multiple muscle types and at least two different maximum power requirements, the skeletal muscle is far more complex than other muscle types. In this context, two conditions will be examined: maximum sustained power, also known as critical power, where muscle contractile power can be sustained for an extended period through the energy conversion of intermediary metabolism, and peak nonsustainable power, where metabolic recovery capacity may be more significant than the sustainable rate of energy conversion. Critical power is a metric that is comparable to the heart's maximal sustained cardiac output. We will be looking for shared characteristics that are present in the majority of skeletal muscle fiber types due to their amazing diversity.

Separate discussions will be held regarding the energy conversion architecture of the heart and skeletal muscle. The heart and skeletal muscle have very different design constraints, so any comparisons between the two will be limited to conditions of maximum sustained power. In order to avoid oversimplifying the overall spectrum of skeletal muscle fiber types, where contractile and metabolic phenotypes may differ, skeletal muscle will be evaluated simply as fast-twitch, glycolytic and slow-twitch, oxidative fiber types, with certain qualifications. The theoretical and historical background of the energy distribution system will also be discussed when particular components, like myoglobin, creatine kinase, and the mitochondrial reticulum, are introduced. This section will provide a more thorough explanation of the general muscle designs. Section four of the review. Lastly, the focus will be on the energy metabolism design of the healthy striated muscle cell, even though it is widely acknowledged that deficiencies in the striated muscle cell's ability to convert energy have been linked to several infections.

2.3.1. Metabolic Homeostasis in Striated Muscle

Converting chemical potential energy into contractile work, the muscle is an amazing machine. In human skeletal muscle operating at about 20% total efficiency, it accomplishes this fairly efficiently. The energy conversion pathways of mitochondrial OxPhos and cytosolic glycolysis, which are carefully regulated to meet the muscular demands for energy, are the main ways that muscle works. It is now widely known that ATP serves as the main energy intermediary in this process, enabling ion transport as well as muscle contraction. It was discovered early on in the process of figuring out the energy sources for muscle contraction that, despite variations in ATP hydrolysis, the concentration of ATP remains remarkably constant within the cell. This is although ATP is clearly the potential energy intermediate between carbon substrates and work. In 1950, Hill expressed his confusion about the function of ATP in intact muscle in his "Challenge to Biochemists" paper. He wrote, "There is no direct evidence that the breakdown of ATP really causes contraction or relaxation, but it may very well be the case, and none will be happier than I to be quit of revolutions." In fact, ATP has never been observed to change in living muscle other than in situations of extreme exhaustion that border on rigor. This can be explained by assuming that ATP is quickly restored to its original form after being broken down into ADP and phosphate. It will be exceedingly difficult to obtain any direct evidence on the subject if this occurs after every stimulus due to the small size and speed of the changes. Hill was concentrating on the Lohmann reaction (creatine kinase), which is covered below, at the time. Ten years later, the Davies laboratory was able to overcome this difficulty by demonstrating a change in ATP with muscular work through the inhibition of both creatine kinase and metabolism. Therefore, the creatine kinase reaction or metabolism can sustain the homeostasis of ATP, as will be further discussed below about the creatine kinase knockout mouse models.

Using traditional freeze-clamp extraction assays, the phenomenon of nearly constant ATP in skeletal muscle under physiological workloads has also been noted for decades in the heart. However, since it was challenging to assay the ADP and phosphate (Pi) using these extraction techniques, it was unclear what was happening to the phosphorylation potential. The extensive investigation of the impact of workload on phosphate metabolites using noninvasive physical methods was made possible by the development of 31P-NMR, a non-invasive technique for measuring intact tissue phosphate metabolites, and the application of enzyme equilibrium measures to estimate the chemical activity of ADP. The freeze-clamp approach is difficult in active tissues because, as respiratory rates approach maximum, the entire pool lifetime of ADP is only 10–170 ms, whereas ATP is 2–10 s and mitochondrial NADH is 70–250 ms. The original finding that the concentration of ATP was exceptionally well maintained in both the heart and skeletal muscle has been well-replicated in the literature. While the concentration of ATP ([ATP]) stays relatively constant below contraction exhaustion levels, most skeletal muscle types exhibit a modest decrease in phosphocreatine (PCr) and an increase in Pi, which are accompanied by an increase in work and a corresponding increase in the calculated ADP and decrease in free energy for ATP hydrolysis. For a brief period, the creatine kinase reaction can use PCr to temporarily sustain ATP, but metabolically produced ATP synthesis is required to sustain muscle [ATP] for prolonged striated muscle work. Therefore, as the Davies laboratory first demonstrated, the regeneration of ATP through intermediary metabolism is essential for preserving ATP levels within the cell. It is noteworthy to mention that certain human subjects have experienced decreases in [ATP] during prolonged, intense exercise, which is linked to a decrease in muscle oxygen content. These findings are consistent with compromised metabolism caused by hypoxia. Metabolic homeostasis in the heart happens under a variety of physiological loads. With an emphasis on in vivo cardiac research, physiological increases in workload are maintained at ^{31}P-NMR sensitivity, maintaining ATP, PCr, and Pi constant until nearly maximum experimental workloads are reached in all mammalian species. These investigations have also been conducted on human participants in good health.

It is now well known that the heart and, to a lesser extent, the skeletal muscle, are capable of maintaining metabolic homeostasis during increases in workload. The wide dynamic range of skeletal muscle energy demands compared with the heart may be the cause of the slight changes seen in even highly aerobic fibers. It is still unclear, nevertheless, how metabolic homeostasis is preserved in every muscle cell. It appears that oxidative respiration and glycolysis cannot be driven by the classical model of a simple feedback of ADP and Pi without significant changes to the kinetics of ATP and Pi utilization or substrate compartmentation. According to some theories, there exist parallel activation schemes in which intracellular calcium may play a role in simultaneously activating muscle contractile activity and metabolism. Though MCU knockout mice are not born at the expected Mendelian ratios and some have in fact reported significant metabolic effects in the MCU knockout mouse, the survival and modest effect of removing the putative mitochondrial calcium transporter (MCU) in heart and skeletal muscle in mice has challenged the dominance of calcium as a parallel regulator of OxPhos. The removal of MCU, creatine kinase, and myoglobin—discussed below—does not, however, affect the mouse whose heart beats at nearly full capacity at rest. Instead, it causes only slight alterations in metabolic regulation, indicating that the signaling network supporting muscle metabolic homeostasis is likely complex and depends on a variety of signaling processes rather than just one or two. It is evident that this rather amazing bioengineering task requires the coordinated modulation of blood flow, substrate entry, substrate oxidation, and the activation of the entire OxPhos cascade.

The metabolic balance observed in muscle cells also impacts the distribution of free energy within the cell. It is essential for the rate at which metabolically converted free energy is distributed to match or exceed the rate of ATP hydrolysis/synthesis in the muscle cell while ensuring that the concentration of ATP remains stable. Difficulties may arise due to the need for proportional changes in concentration gradients with changes in metabolite diffusion rates, although factors such as small diffusion distances, facilitated diffusion, and specialized gradient barriers can help explain some aspects of this process. Despite significant changes in ATP, ADP, and Pi flux in muscle cells, the concentrations of these metabolites remain relatively constant, leading to questioning the role of metabolite diffusion in regulating overall energy conversion rates. This review will focus on hypotheses suggesting the presence of a mitochondrial reticulum for the distribution of free energy in the form of the mitochondrial membrane potential, which could rapidly travel through the muscle cell via a regulated mitochondrial reticulum, thus reducing the need for significant metabolite diffusion.

2.3.2. Metabolic Support Design of the Muscle Cell

The heart must be able to beat steadily under a variety of workloads and corresponding metabolic rates. The small energy conversion capacity of glycolysis in the heart serves as an example of how almost exclusively this steady-state work is supported by the energy conversion occurring in OxPhos. Given this restriction, the highest rate of ATP synthesis by OxPhos ought to correspond with the highest requirement for energy conversion to facilitate prolonged myocardial contraction (i.e., muscle contraction) and regulation (i.e., ion transport) in addition to the myocyte's basal maintenance. This idea is supported by the fact that the maximum rate of respiration found in the exercising animal nearly matches the heart's maximum rate of mitochondrial OxPhos, which is estimated from cytochrome oxidase (COX) content. These findings imply that the heart's architecture allows substrates, such as carbon and oxygen metabolites, to be delivered at maximal rates without significantly reducing OxPhos reserve capacity.

A mammalian skeletal muscle that contracts intermittently places more emphasis on maximal contractile power at the expense of reduced oxidative energy metabolism than does cardiac muscle, which is designed to maintain energy homeostasis across nearly the entire range of contractile demands in the constantly beating heart. Consistently, lower capillary densities and larger cell sizes in skeletal muscle fibers contribute to larger and more dynamic oxygen gradients from the capillary to the mitochondrion, whereas high capillarization, relatively smaller cell sizes, and stable pO2 gradients in the heart make oxygen delivery largely nonlimiting under physiological conditions as previously discussed. Because of this, skeletal muscle cells and glycolytic muscle fibers are much more likely to experience limitations in oxygen delivery than oxidative muscle fibers. Indeed, it has been observed that training in endurance exercises doubles the amount of mitochondria in skeletal muscle in both humans and rodents, but only modifies maximal oxygen uptake by about 15%. According to these findings, mitochondrial content does not seem to be a significant barrier to the maximum oxygen uptake by the skeletal muscle cell, even though it does correlate favorably with performance on submaximal endurance tests. The precise roles that particular limiting factors play in achieving maximum oxygen uptake, however, are still up for dispute. It is noteworthy that critical power, which refers to the maximum sustainable work rate of skeletal muscle, typically transpires at approximately 70–80% of the maximal oxygen uptake rate in humans. Consequently, it may not encounter the same constraints regarding oxygen supply. The following section will cover the main elements of the oxygen delivery system that interact directly with the muscle fiber, capillaries, and myoglobin. You can locate more recent, in-depth analyses of the pathways by which oxygen is delivered upstream from the capillaries elsewhere.

2.3.2.1. Major Muscle Cell Energy Conversion Processes

Evaluation of the sources of energy conversion to ATP and the topology of these sites in the cell is necessary to comprehend the distribution of potential energy throughout the muscle. During muscle contraction, OxPhos, glycolysis, and creatine kinase are the main sources of ATP (Figure 2.7). This section will mostly focus on glycolysis and OxPhos, which supply the majority of ATP during contractions longer than a few seconds.

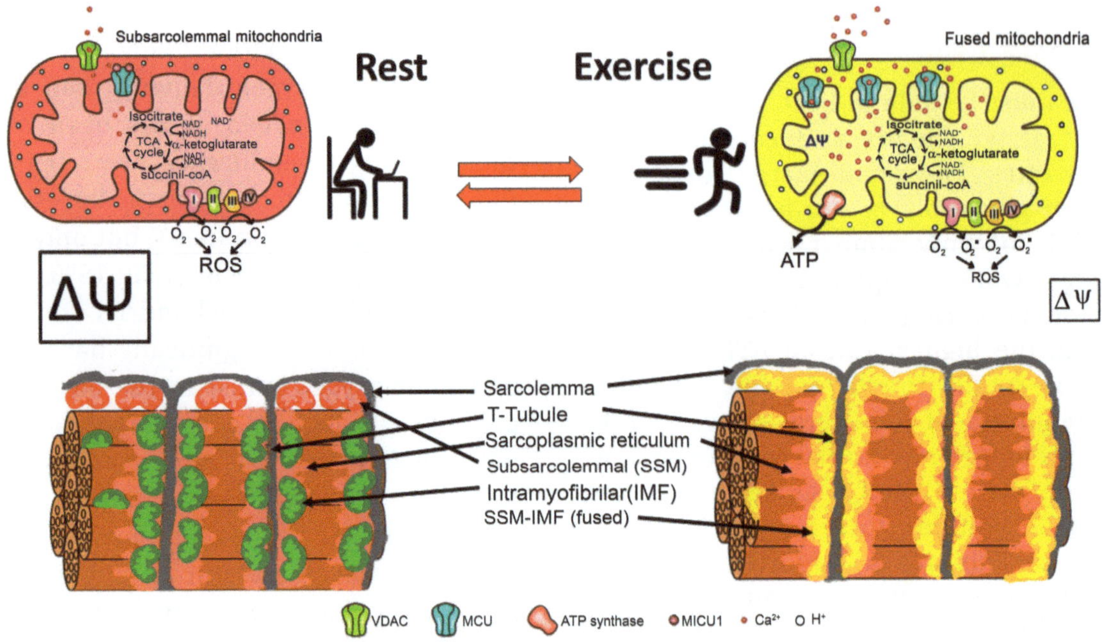

Figure 2.7. *Major adenosine triphosphate (ATP) production and utilization processes in striated muscle.*

Source: Espinosa A, Casas M, Jaimovich E. energy (and reactive oxygen species generation) saving distribution of mitochondria for the activation of atp production in skeletal muscle. Antioxidants. 2023; 12(8):1624. https://doi.org/10.3390/antiox12081624.

The two main activities in striated muscle cells that use ATP are the contraction of muscles and the preservation of ion gradients across membranes. Energy conversion pathways including oxidative phosphorylation, glycolysis, and creatine kinase produce ATP, which maintains metabolic homeostasis.

With regard to the enzymes involved in the major energy conversion processes, it is reasonable to assume that the protein content of an enzyme is a reflection of its relative maximum velocity based on the simplified Michaelis-Menten kinetics, where V_{max} is assumed to be proportional to the concentration of the enzyme as $V_{max} \sim k_{cat}$ [E], where k_{cat} is the enzyme rate constant that can depend on many parameters including pH, ions, allosteric interactions, and posttranslational modifications. However, with all of these modulators being equal, the enzyme concentration can be used to estimate the "potential" V_{max} of the system. This is important for this review to understand the relative capacity of the different muscles to produce ATP together with the localization within the cell.

In the past, the maximum ATP production of glycolysis has been estimated using the maximum velocity of enzymes, particularly putative rate-limiting enzymes such as phosphofructokinase, enolase, and glyceraldehyde-3-phosphate dehydrogenase. Essentially irreversible phosphofructokinase continues to be the main contender as a rate-limiting step, despite some models indicating other glycolytic enzymes might also be involved. It does not seem to be a single rate-limiting enzyme for OxPhos, despite estimates of OxPhos being made from enzymes of the citric acid cycle (oxoglutarate dehydrogenase) or the electron transport chain (cytochrome oxidase). Rather, almost all of the enzymes share control over flux through the OxPhos process. It is crucial to remember that estimating V_{max} using enzyme concentrations assumes that the k_{cat} is the same for all tissues at workloads that are maximally stimulated. However, this is frequently complicated by the artificial environment that an enzyme is exposed to during in vitro studies, as well as different tissue isoforms with different kinetic properties. Nevertheless, a wealth of research on the protein makeup and enzyme activities of muscle tissues has been produced, demonstrating the value of this kind of data in the literature.

Relying on the comparatively simple enzymatic activity of tissue extracts instead of the more challenging determination of absolute protein content has proven to be a challenge in the field. We have chosen to use protein content measured with quantitative antibody or, preferably, physical measures like mass spectrometry or optical spectroscopy to characterize the flux capacity of various muscle systems because enzyme activity depends on the assay conditions and purification conditions. A relational quantitative study of the protein content in the three muscle types we are considering in this review—heart, slow-twitch, and fast-twitch muscles from a single species—has not been published in the literature, despite the substantial work on muscle protein content. We developed a relational database of the proteins of the rabbit heart, soleus (98% slow-twitch), and gracilis (99% fast-twitch) muscles using common modern mass spectrometry labeling techniques to aid our analysis in assimilating data from numerous sources.

2.3.2.2. Glycolysis

Glycolysis is a crucial source of energy because it produces ATP and pyruvate, which OxPhos uses. The glycolytic enzyme baseline concentrations supplied by Maughan et al. (135) of the free cytosolic proteins in the rabbit's fast-twitch psoas muscle can be referred to in Tablle 2.1.

Table 2.1. *Mitochondrial Modulators*

	Compounds	**Model**	**Dose**	**Mechanisms**
1.	Quercetin	PC12 cells Wistar rats	1–100 µM 2–100 mg/kg	↓ROS, ↓LPO, ↑SOD, ↑GSH, ↑CAT, ↓Apoptosis, ↑MMP, ↑ATP, ↑Nrf2 ↑AMPK, ↑PGC-1α, ↑SIRT1, Restored Mt morphology, ↑PINK1 and ↑Parkin
2.	Baicalein	SH-SY5Y cells V79-4 cells	10–25 µM 10 µg/mL	↓ROS, ↓LPO, ↑SOD, ↓Bax, ↑Bcl-2, ↓Cyt c, ↓Caspase-3 ↓Ca^{2+}, ↑Nrf2, ↑MMP
3.	Kaempferol	HUVECs cells L2 cells	10–40 µM	↓ROS, ↓LPO, ↑SOD, ↑GSH, ↑GPx, ↓Bax, ↑Bcl-2, ↓Cyt c, ↓Caspase-3 ↑MMP, mPTP blockage, ↑ATP, ↑SIRT1
4.	Fisetin	Wistar rats	15 and 20 mg/kg	↓ROS, ↓LPO, ↑SOD, ↑GSH, ↑CAT, ↑MMP, ↓Caspase-3, ↑ATP, ↑Complex I

5.	Luteolin	C57BL/6 mice	10 μg/kg	↓ROS, ↓LPO, ↑MMP, ↓Caspase-3, -9, ↑ATP, ↑AMPK, ↑Complexes I, II, III, IV, and V
6.	7,8-dihydroxyflavone	Wistar Rat H92c cells	5–20 mg/kg 100 μM	↓ROS, ↓LPO, ↑SOD, GSH, CAT, GPx ↑MMP, ↑Complexes I, II, III, IV
7.	Naringenin	SH-SY5Y cells	10–80 μM	↓ROS, ↓LPO, ↑SOD, ↑GSH, ↑CAT, ↑PI3K/Akt/GSK-3β, ↑MMP, ↑ATP, ↑Nrf2, ↑Complexes I, V
8.	Genistein	C57/BL6J mice H9c2 cells	2.5–10 mg/kg 10 pM–1 μM	↓ROS, ↓LPO, ↑SOD, ↑GSH, ↑CAT ↑GPx ↑MMP, ↓Cyt c, ↓Caspase-3, ↑Nrf2
9.	Icariin	Human NP cells	10 μM	↓ROS, ↓Bax, ↑Bcl-2, ↓Cyt c, ↓Caspase-3, ↑MMP, ↑Nrf2
10.	Catechin	EA.hy926 cells HepG2 cells	4 mM 10 μM	↓ROS, ↓LPO, ↑SOD, ↑CAT, ↑MMP, Restored Mt morphology, ↑SIRT1, ↑Complex I, ↑ATP
11.	Epicatechin	MRC-5 cells BV2 cells	10 μM 100 μM	↓ROS, ↓LPO, ↑SOD, ↑CAT, ↑MMP Restored Mt morphology, ↑AMPK, ↑SIRT1, ↑Complex I, ↑ATP
12.	Epigallocatechin gallate	HLE B-3 cells	50 μM	↓ROS, ↓LPO, ↑SOD, ↑GSH, ↑CAT ↑GPx, ↓Bax, ↑Bcl-2, ↓Cyt c, ↓Caspase-3, -9, ↑MMP, ↑ATP
13.	Hesperidin	Mice	25–50 mg/kg	↑SOD, GSH, CAT, GPx, ↓Caspase-3, -9, ↑MMP, ↑ATP, ↑Complexes I, II, IV, V
14.	Resveratrol	Wistar rats C57BL/6 mice MC3T3-E1 cells	20 mg/kg 40 mg/kg 25 μM	↓ROS, ↑SOD,↑Bcl-2, ↓Cyt c, ↑SIRT1-AMPK-PGC-1α, ↑PINK1 ↑MMP, ↑Nrf2, ↑ATP, ↑Complex I, CypD
15.	Tyrosol	CATH.a cells SH-SY5Y cells	50–200 μM	↓ROS, ↑MMP ↓Bax, ↑Bcl-2, ↓Cyt c, ↓Caspase-3, -9, ↑ATP
16.	Hydroxytyrosol	ARPE cells HCN-2 cells	100 μM 30 μM	↓ROS ↓LPO, ↑SOD, GSH, CAT, GPx ↓Ca^{2+}, ↑Nrf2, ↑MMP, ↑Complexes I, II, V
17.	Curcumin	SH-SY5Y cells	5 μM	↓ROS, ↓LPO, ↑GSH, ↑GPx, ↑MMP, ↑ATP, ↓Ca^{2+}, ↓Caspase-3, -9, ↑Complexes II, IV
18.	Esculetin Mito-esculetin	C_2C1_2 cells HAEC cells	5 μM 2.5 μM	↓ROS, ↑GSH, ↑MMP, ↑Nrf2 ↓Caspase-3, -8, ↑AMPK/SIRT3/ PGC1α
19.	Protocatechuic Acid	PC12 cells Human Platelets	0.1–1.2 mM	↓ROS, ↓LPO, ↑GSH, ↑GPx, ↑MMP ↓Bax, ↑Bcl-2, ↓Cyt c, ↓Caspase-3, -9, ↓PI3K/Akt/ GSK-3β

20.	Salvianic acid A	SH-SY5Y cells SD Rat	1–100 μg/mL 52 μg/mL	↓ROS, ↓LPO, ↑MMP ↓Bax, ↑Bcl-2, ↓Cyt c, ↓Caspase-3
21.	Sesamin	BEAS-2B cells	40 μM	↓ROS, ↓LPO, ↑SOD, ↑CAT, ↓Bax, ↑Bcl-2, ↓Caspase-3 ↑MMP, ↑Nrf2, ↓PINK1, Parkin
22.	α-Arbutin	SH-SY5Y cells	1–100 μM	↓ROS, ↑SOD, ↑GSH, ↑MMP, ↑ATP, ↓AMPK
23.	Ellagic acid	Wistar rats C57BL/6 mice SH-SY5Y cells	10–100 mg/kg 20 μM	↓ROS, ↑SOD↑, MMP, ↑Nrf2 mPTP blockage, ↓Cyt c, ↑ATP, ↑Sirt3 ↑Complexes I, II, III, and IV
24.	Mangiferin	SH-SY5Y cells C57BL/6 mice	10–50 μM 10–50 mg/kg	↓ROS, ↓LPO, ↑SOD, ↑GSH ↑CAT, ↑GPx, ↓Bax, ↑Bcl-2, ↓Cyt c, ↓Caspase-3, -9, ↑Nrf2, ↑MMP, ↑ATP, ↑Complex I
25.	Panduratin A	RPTEC/TERT1	5 μM	↓ROS, ↑MMP, ↑Bcl-2, ↓Cyt c, ↓Caspase-3
26.	α-Mangostin	SH-SY5Y cells	0.03–0.3 μM	↓ROS, ↑MMP, ↑ATP, ↓Caspase-3, -8
27.	Rosmarinic acid	H9c2 cells SH-SY5Y cells Zebra fish C57BL/6 Mice	1–200 μM 20–80 mg/kg	↓ROS ↑GSH, ↑Nrf2, ↑MMP, ↑SIRT1/PGC-1a ↑PI3K/Akt Restored Mt Morphology, ↑ATP
28.	Chlorogenic acid	HUVECs cell Albino mice	25–160 μM 50 mg/kg	↑SOD, ↑GSH, ↑MMP, ↑ATP, ↑SIRT1 ↓Caspase-3, ↑Complexes I, II, III, IV, and V
29.	Theaflavin	TCMK-1 cells	2–10 μM	↓ROS, ↓LPO, ↑SOD, ↑MMP, ↑Nrf2, ↓Bax, ↑Bcl-2, ↓Caspase-3 ↑ATP, Restored Mt morphology
30.	Salvianolic acid A	Cardiomyocyte 3T3-L1 cells	12.5–50 μg/mL 1–100 nM	↓ROS, ↓Bax/Bcl-2 ratio, ↓Caspase-3, ↑Akt/GSK-3β, ↑MMP mPTP blockage, ↑ATP, ↑PGC-1α, ↑Complexes III and IV
31.	Salvianolic acid B	HL-7702 cells IEC-6 cells	50–200 μM 2.5–40 μM	↓ROS, ↓LPO, ↑SOD, ↑CAT, ↑MMP, ↑PI3K/Akt/GSK-3β, ↑ATP Restored Mt morphology, ↑AMPK/Sirt3
32.	Sarain A	SH-SY5Y cells	0.01–10 μM	↓ROS, ↑SOD, ↑Nrf2, ↑MMP, mPTP blockage, ↓Cyp D, ↑ATP
33.	Sarain 2	SH-SY5Y cells	10 μM	↓ROS, ↑MMP
34.	Piperine	Wistar rats	10 mg/kg	↓ROS, ↓LPO, ↑GSH, ↑MMP, ↑Bax/Bcl-2, ↓Cyt c, ↓Caspase-3, -9 ↑Complexes I, II, and II
35.	Caffeine	SH-SY5Y cells SD rats APPsw rats	1–100 μM 40 mg/kg 120 mg/L	↓ROS, ↑MMP, ↑ATP ↓Bax/Bcl-2, ↓Cyt c, ↓Caspase-3, -6 ↑PI3K/Akt, ↑Complexes I, II, and III

36.	Celastrol	C57BL6/J mice SD rats	100 µg/kg 1–3 mg/kg	↓ROS, ↑GSH, ↑MMP, ↑ATP ↑AMPK/SIRT1/ PGC1α, ↑Complexes I, and III
37.	Boswellic acid	Albino rats	100–250 mg/kg	↓ROS, ↓LPO, ↑SOD, ↑GPx, ↑CAT, ↑Nrf2, ↓Caspase-3 ↑Complexes I, II, III, and IV
38.	Asiatic acid	SH-SY5Y cells	10 nM	↓ROS↑, MMP, ↓Bax, ↑Bcl-2, ↓Cyt c, ↓Caspase-3, -8, -8, -9
39.	Peoniflorin	SD rats, PC12 cells	25–100 µM	↓ROS, ↑MMP, ↑ATP, ↓Bax, ↑Bcl-2, ↓Cyt c, ↓Caspase-3, -9
40.	Isolongifolene	Rats SH-SY5Y cells	10 mg/kg 10 µM	↓ROS, ↓LPO, ↑SOD, GSH, CAT, GPx, ↑Bax, Bcl-2, ↓Cyt c, ↓Caspase-3, -6, -8, -9, ↑PI3K/Akt/ GSK-3β, ↑MMP
41.	Lycopene	SD rats	5 µM	↓ROS, ↑MMP, mPTP blockage, ↑ATP, ↓Bax, ↑Bcl-2, ↓Bax/Bcl-2 ratio, ↓Cyt c, ↓Caspase-3, -9, ↑PGC1α, ↑Complexes I, II, III, IV
42.	Auraptene	SN4741 cells bEnd.3 cells	10 µM 1 µM	↓ROS, ↑MMP, ↑Nrf2
43.	Astaxanthin	LO2 cells	30–90 µM	↓ROS, ↑MMP, ↑ATP, ↓Bax, ↓Caspase-3, ↑PGC1α, Restored Mt morphology
44.	Allicin	PC12 cells	0.01–1 µg/mL	↓ROS, ↑MMP, ↑PGC1α, ↓Bax, ↑Bcl-2, ↓Cyt c, ↓Caspase-3
45.	Fucoidan	SH-SY5Y cells HPBM cells	50 µg/mL 20 and 50 µM	↓ROS, ↑MMP, ↓Bax, ↑Bcl-2, ↓Caspase-3 ↑Complexes I and IV, ↑AMPK/ PGC1α
46.	Sulforaphane	HHL-5 cells	10 and 250 µM	↓ROS, ↓LPO, ↑SOD, ↑GSH, ↑Nrf2, ↑MMP, ↑ATP, ↓Apoptosis, ↑PGC1α, ↓Ca^{2+}, ↑Complexes I and IV
47.	β-Lapachone	MELAS cells	1 µM	↓ROS, ↑MMP, ↑ATP
48.	Melatonin	Porcine oocytes	500 nM	↓ROS, ↑MMP, ↑ATP,↓Caspase-3 ↑PGC1α/SIRT1
49.	Ligustilide	HT-22 cells, SD rats	20 µM, 10, 20 mg/kg	↓ROS, ↑MMP, ↑PINK1/Parkin
50.	Xyloketal B	PC12 cells	100–250 µM	↓ROS, ↑GSH, and ↑MMP Restored Mt morphology
51.	Osthole	PC12 cells SD rats	7 µg/cc 50 mg/kg	↓ROS, ↑MMP, ↑ATP, ↓Bax, ↑Bcl-2, ↓Bax/Bcl-2 ratio, ↓Cyt c, ↓Caspase-3, -9, ↑Complexes I, II, III and IV
52.	Cinnamic Acid	H9c2 cells	100–500 nM	↓ROS, ↓LPO, ↑SOD, ↑GSH, ↑MMP, ↓Bax, ↑Bcl-2, ↓Caspase-3

53.	DL0410	SH-SY5Y cells	1–10 μM	↓ROS, ↓LPO, ↑Nrf2, ↑MMP, ↓Bax, ↑Bcl-2, ↓Cyt c, ↓Caspase-3
54.	Mito-Q	NP cells	500 nM	↓ROS, ↓LPO, ↑SOD, ↑GSH, ↑Nrf2, ↑MMP, ↓PINK1/Parkin
55.	FLZ	SH-SY5Y cell	100 μM	↓ROS, ↑GSH, ↑MMP, mPTP blockage, ↑Complexes IV
56.	MHY-1684	hCPCsc-$^{kit+}$	1 μM	↓ROS, ↑AKT signaling, ↓Apoptosis
57.	Diphenyl diselenide	HT22 cells LDLr$^{-/-}$ mice	2 μM 1 mg/kg	↓ROS, ↓LPO, ↑SOD, ↑GSH, ↑GPx, ↑MMP ↑Complexes I and II
58.	Rasagiline	SH-SY5Y cells Rat mitochondria	100 nM 1–10 μM	↓ROS, ↑SOD, ↑GSH, ↑MMP, ↓Cyt c, ↑ATP
59.	Succinnobucol	SH-SY5Y cells	3 μM	↓ROS, ↑GSH, ↑MMP, ↓Cyt c, ↑ATP
60.	FMU200	SH-SY5Y cells	0.1 and 1 μM	↓ROS, ↑MMP
61.	CNB-001	C57BL/6 mice SK-N-SH cells	6–48 mg/kg 2 μM	↓ROS, ↓LPO, ↑SOD, ↑GSH, ↑GPx,↑CAT, ↑MMP ↓Bax, ↑Bcl-2, ↓Cyt c, ↓Caspase-3

Source: *Makinde E, Ma L, Mellick GD, Feng Y. Mitochondrial Modulators: The Defender.* Biomolecules. *2023; 13(2):226. https://doi.org/10.3390/biom13020226.*

When we calculate the total mass of these proteins in grams of protein per liter cell, we discover that the soleus and heart muscles have only 9 and 10 g/L of protein per liter cell devoted to glycolysis, respectively, whereas the gracilis muscle has over 60 g. With a protein density of 1.37% per milliliter, this means that approximately 9% of the gracilis muscle's cell volume is dedicated to glycolytic enzymes, compared to 1–2% of the soleus and heart's cell volume. Keep in mind that the sarcoplasmic reticulum (SR), myofilaments, and mitochondria—which are covered in more detail below—take up the majority of the remaining space. Compared to soleus or heart muscle, these relatively large differences show the known heavy dependence of the gracilis, a glycolytic fast-twitch muscle, on the production of ATP from glycolysis.

2.3.2.3. Oxidative Phosphorylation

The heart has a far higher concentration of mitochondrial protein than the other muscle tissues. When we add up all of the mitochondrial proteins, we discover that for the 304 mitochondrial proteins with the highest abundance, the ratio of mitochondrial proteins to the heart was, for the heart/gracilis, 36 ± 2 and, for the heart/soleus, 4 ± 0.1, respectively. The protein content for OxPhos has been reduced to the levels of COX, the only irreversible step in the entire cascade from NADH to the terminal reduction of oxygen to water, because of the striking consistency in the ratios across tissues for these mitochondrial enzymes. Thus, a system's OxPhos capacity can be roughly estimated from its COX content.

2.3.2.4. Specific Power of Energy Conversion Processes in Muscle

Muscle is a moving organic system, so the weight efficiency—or specific power—of the energy conversion process used is crucial because it adds to the muscle's workload to move the energy conversion system's "weight." Therefore, the muscle can perform work more effectively with the higher the specific power of the energy conversion system. For instance, airplane flight was made possible by the internal combustion engine's higher specific power compared to the steam engine.

We can calculate the total glycolysis enzymes for ATP production using the rabbit heart's data, which comes out to be about 10 mg/g wet weight. Additionally, our relational proteomic data supports a realized rate of 5 μmol ATP/min/g heart, which equals 0–5 mmol ATP/min/g glycolytic enzymes.

The maximum rate of ATP production by OxPhos per gram of mitochondria (including associated water) can be estimated from the cytochrome oxidase (COX) content and maximum activity in intact heart mitochondria of approximately 700 nmol O_2/nmol COX/min, or assuming 5.6 ATP/O_2 then approximately 4 μmol ATP/nmol COX/min, which correlates with maximum in vivo rates of canines.

How does this compare with the weight/volume efficiency of OxPhos? About 1 nmol of COX per milligram of heart mitochondria produces 4 μmol of ATP per milligram of heart mitochondrial protein. Unlike glycolysis, which depends on an intact compartmentalized structure to function, the mass of mitochondrial lipids, water, and solutes must be taken into consideration to determine the wet weight of mitochondria. Since 25% of the mass of mitochondria is made up of protein, 1 mg of protein is equal to 4 mg of wet weight of mitochondria. In comparison to the previously calculated 0.5 mmol ATP/min/g for glycolysis, this yields 1 μmol ATP/min/mg wet weight or 1 mmol ATP/min/g. These values translate to specific powers (kW/kg) of 1.1 and 0.5, respectively, for aerobic respiration and glycolysis in the heart, assuming free energy of hydrolysis (ΔGATP) of −64 kJ/mol of ATP. Skeletal muscle computations show that the specific powers of aerobic respiration (1.7 kW/kg) and glycolysis (3.8 kW/kg) are comparable; however, glycolysis seems to have a higher specific power than OxPhos in the skeletal muscle.

A V8 internal combustion engine's specific power is approximately 0.65 kW/kg, which is comparable to the specific power of the heart's glycolysis. Taking into consideration the possible errors in this kind of computation, such as ignoring the water space associated with glycolysis, the weight efficiency of OxPhos and glycolysis is evidently very close, within a factor of 3. So why choose more widely distributed glycolysis over localized mitochondrial OxPhos, or vice versa? The choice of energy source is far more intricate than the basic specific power of the enzyme system.

The entire process of converting glucose to CO2 maximizes the utilization of glucose entry and prevents the production of lactate, a metabolic end product with a high potential that must be replenished in the liver and kidney at the expense of the animal's overall energy balance. That is, the body would lose four ATP for every oxidized glucose if the muscles only used glycolysis and the lactate was recycled back into glucose in the liver and kidney for later use. This would not be sustainable. To make up for this significant loss of potential energy, lactate must either be eliminated or used as reducing equivalents for OxPhos in other parts of the body. This latter restriction is probably the cause of the heart's preference for plasma lactate oxidation over practically all other substrates when blood levels of the substance are high. The structural differences between OxPhos and glycolysis may be another factor. Though it is in the freely soluble cytosolic fraction, glycolysis is undoubtedly partially compartmentalized and allows for tight packing within the myofilaments. Furthermore, because they are free in the cytosol, the mitochondria are less vulnerable to the internal shear forces of the muscle, which could otherwise damage them as complex organelles. Shear on the highly compliant mitochondria may be generated in both the short and long axis during muscle contraction as the muscle thickens and decreases in longitudinal length.

Placing mitochondria in areas of the cell such as the I-band, Z-disk, or subsarcolemmal regions—where internal shear is reduced—is one compensatory mechanism. A different method involves having the mitochondria move in tandem with the myofilaments in both dimensions. This allows the mitochondria to thicken and shorten with each contraction. Heart mitochondria have been shown to stay connected to the sarcomere, growing and contracting with each contraction while maintaining their bond with the sarcomere.

The desmin and plectin intermediate fibers may serve as the pathway for the connection to the sarcomere. Not much research has been done on how this remodeling of the mitochondria affects each contraction. All things considered, the mitochondria need their own space, which is hard to find within the muscle without sacrificing the cross-sectional area of the contractile apparatus that is necessary to maximize power.

Furthermore, the placement of the mitochondria may expose them to the previously mentioned shear forces. In addition, myofibrils or other cellular structures must be moved to make room for lipid droplets, which are frequently tightly coupled to mitochondria, when OxPhos is produced by fatty acid fuel sources, as is most frequently seen in the heart.

2.3.3. Energy Distribution Processes of the Muscle Cell

The distribution of the inputs, intermediates, and outputs involved in the energy conversion processes must be considered in the energetic design of a cell in addition to the content and composition of the processes as discussed above. The distances between the various structures as well as the mechanisms controlling the flow of metabolites and ions between them, therefore, are particularly significant in defining the energetic support capacity of the relatively large and densely packed muscle cell. We will concentrate on three main processes in this review section: the transfer of electrical potential energy within mitochondria, the delivery of oxygen from the capillary to mitochondria, and the transfer of ATP from mitochondria to cellular ATPases. You can find a detailed explanation of substrate metabolism in muscle cells elsewhere.

2.3.3.1. Capillary Structure and Blood Flow

Providing oxygen is one of the main needs for OxPhos to function. The heart is highly vascular, with an astounding density of capillaries between 2,500 and 4,500 capillaries/mm^2, nearly evenly spaced every 12 to 22 μm, consistent with the average diameter of a heart cell, to support the supply of oxygen. These densities imply that at least one supporting capillary is in contact with every heart cell. This is in line with studies using three-dimensional electron microscopy that show that most cardiac myocytes have a capillary-associated region. Although they are not as well developed as those in skeletal muscle, the paravascular pool contains a slightly higher density of mitochondria next to these capillaries. As a result, the capillary network is optimally shaped to supply blood, along with related substrates and oxygen, to nearly every cell in the heart wall. The coronary blood flow is relatively high and linearly balanced, with the workload sustaining a low venous pO2 (~18

Torr) over a large portion of the workload range, to support the high level of OxPhos.

A fundamental question in cardiac physiology is how coronary flow is precisely matched to oxygen demand. Multiple, redundant mechanisms operating at different spatial scales are likely involved in this vitally important bodily and cardiac function. The end effect is a highly dynamic system that meets the heart's oxygen delivery needs through a dense feeding capillary network, maintains a nearly constant venous pO_2, and supplies an adequate amount of oxygen.

Since August Krogh's Nobel Prize-winning research on the control of oxygen diffusion in muscles approximately a century ago, the ability of capillaries to supply oxygen to skeletal muscles has been of great interest. Skeletal muscle capillary density ranges widely from approximately 250 to 1,500/mm^2 of muscle volume, with oxidative muscles having up to twice as many capillaries per unit volume and approximately 33% greater capillary-to-muscle fiber ratio (~2.0 vs. 1.5).

Diffusion capacity between these structures is largely determined by the way the capillary interacts with the muscle fiber, even though capillary-to-fiber ratio and capillary density have been routinely measured on 2-D images for decades and frequently, though not always, correlate well with muscle oxidative capacity. As a matter of fact, measurements that take into account the geometry of capillary-fiber interactions in two or three dimensions have proliferated and exhibit a stronger correlation with mitochondrial content in both oxidative and glycolytic muscle types under diverse circumstances. Therefore, three factors determine the total structural capacity for oxygen delivery from capillaries to the skeletal muscle fiber: 1) the number of capillaries close to the cell, 2) the area of direct surface contact between the capillaries and the muscle fiber, and 3) the cell's cross-sectional area. More oxidative muscles are smaller, have higher capillary densities, and have more capillary surface area contact than more glycolytic muscles, as was previously mentioned. However, the majority of muscles, especially those found in humans, are made up of diverse groups of both oxidative and glycolytic muscle fibers, and the relative amounts of each determine the overall metabolic phenotype of the entirety of the muscle. This heterogeneity causes multiple glycolytic and oxidative muscle fibers to surround a single oxidative muscle fiber, and it also causes these muscle fibers to have differing needs for oxygen delivery along their shared borders.

By arranging capillaries in grooves in the sarcolemma of the more oxidative cell, it may be possible to meet the oxygen demand of oxidative fibers next to glycolytic fibers, which is inconsistent. Another level of control is available when designing the structural capacity for oxygen delivery to the muscle cell within heterogeneous tissues, as it is possible to increase the capillary surface area contact to one fiber but not the other by embedding capillaries atop only one of the two adjacent fibers. There is still a great deal to learn about these capillary grooves, including when and how they form during muscle growth and how exactly they affect the ability of muscle cells to receive oxygen.

Though sarcolemmal grooves are still visible in isolated live muscle fibers even after the adjacent capillaries are removed, it is evident that these grooves in the sarcolemma are real physical structures rather than merely the product of capillary compression of the cell membrane (Acín-Pérez et al., 2004; Acín-Pérez et al., 2008) (Figure 2.8).

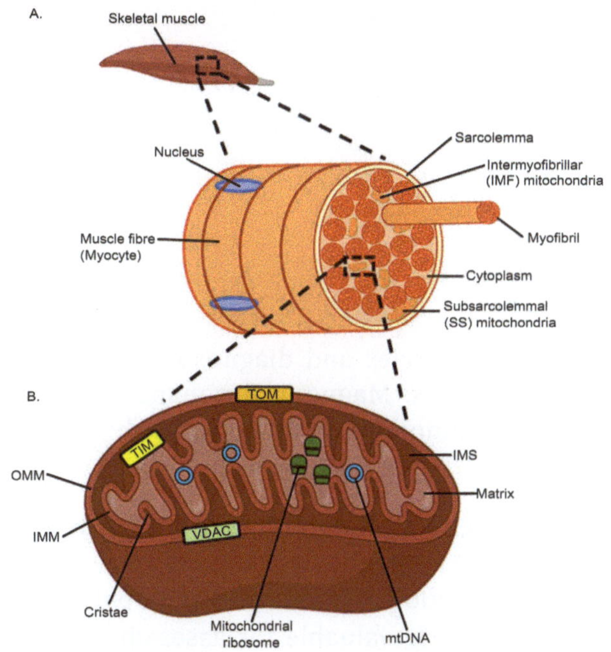

Figure 2.8. *(A) Structure of a human muscle fiber or myocyte. (B) Structure of the mitochondria. TOM; translocase of the outer membrane.*

TIM; translocase of the inner membrane. VDAC; voltage-dependent anion channel. IMM; inner mitochondrial membrane. IMS; inner membrane space. OMM; outer mitochondrial membrane. mtDNA; mitochondrial DNA.

Source: Taylor DF, Bishop DJ. Transcription Factor Movement and Exercise-Induced Mitochondrial Biogenesis in Human Skeletal Muscle: Current Knowledge and Future Perspectives. International Journal of Molecular Sciences. 2022; 23(3):1517. https://doi.org/10.3390/ijms23031517.

The rate of blood flow can increase more than an order of magnitude from rest to exercise, much like the dynamic nature of skeletal muscle contraction. It does so quickly enough that, in healthy populations, oxygen delivery to the muscle does not appear to be limited at the beginning of exercise. The increased contractile rate of the muscle cells during even moderate exercise causes a fall in the mean pO2 in both the capillaries (~35 to 24 Torr) and the interstitial space between capillaries and muscle fibers (~16 to 7 Torr), despite the large, rapid increase in oxygen delivery at the onset of exercise. It has been proposed that exercise does not change the oxygen pressure gradient from the capillary to mitochondria as previously believed, along with the similar magnitude fall in intramuscular pO2 that has been observed, from roughly 10–15 Torr at rest to 2–4 Torr at exercise intensities ranging from moderate to severe. Rather, the increased oxygen flux appears to be accounted for by a multiplication of the diffusion constant for oxygen (DO2), which is similar to its conductance; however, the exact mechanisms underlying this change are still unknown. It is evident that many connected, possibly overlapping processes closely regulate blood flow to the skeletal muscle. These mechanisms offer fine-grained control over oxygen delivery across the broad spectrum of skeletal muscle contractile demands.

2.3.3.2. Cytosolic Facilitated Diffusion Processes

It has frequently been suggested that simple metabolite diffusion is insufficient to support this highly active structure because of the metabolic rates and unique compartmentation of the ATP-utilizing and -producing machinery in muscle, as well as the observed metabolic homeostasis limiting large metabolite gradients. The two main cytosolic facilitated diffusion systems, myoglobin for oxygen and creatine kinase for ATP and ADP, have been the subject of intense research.

A Closer Look

Muscle Imaging Techniques

Various imaging techniques play a crucial role in visualizing muscles and diagnosing injuries or abnormalities, each offering unique advantages and applications. Magnetic Resonance Imaging (MRI), Computed Tomography (CT) scans, and ultrasound are among the most commonly utilized modalities in musculoskeletal imaging.

MRI is a non-invasive imaging technique that provides high-resolution images of soft tissues, including muscles, tendons, ligaments, and nerves. It uses strong magnetic fields and radio waves to generate detailed cross-sectional images, allowing for the visualization of muscle anatomy, pathology, and injuries with excellent contrast resolution. MRI is particularly valuable for assessing muscle tears, strains, and inflammation, as well as detecting tumors or other soft tissue abnormalities. Additionally, MRI can differentiate between acute and chronic muscle injuries, aiding in treatment planning and prognosis.

CT scans utilize X-rays to produce cross-sectional images of the body, offering excellent spatial resolution and detailed visualization of bony structures. While CT is not the primary modality for evaluating soft tissues like muscles, it can be valuable in certain cases, such as assessing muscle calcifications, detecting foreign bodies, or evaluating traumatic injuries where bone involvement is suspected. CT scans can also provide complementary information in conjunction with MRI in complex cases, offering a comprehensive assessment of musculoskeletal injuries.

Ultrasound imaging employs high-frequency sound waves to generate real-time images of the body's internal structures, including muscles, tendons, and ligaments. Ultrasound is particularly useful for assessing muscle morphology and dynamic function, and guiding interventional procedures such as injections or biopsies. It offers advantages such as portability, cost-effectiveness, and the absence of ionizing radiation, making it suitable for point-of-care evaluation and follow-up assessments. Ultrasound can detect muscle tears, tendonitis, fluid collections, and muscle hernias, providing valuable information for diagnosing and monitoring musculoskeletal conditions.

Each imaging modality has its strengths and limitations, and the choice of technique depends on factors such as the suspected pathology, clinical indication, patient characteristics, and availability of resources. Integrating information from multiple imaging modalities can enhance diagnostic accuracy and improve patient management in cases of complex musculoskeletal conditions. As technology continues to advance, imaging techniques are evolving to provide even greater precision, sensitivity, and accessibility in the evaluation of muscle injuries and abnormalities, ultimately contributing to improved patient outcomes and quality of care.

Summary

- Muscle metabolism refers to the intricate biochemical processes that occur within muscle cells to generate energy, facilitate muscle contraction, and maintain cellular functions. These processes are essential for activities ranging from simple movements to intense physical exertion.
- Cellular respiration is the process by which ATP is obtained from energy-rich molecules. Several major metabolic pathways are involved, some of which require the presence of oxygen.
- Aerobic respiration can sustain muscular activity from intrinsic muscular sources of metabolites until the supply of intramuscular glycogen and some lipids runs out. At that point, the muscles must get their energy sources from elsewhere in the body, especially the liver, via the blood.
- Nutrient utilization in muscle metabolism is a complex process whereby muscle cells harness the energy stored in various nutrients to fuel contraction, maintain cellular functions, and support exercise performance.
- Muscle metabolism plays a critical role in determining exercise performance by regulating energy production, substrate utilization, and metabolic adaptations in response to physical activity. The efficiency and flexibility of muscle metabolism influence an individual's capacity for endurance, strength, and power output during exercise.
- Skeletal muscle hypertrophy is a culmination of catabolic and anabolic processes that are interwoven into major metabolic pathways, and as such modulation of skeletal muscle metabolism may have implications on animal growth efficiency.
- Skeletal muscle has the remarkable ability to adjust its energy expenditure according to energy demands. Within milliseconds, a muscle can increase its energy expenditure 100-fold to transition between resting and active states.
- Glycolysis converts glucose into pyruvate through a series of enzymatic reactions and can produce ATP 100 times faster than oxidative phosphorylation (OxPhos). Large glycogen stores in muscle allow for rapid mobilization of glucose-1-phosphate by glycogen phosphorylase to fuel glycolysis, which is the predominant energy source during high-intensity exercise.
- In skeletal muscle, mitochondria morphology and functions are quite responsive to a range of intermittent and continuous stimuli including exercise, nutritional factors, aging, and disease.
- Mitochondrial dynamics also permit a fluid response to changing nutritional factors. For example, muscle cells isolated from the extensor digitorum longus (EDL) incubated in media containing acetoacetate for 24 hours, an oxidative substrate, have more extensive (fused) mitochondrial networks than those treated with glucose for the same amount of time.
- Myostatin is a negative regulator of muscle growth. Natural mutations of the myostatin gene have been discovered in sheep, cattle, dogs, and humans that result in gene disruption and a subsequent increase in muscle mass.

- Adult skeletal muscle contains a heterogeneous population of stem cells, known as satellite cells (SC, that contribute to postnatal muscle growth, maintenance, and repair.
- The design of the energy metabolism system in striated muscle remains a major area of investigation. To understand the design of energy conversion and distribution in the muscle cell, the entire process needs to be evaluated as it pertains to its physiological function.

References

1. Abreu, P., Serna, J. D. C., Munhoz, A. C., & Kowaltowski, A. J. (2020). Calorie restriction changes muscle satellite cell proliferation in a manner independent of metabolic modulation. *Mechanisms of Ageing and Development, 192*, 111362. https://doi.org/10.1016/j.mad.2020.111362.
2. Acín-Pérez, R., Bayona-Bafaluy, M. P., Fernández-Silva, P., Moreno-Loshuertos, R., Pérez-Martos, A., Bruno, C., Moraes, C. T., & Enríquez, J. A. (2004). Respiratory complex III is required to maintain complex I in mammalian mitochondria. *Molecular Cell, 13*(5), 805–815. https://doi.org/10.1016/s1097-2765(04)00124-8.
3. Acín-Pérez, R., Fernández-Silva, P., Peleato, M. L., Pérez-Martos, A., & Enríquez, J. A. (2008). Respiratory active mitochondrial super complexes. *Molecular Cell, 32*(4), 529–539. https://doi.org/10.1016/j.molcel.2008.10.021.
4. Ahn, C. S., & Metallo, C. M. (2015). Mitochondria as biosynthetic factories for cancer proliferation. *Cancer & Metabolism, 3*, 1. https://doi.org/10.1186/s40170-015-0128-2.
5. Amirouche, A., Durieux, A. C., Banzet, S., Koulmann, N., Bonnefoy, R., Mouret, C., Bigard, X., Peinnequin, A., & Freyssenet, D. (2009). Down-regulation of Akt/mammalian target of rapamycin signaling pathway in response to myostatin overexpression in skeletal muscle. *Endocrinology, 150*(1), 286–294. https://doi.org/10.1210/en.2008-0959.
6. Aon, M. A., Cortassa, S., & O'Rourke, B. (2010). Redox-optimized ROS balance: A unifying hypothesis. *Biochimica et Biophysica Acta (BBA)–Bioenergetics, 1797*(6–7), 865–877. https://doi.org/10.1016/j.bbabio.2010.02.016.
7. Apaoblaza, A., Gerrard, S. D., Matarneh, S. K., Wicks, J. C., Kirkpatrick, L., England, E. M., Scheffler, T. L., Duckett, S. K., Shi, H., Silva, S. L., et al. (2020). Muscle from grass- and grain-fed cattle differs energetically. *Meat Science, 161*, 107996. https://doi.org/10.1016/j.meatsci.2019.107996.
8. Arnold, D. L., Matthews, P. M., & Radda, G. K. (1984). Metabolic recovery after exercise and the assessment of mitochondrial function in vivo in human skeletal muscle by means of 31P NMR. *Magnetic Resonance in Medicine, 1*(3), 307–315. https://doi.org/10.1002/mrm.1910010303.
9. Averous, J., Gabillard, J. C., Seiliez, I., & Dardevet, D. (2012). Leucine limitation regulates myf5 and myoD expression and inhibits myoblast differentiation. *Experimental Cell Research, 318*(2), 217–227. https://doi.org/10.1016/j.yexcr.2011.10.015.
10. Banerjee, P. S., Ma, J., & Hart, G. W. (2015). Diabetes-associated dysregulation of O-GlcNAcylation in rat cardiac mitochondria. *Proceedings of the National Academy of Sciences of the United States of America, 112*(19), 6050–6055. https://doi.org/10.1073/pnas.1424017112.
11. Battistuzzi, G., D'Urso, M., Toniolo, D., Persico, G. M., & Luzzatto, L. (1985). Tissue-specific levels of human glucose-6-phosphate dehydrogenase correlate with methylation of specific

sites at the 3' end of the gene. *Proceedings of the National Academy of Sciences of the United States of America, 82*(5), 1465–1469. https://doi.org/10.1073/pnas.82.5.1465.

12. Bentzinger, C. F., Romanino, K., Cloëtta, D., Lin, S., Mascarenhas, J. B., Oliveri, F., Xia, J., Casanova, E., Costa, C. F., Brink, M., et al. (2008). Skeletal muscle-specific ablation of raptor, but not of rictor, causes metabolic changes and results in muscle dystrophy. *Cell Metabolism, 8*(5), 411–424. https://doi.org/10.1016/j.cmet.2008.10.002.

Chapter

SKELETAL MUSCLE MECHANICS

3

Contents

Introduction

The skeletal muscles are the organs of the vertebrate muscular system. Normally, tendons connect the skeletal muscles to the skeleton's bones. Known as muscle fibers, the muscle cells found in skeletal muscles are notably longer than those found in other forms of muscle tissue. Because of how the sarcomeres are arranged, the muscle tissue of skeletal muscles has a striped appearance. Voluntary muscles controlled by the somatic nervous system are known as skeletal muscles. There are two other types of muscle: striated cardiac muscle and non-striated smooth muscle. Both of these muscle types are categorized as involuntary, meaning they are controlled by the autonomic nervous system. There are numerous fascicles, or bundles of muscle fibers, within a skeletal muscle. Fascia is a type of connective tissue layer that envelops every single fiber and muscle in the body. In a process known as myogenesis, developing myoblasts fuse to form long, multinucleated cells that eventually become muscle fibers. The nuclei of these cells are situated inside the cell membrane and are referred to as myonuclei. Muscle fibers possess multiple mitochondria to fulfill their energy requirements.

Myofibrils are the building blocks of muscle fibers. The fundamental functional, contractile units of the muscle fiber required for muscle contraction, sarcomeres, are repeating units of actin and myosin filaments, or myofilaments, which make up myofibrils. Although the oxidation of fats and carbohydrates powers muscles primarily, anaerobic chemical reactions also power muscles, especially in the case of fast twitch fibers. Adenosine triphosphate (ATP), which powers the movement of the myosin heads, is produced by these chemical reactions. Human skeletal muscle makes up approximately 35% of the body weight. Skeletal muscle is responsible for generating movement, preserving posture, regulating body temperature, and stabilizing joints. Additionally, skeletal muscle is an endocrine organ. Skeletal muscle secretome contains subsets of 654 distinct proteins, lipids, amino acids, metabolites, and small RNAs under various physiological conditions.

Skeletal muscles do, however, also contain a sizable population of resident and infiltrating mononuclear cells. Myocytes comprise the vast majority of skeletal muscle in terms of volume. Skeletal muscle myocytes typically measure 2–3 cm in length and 100 μm in diameter, making them incredibly large cells. Muscle cells have much smaller mononuclear cells in contrast. A few of the mononuclear cells found in muscles are neutrophils (12–15 μm in diameter), macrophages (21 μm in diameter), and endothelial cells (about 50–70 μm long, 10–30 μm wide, and 0.1–10 μm thick). Myocyte nuclei, however, might only make up half of the nuclei found in skeletal muscle; the other half would come from resident and infiltrating mononuclear cells.

Orientation and Directional Terms:

Term	Definition	Illustration
Actin proteins	A family of globular multi-functional proteins that form microfilaments in the cytoskeleton, and the thin filaments in muscle fibrils.	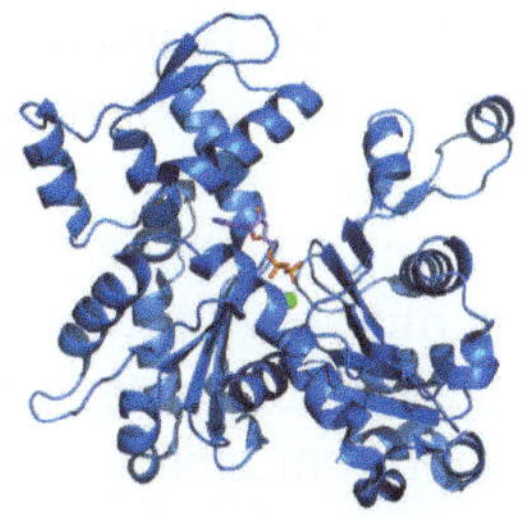
Elastic tissue	A type of dense connective tissue. They provide tensile strength and resistance to stretching. They contain both elastin and collagen fibres called fibroblasts. The elastin fibres give it a property of elasticity so that a structure can return to its original position even after stretching.	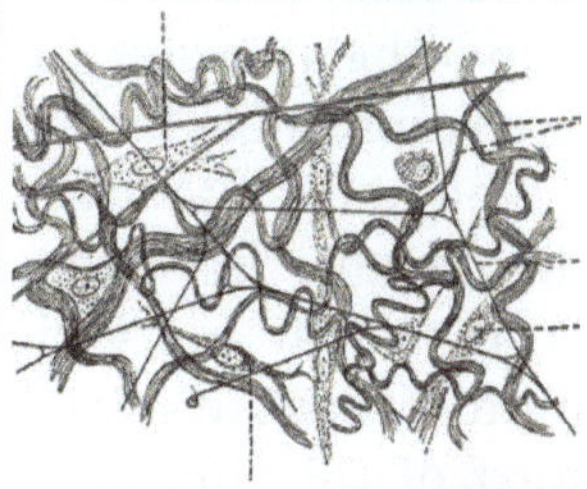
Endomysium	Endomysium is the deepest and smallest component of muscle connective tissue. This thin layer helps provide an appropriate chemical environment for the exchange of calcium, sodium, and potassium, which is essential for the excitation and subsequent contraction of a muscle fiber.	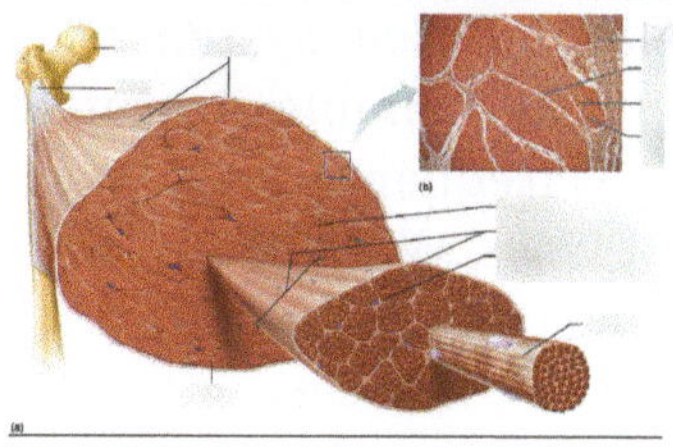
Limb muscles	A jointed, muscled appendage of a tetrapod vertebrate animal used for weight-bearing, terrestrial locomotion and physical interaction with other objects.	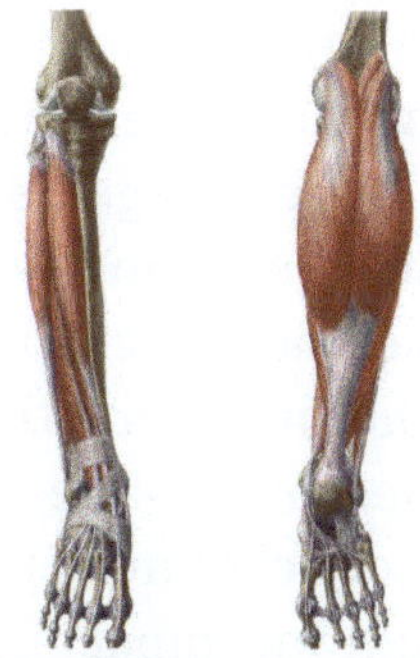
Myofibril	The myofibrils are bundles of interconnected protein filaments of striated muscles. The filaments (myofilaments) included in the myofibrils are mainly thick filaments (myosin), and thin filaments (actin). The contractile functional unit of the myofibril is called the sarcomere.	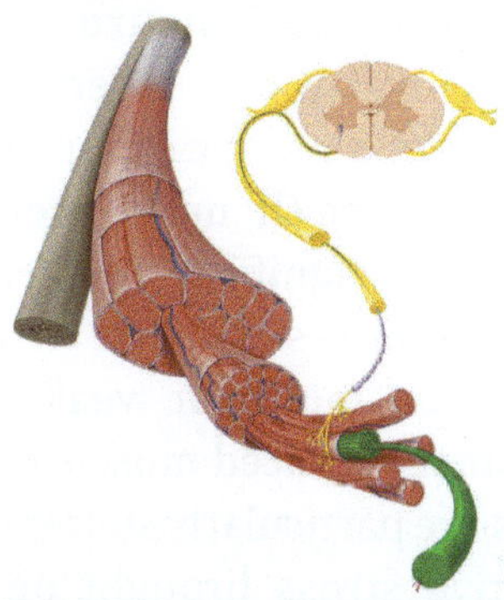

3.1. Basics of Skeletal Muscle

Since the skeletal muscles make up approximately half of a mammal's body weight, they are subjected to disproportionately high dosages of chemicals. A multitude of chemicals can target skeletal muscle, and the harmful or toxic effects can vary from mild pain or weakness to total paralysis. The only organ more sensitive to the toxicity of organophosphate (OP) nerve agents than the skeletal muscles is the brain. The effects of these compounds on skeletal muscles in general and the muscles of respiration in particular are responsible for the morbidity and mortality linked to OP intoxication. Respiratory paralysis that results from the depolarization of the neuromuscular blockade is one factor contributing to overdose deaths from opioids. In the context of OP poisoning, knowledge of the skeletal muscle system is crucial, but it is also extremely complex because various muscle fiber types frequently react to OP compounds in different ways. What makes skeletal muscles so fascinating to study are the differences between slow and fast muscles.

Both cholinergic and noncholinergic components that are either directly or indirectly regulated by OP nerve agents are abundant in skeletal muscles. Neuromuscular activity is one of the many skeletal muscle properties that are regulated by motor innervation. Modifications in the activities of choline acetyltransferase (ChAT) and acetylcholinesterase (AChE) seem to have a significant impact on neuromuscular transmission and neuromuscular activity. Acetylcholine (ACh) is taken out of the synaptic cleft at the cholinergic synapse in part by AChE. Compounds like OP nerve agents, which inhibit this enzyme, significantly alter neuromuscular transmission, resulting in twitch potentiation, fasciculation, muscular weakness, and necrosis or apoptosis-induced muscle cell death. Skeletal muscles are particularly susceptible to oxidative/nitrosative stress brought on by OP because of their high metabolism, which produces an excessive amount of free radicals. Skeletal muscle has garnered increased attention in the last twenty years due to its role in intermediate syndrome (IMS) and tolerance development resulting from OP pesticide toxicity. Effects of OP on skeletal muscles can happen at one or more of the following sites: the motor endplate, the junctional cleft, the nerve fiber, the nerve terminal, and the myofibrils.

Each skeletal muscle is an organ composed of various tissues like connective tissue, blood vessels, nerve fibers, and skeletal muscle fibers. Three layers of connective tissue, called mysia, surround each skeletal muscle, providing structure and compartmentalizing the muscle fibers (Figure 3.1). The epimysium, a sheath of dense, asymmetric connective tissue, envelops every muscle and permits it to contract and move forcefully without compromising its structural integrity. Moreover, the epimysium permits muscle to move independently by dividing it from nearby tissues and organs.

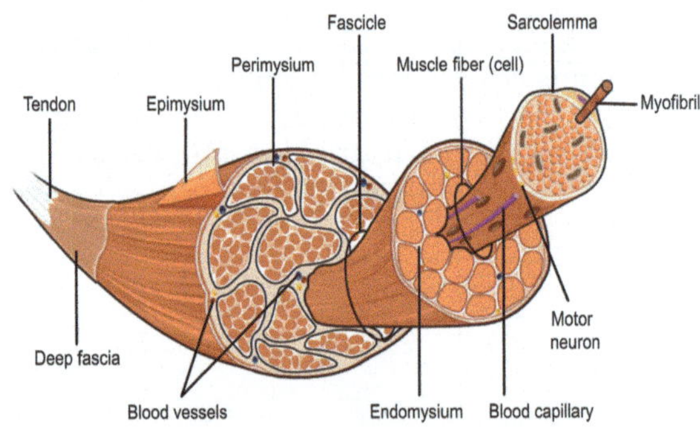

Figure 3.1. *The three connective tissue Layers: bundles of muscle fibers, called fascicles, are covered by the perimysium. Muscle fibers are covered by the endomysium.*

Source: https://open.oregonstate.education/app/uploads/sites/157/2019/07/1001_Muscle_Tissue_revised-768x387.png.

Muscle fibers in skeletal muscles form fascicles surrounded by perimysium, a connective tissue layer. This organization in limb muscles allows the nervous system to trigger specific muscle movements by activating certain fibers in a fascicle. The endomysium, a thin layer of collagen and reticular fibers that surrounds each muscle fiber inside a fascicle. The endomysium, which envelops the cells' extracellular matrix, aids in the force transmission from the muscle fibers to the tendons. The collagen in the three layers of connective tissue intertwines with that of a tendon in skeletal muscles, pulling on bones in unison. The tendon merges with the periosteum covering the bone at the other end. Muscle fiber contraction generates tension, transmitted through the layers of connective tissue, tendon, and periosteum to move the skeleton. In other places, the mysia may join with fascia, the connective tissue between the skin and bones, or with an aponeurosis, a broad sheet similar to a tendon. An example of an aponeurosis is the broad sheet of connective tissue in the lower back where the latissimus dorsi muscles, also called the "lats," merge.

Moreover, blood vessels supply each skeletal muscle with plenty of nutrients, oxygen, and waste removal agents. Also, the axon branch of a somatic motor neuron supplies each muscle fiber in skeletal muscle, signaling the fiber to contract. Skeletal muscle can only contract functionally through nerve system signals, unlike cardiac and smooth muscle. Similar to the appendicular and axial skeletons, skeletal muscle is a contractile, excitable tissue that helps maintain posture and move the orbits. Tendons are used to connect it to the orbits and bones. Excitable tissue uses electrical signals to react to stimuli. Contractile tissue can produce tension. Additionally, skeletal muscle tissue is extensible and elastic. Elastic tissue can revert to its original shape after distortion, while extensible tissue can be stretched.

3.1.1. Muscle Fibers

Skeletal muscle cells are often referred to as muscle fibers (or myofibers) because they are long and cylindrical. In comparison to other cells, skeletal muscle fibers can reach lengths of up to 30 cm (11.8 in) and diameters of up to 100 μm in the upper leg's Sartorius. Large, protein-rich cells with multiple nuclei can efficiently produce the proteins and enzymes needed for their functions. Skeletal muscle fibers contain organelles like mitochondria, endoplasmic reticulum, and nuclei, which are unique to these cells. The sarcoplasmic reticulum (SR), a specialized smooth endoplasmic reticulum, stores, releases, and retrieves calcium ions (Ca^{++}).

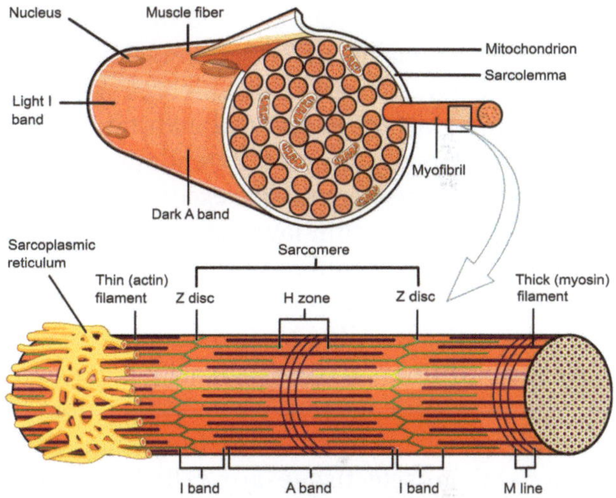

Figure 3.2. *Muscle fiber: A skeletal muscle fiber is surrounded by a plasma membrane called the sarcolemma, which contains sarcoplasm, the cytoplasm of muscle cells. A muscle fiber is composed of many myofibrils, which contain sarcomeres with light and dark regions that give the cell its striated appearance.*

Source: https://open.oregonstate.education/app/uploads/sites/157/2021/02/1022_Muscle_Fibers_small_revised-1-768x620.png

Sarcolemma, the name for the plasma membrane of muscle fibers, comes from the Greek word sarco, which means "flesh," and sarcoplasm is the name for the cytoplasm (Figure 3.2). Sarcomeres connected in series are found within myofibrils, organelles made of proteins that run the length of a muscle fiber. One muscle fiber can have hundreds to thousands of myofibrils, each containing thousands of sarcomeres, as myofibrils are only about 1.2 μm in diameter. The skeletal muscle fiber's smallest functional unit is called a sarcomere, which is made up of a highly ordered arrangement of structural, regulatory, and contractile proteins. The contraction of individual skeletal muscle fibers (and eventually the entire muscle) is caused by the shortening of these individual sarcomeres.

3.1.1.1. Structure

A group of muscle fibers encased in connective tissue sheaths makes up skeletal muscle tissue. Connective tissue sheaths come in three varieties, each named after its natural habitat. Every muscle fiber is surrounded by endomysium. It functions as a site of metabolic exchange because it is composed of a thin layer of reticular fibers and only allows capillaries and nerve fibers with small diameters. A slightly thicker layer of connective tissue called perimysium envelops a collection of fibers and is primarily composed of type I and III collagen. We call this group of fibers a fascicle or bundle. The functional units of skeletal muscle tissue are called fascicles. Blood vessels and nerve fibers passing through the perimysium are marginally bigger than those passing through the endomysium. An individual muscle's entire fascicle collection is surrounded by its epimysium. The neurovascular supply to the muscle is found in this dense connective tissue, which is primarily composed of type I collagen.

3.1.1.2. Types

There are three types of skeletal muscle fibers: Type I, Type IIa, and Type IIb.

- Type I muscle fibers, also called slow oxidative fibers, are specialized for aerobic activity. They are small, contain a high amount of myoglobin, and appear red in fresh tissue. A muscle twitch is a single contraction of a muscle. Type I fibers make up slow-twitch, fatigue-resistant motor units. Muscles of the deep back responsible for maintaining posture are mostly made up of Type I slow oxidative fibers.
- Type IIa muscle fibers are also known as fast oxidative glycolytic fibers. These fibers appear slightly lighter than Type I in fresh tissues. They contain many mitochondria and have a higher myoglobin content than type IIb fibers. Unlike Type I fibers, Type IIa fibers have high amounts of glycogen. Because of this, they are capable of anaerobic glycolysis and make up fast-twitch, fatigue-resistant motor units. Type IIa fibers are more fatigue-resistant than Type IIb fibers and are used in movements that require high sustained power. Many athletes have high amounts of these fibers, especially competitive swimmers.
- Type IIb muscle fibers are also referred to as fast glycolytic fibers. They are large fibers and appear light pink in fresh tissues. Type IIb fibers contain fewer mitochondria and a lower amount of myoglobin. Although they contain a low level of oxidative enzymes, they show high anaerobic enzyme activity and contain a high amount of glycogen. Type IIb fibers are more prone to fatigue than Type I and Type IIa fibers and make fast-twitch, fatigue-prone motor units. Type IIb fibers have the fastest rate of ATPase activity and are found in muscles used for short, rapid

bursts of contraction such as the gastrocnemius, a muscle in the leg that is used in jumping.

3.1.2. The Sarcomere

The region of a myofibril that lies between two cytoskeletal structures known as Z-discs (also known as Z-lines or Z-bands) is known as a sarcomere. The arrangement of the thick and thin myofilaments within each sarcomere is what gives skeletal muscle fibers their striated appearance (Figure 3.2). The thick myosin-containing filaments that cross the sarcomere's center and extend toward the Z-discs make up the dark, striated A band. A protein known as myomesin anchors the thick filaments at the M-line, which is the center of the sarcomere. A protein known as α-actinin anchors thin actin filaments at the Z-discs in the lighter I band regions. The thin filaments cross over with thick filament regions as they move into the A band in the direction of the M-line. Because the myosin filaments overlap with the actin filaments and are thicker, the A band appears darker. Because it only contains the part of the thick filaments that do not overlap with the thin filaments, the H zone in the center of the A band has a slightly lighter color, i.e., the H zone is not penetrated by the thin filaments. A single sarcomere has one dark A band with half of the lighter I band on each end since Z-discs define sarcomeres (Figure 3.2). The myofilaments themselves do not lengthen during contraction; instead, they slide across one another, shortening the distance between the Z-discs and the sarcomere. The H zone and I band regions contract, but the length of the A band stays the same due to the constant length of the thick myosin filament. These regions show the places where the filaments do not overlap; during contraction, these regions of no overlap decrease as filament overlap increases.

The skeletal muscle cell's functional unit is called a sarcomere. The length of each sarcomere is approximately 2.5 micrometers. It is composed of numerous parallel-oriented myosin and actin filaments. Actin and myosin filaments overlap in specific locations to form multiple bands and zones. The sarcomere's perimeter is formed by a Z disc on either side. Actin filaments that are thin extend from a Z disc in both directions, but they do not go across the whole length of the sarcomere. With a diameter of nearly 8 nm, they are composed of tightly bound regulatory proteins known as troponin and tropomyosin. Actin filaments are absent from the sarcomere center, which is known as the H zone. Perpendicular to the filaments, an M line passes through the center of the H zone. In between the actin filaments are thick myosin filaments. Their globular head region, which consists of both heavy and light chain, has a diameter of roughly 15 nm. This head can attach to an actin filament, move along it, and exhibit ATPase activity. They travel through the H zone but are not attached to the Z discs. There are three bands that separate the sarcomere. The middle band, or A band, represents the myosin filaments along with the thin filaments that overlap at both ends. The region where only actin filaments are present is represented by the two I bands that are present on either side of the A band.

3.1.2.1. Sarcoplasmic Structures

- Ø Sarcolemma – cell plasma membrane of a muscle cell
- Ø Sarcoplasmic reticulum – modified endoplasmic reticulum. The sarcoplasmic reticulum resembles a piece of lace that surrounds the myofibril. It is made up of a network of tubules with a reservoir at either end. This reservoir is referred to as the terminal cisterna.
- Ø Terminal cisterna – enlarged regions

on either end of the sarcoplasmic reticulum. The terminal cisternae sequester calcium to be used in the contraction cycle. There is a terminal cisterna on either side of a t-tubule. Altogether they are called a triad.

Ø T-tubules – also called transverse tubules. The t-tubules are pits along the surface of the muscle cells. Their walls are continuous with the sarcolemma, meaning the internal surface of the t-tubule is exposed to the extracellular matrix. The t-tubules are responsible for moving action potentials to the inner region of the muscle cell.

3.1.3. Accessory Proteins

The thick and thin filaments in the myofibrils are supported by accessory proteins. These proteins maintain the speed and alignment of filaments during the contraction cycle. Some of them are described below.

- Titin is a large, elastic protein that anchors thick filaments to Z lines to prevent excessive stretching of the myofibril.
- Tropomodulin acts like an actin cap. It attaches to the free end of an actin filament to maintain its length.
- α-Actinin is a short, rod-shaped protein that arranges thin filaments into parallel bundles and anchors them to the Z line.
- Desmin is an intermediate filament that forms a lattice surrounding the sarcomere near the Z lines to attach them to each other and the plasma membrane.
- Nebulin is a thin, elongated protein running parallel to thin filaments. It assists α-Actinin in binding the thin filaments to the Z line and is thought to be important during the development of muscle tissue
- Dystrophin is thought to link actin filaments to the external lamina of the muscle cell.
- Myomesin anchors thick filaments to the M line.

3.1.4. Neuromuscular Junction

A motor nerve ending and a muscle cell synapse at a place known as a neuromuscular junction, or NMJ for short. Acetylcholine is released by motor neurons into the neuromuscular junction's synaptic cleft. After passing through the synaptic cleft, the acetylcholine molecules attach to receptors on the muscle fiber membrane. The muscle cell depolarizes as a result, contracting later on (Figure 3.3).

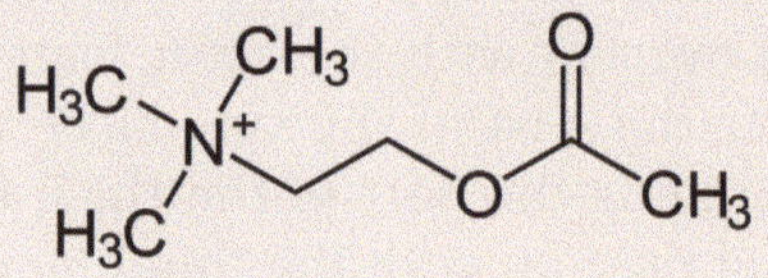

Figure 3.3. *Acetylcholine.*

Source: By NEUROtiker Own work, Public Domain, https://commons.wikimedia.org/w/index.php?curid=2125698.

A beta-motor neuron innervates skeletal muscle, inducing contractions in its fibers. Alpha-motor neurons' cell bodies can be found in the motor nuclei of the brainstem (for head and face muscles) or the ventral horn of the spinal cord (for limbs and trunk muscles). The collection of individual muscle fibers innervated by an alpha-motor neuron is referred to as a motor unit. Depending on the type of muscle, a single alpha-motor neuron can innervate multiple muscle fibers, but only one alpha-motor neuron can innervate a single muscle fiber.

3.1.5. Contraction

The sliding filament theory is the name given to the mechanism underlying muscle contraction. Actin and myosin filaments slide past one another during this process, shortening the sarcomere. Adenosine triphosphate (ATP) molecules must hydrolyze for the sliding filament mechanism to work, and myosin heads on actin filaments must bind and release.

- Following excitation by a motor nerve ending, ATP binds to myosin, decreasing the affinity of actin to myosin. Myosin releases actin.
- Myosin hydrolyzes ATP to adenosine diphosphate (ADP) and a phosphate molecule. This provides the energy needed for the myosin head to rotate to a 90° angle and reattach to a new actin.
- Power stroke – A troponin molecule partially blocks the myosin binding site when the muscle is not contracting. When myosin binds more tightly and releases a phosphate during contraction, calcium binds to troponin, decreasing its affinity to the myosin binding site and uncovering it. The attached actin filament slides along with the myosin head as it swings toward the M line as a result of the phosphate release.
- At the end of the power stroke, myosin releases the ADP molecule. The head returns to its original position and is ready to begin the cycle again.

3.1.6. Skeletal Muscle Contraction

A specialized synapse that connects a skeletal muscle fiber and an α-motor neuron is known as a neuromuscular junction. Voltage-gated calcium ion channels open in response to an action potential that occurs at the neuromuscular junction, which causes skeletal muscle contraction.

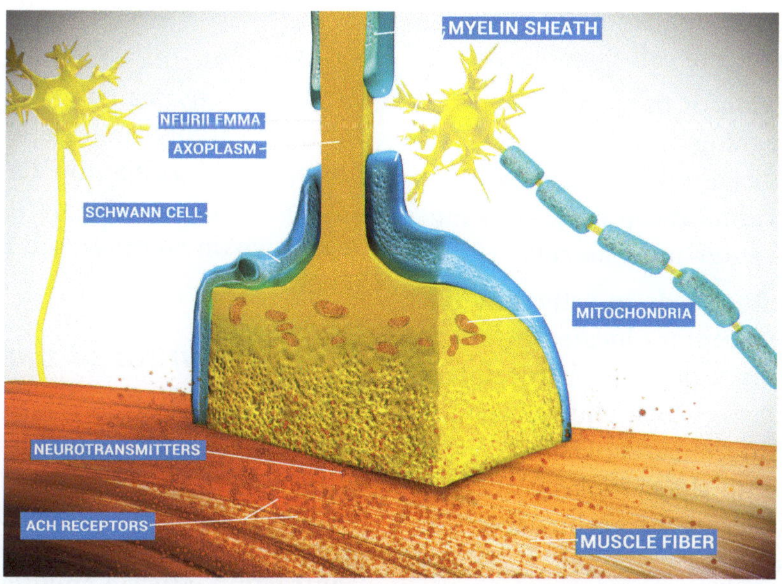

Figure 3.4. *Diagram of a neuromuscular junction.*

Source: By Doctor Jana – https://docjana.com/neuro-muscular-junction/, CC BY 4.0, https://commons.wikimedia.org/w/index.php?curid=46835961.

The release of acetylcholine (ACh) from vesicles into the synaptic cleft is caused by the subsequent rise in intracellular Ca2+. The muscle fiber's plasma membrane contains ligand-gated ion channels called nicotinic ACh receptors, which are activated by ACh. This causes an influx of sodium ions and a depolarization of the muscle fiber membrane potential. The skeletal muscle fiber generates an action potential as a result of this local depolarization activating voltage-sensitive sodium channels (Figure 3.4).

ACh is then rapidly broken down (hydrolyzed) in the synaptic cleft by the enzyme acetylcholinesterase to terminate signal transmission and allow membrane repolarization.

Excitation-Contraction Coupling

Excitation-contraction coupling describes the process whereby an action potential triggers a skeletal muscle fiber to contract.

1. Action potentials generated at the neuromuscular junction travel along the sarcolemma and down into the transverse tubule (T-tubule) system to depolarize the cell membrane.
2. Depolarization of the sarcolemma triggers opening of voltage-gated L-type Ca^{2+} channels (also known as dihydropyridine receptors), allowing calcium to enter into the cell.
3. Calcium influx leads to activation of ryanodine receptors located in the sarcoplasmic reticulum (intracellular calcium store), which allows calcium to flow from the sarcoplasmic reticulum into the cytoplasm and further increases intracellular calcium concentration.
4. Calcium binds to troponin-C, inducing a conformational change which reveals a binding site on actin for the myosin head.
5. This binding results in ATP hydrolysis, providing energy for the actin and myosin filaments to slide past each other and shorten the sarcomere length, thereby initiating muscle contraction (Figure 3.5).

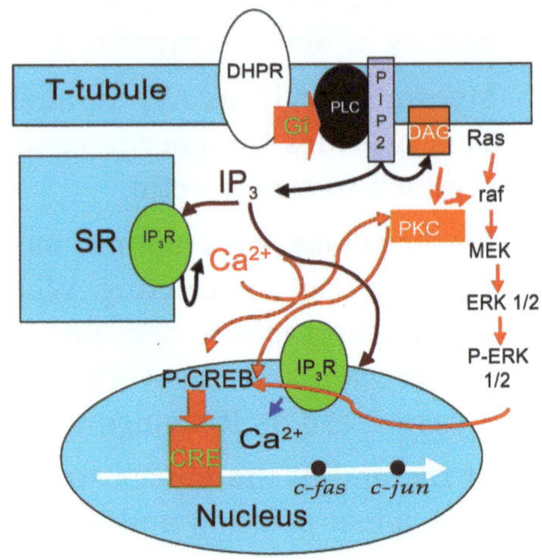

Figure 3.5. *Diagram of excitation-contraction coupling.*

Relaxation of the muscle fiber is facilitated by calcium being pumped back into the sarcoplasmic reticulum by the sarco/endoplasmic reticulum Ca^{2+}-ATPase (SERCA), reversing the conformational change in the tropomyosin complex and restoring sarcomere length.

3.1.6.1. Control of the Skeletal Muscle Contraction

Two main proprioceptors influence the strength and duration of muscle contraction: Golgi tendon organs and muscle spindle fibers. Golgi tendon organs relay information about the force of contraction. Muscle spindles detect changes in muscle length.

3.1.6.2. Golgi Tendon Organs

Receptors called Golgi tendon organs are located where myofibrils and tendons meet. The collagenous fibers of a tendon are entangled with the receptor endings of a Golgi tendon organ. The tendon stretches and the receptors in a web of connective tissue are compressed when a muscle contracts. The pressure causes the nerve ending to undergo an action potential, which then sends a signal to the central nervous system. The Golgi tendon organ's function is to stop muscles from contracting excessively.

3.1.6.3. Muscle Spindle Fibers

Muscle spindles track variations in muscle velocity, position, and length. The long, thin encapsulated fibers that make up muscle spindle fibers are arranged parallel to myofibrils. Extrafusal fibers are found outside the spindle capsule, whereas intrafusal fibers are also referred to as muscle fibers. Because the ends of the intrafusal muscle fibers are joined to myofibrils, the muscle spindle fibers also stretch in tandem with the muscle when the muscle is stretched. The spindle depolarizes when it is stretched, transmitting information via the spinal cord.

3.1.7. Myofilament Components

Actin proteins are assembled into two filamentous actin chains (F-actin) to form the thin filaments (Figure 3.6). These tiny filaments reach the sarcomere's center after being secured at the Z-disc. Every globular actin monomer (G-actin) in the filament has a myosin binding site and is connected to the regulatory proteins troponin and tropomyosin. Tripeptides make up the troponin protein complex. Actin, tropomyosin, and calcium ions are the binding sites for troponin I (TnI), troponin T (TnT), and troponin C (TnC). Along the actin filaments, troponin and tropomyosin regulate the timing of the actin binding sites' exposure for myosin binding. Myosin protein complexes, consisting of two heavy chains and four light chains, are the building blocks of thick myofilaments. The tail region, flexible hinge region, and globular head, which has binding sites for both actin and the high-energy molecule ATP, are the components that make up the heavy chains. While the light chains regulate at the hinge region, the primary force-generating factor is the heavy chain head region, which interacts with actin. With heads extending toward the Z-discs and tails pointing toward the M-line, hundreds of myosin proteins are grouped into each thick filament. Several structural proteins are connected to the sarcomere but are not directly involved in the generation of active force. Adding an elastic element to the sarcomere and aiding in the alignment of the thick filament is titin, the largest known protein. Titin is attached to the M-line, travels through myosin, and ends at the Z-disc. The stabilizing protein nebulin, which extends the length of the thick filaments, is also present in the thin filaments (Gomes et al., 2002; Frontera & Ochala, 2015; Bordoni et al., 2023).

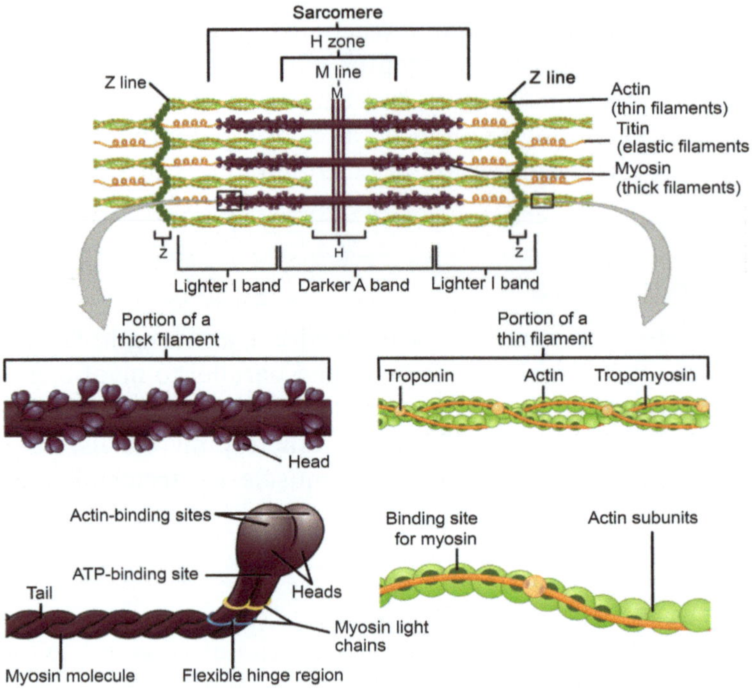

Figure 3.6. *The Sarcomere: the region from one Z-disc to the next Z-disc, is the functional unit of a skeletal muscle fiber.*

Source: https://open.oregonstate.education/app/uploads/sites/157/2021/02/1003_Thick_and_Thin_Filaments_revised-768x693.png.

3.2. Physiology – Skeletal Muscle

In the human body, there are three different types of muscles: visceral, cardiac, and skeletal. Skeletal muscles are defined, characterized, and discussed in detail in this lesson, along with their properties, functions, and types. The muscle tissue known as skeletal muscle is affixed to the bones and plays a vital role in the operation of various body parts.

Because the nervous system in the body is in charge of these muscles, they are also referred to as voluntary muscles. Skeletal muscle can contract in response to external stimuli and is distributed throughout the body. A person's skeletal muscle is used to produce movement, maintain posture and position, regulate body temperature, store nutrients, and stabilize joints, among other functions. Most skeletal muscle contraction is voluntary, as it is controlled by neural inputs that enable conscious control of muscles, in contrast to cardiac and smooth muscle contraction. Between 50 and 75% of all body proteins are found in skeletal muscle, which makes up about 40% of the human body weight. Usually, skeletal muscle diseases show up as muscular weakness. Numerous skeletal muscle disorders, such as muscular dystrophies, congenital myopathies, inflammatory disorders, and diseases affecting the neuromuscular junction, have been studied.

3.2.1. Cellular Level

Muscle fiber bundles called myofibers, which are made up of multiple myofibrils, make up the highly ordered tissue that is skeletal muscle. Every muscle cell, represented by a myofiber, has a sarcomere as its fundamental cellular unit. Myofiber bundles form fascicles, which in turn form bundles of muscle tissue. Skeletal muscle fibers are multinucleated, striated cells that have a diameter of 10–100 micrometers and a length of several centimeters. The nuclei are situated close to the sarcolemma on the outer edge of the cell. Each muscle fiber is enclosed and defined by the tubular sheath known as the sarcolemma, which acts as a partition between the extracellular and intracellular compartments. The plasma membrane and the polysaccharide coating unite with the tendon fibers to form the sarcolemma. Transverse tubules, or T tubules, are invaginations found in the sarcolemma and are a key site of ion exchange. Skeletal muscle fibers, which cover the sarcolemma, are composed of endomysium, perimysium, and epimysium. The endomysium is a layer of connective tissue present in every muscle fiber. The endomysium contains nerve tissue and capillaries that supply the individual muscle fibers. A second layer of connective tissue called the perimysium envelops the fascicles formed when multiple muscle fibers unite to form them. A perimysium may envelop ten to one hundred fascicles. An additional layer of muscle fascicles forms a muscle, which is surrounded by an envelope of fibrous tissue known as the epimysium. Numerous hundred to several thousand myofibrils make up each muscle fiber. Actin (thin filaments), myosin (thick filaments), and support proteins make up myofibrils. Sarcomeres are functional units in skeletal muscle that are created by the arrangement of actin and myosin, giving the muscle its microscopic striated appearance. Sarcomeres are arranged longitudinally and include the M line, Z disk, H band, A band, and I band when observed under electron microscopy.

The sarcomere's terminal boundary, known as the Z line or Z disk, is where alpha-actinin serves as an anchor for the actin filaments. Myosin filaments are bound together by binding sites found in the myosin filaments at the M line, which is the central line of the sarcomere. The M line is located in the H band, which is the part of the sarcomere that is entirely made up of myosin filaments. Actin and myosin overlap areas are present in the A band, a larger section of the sarcomere that houses all of the myosin fibers. Actin filaments are the only structure found in the I band, which spans the terminal regions of two neighboring sarcomeres. When muscles contract, the H and I bands get shorter, but the A band stays the same length. Monomeric G-actin units combine to form filamentous-actin (F-actin), double-helical structures that make up actin filaments. Within the sarcomere, polar G-actin forms a positive and negative end, with the positive end located closer to the terminal end of the sarcomere. A helical protein called tropomyosin travels through the actin double helix's groove. Troponin, which is made up of troponin-C (Tn-C), troponin-I (Tn-I), and troponin-T (Tn-T), binds tropomyosin by forming a troponin complex at every seven actin monomers. Actin and myosin binding is inhibited by Tn-I, calcium is bound by Tn-C, and tropomyosin is bound by Tn-T. Light and heavy meromyosin are the two regions that make up myosin proteins. To anchor myosin at the M line, light meromyosin binds to other light meromyosin regions. The two regions that make up heavy meromyosin are the S-1 portion, also known as the myosin head, which binds actin and has an ATPase portion, and the S-2 portion, which houses the power stroke.

The support proteins of the sarcomere include plectin, titin, desmin, myomesin, C protein, and nebulin. Adjacent myofibrils' Z disks are connected to one another by plectin. Desmin connects to the cytoskeleton and other structural components of the cell, aids in maintaining the alignment of myofibrils, and distributes contraction force. Myosin-binding proteins like myomesin and C protein tether and stabilize myosin at the M line. At the Z disk, myosin is longitudinally anchored by titin within the sarcomere. Three categories apply to the different types of muscle fibers.

Slow oxidative fibers, also known as type I fibers, have a slow twitch. They are the tiniest fiber type and contain very little glycogen. Because of their low myosin ATPase activity, slow contractile speed, and low rate of fatigue, type I fibers are best suited for endurance types of contraction, like running marathons and maintaining posture. Fast oxidative fibers, sometimes known as type IIa fibers, exhibit an intermediate rate of fatigue and a high myosin ATPase activity. They also twitch quickly. Walking and bicycling are among the medium-duration, moderate-movement activities that are most appropriate for them. The term "red fibers" refers to type I and IIa fibers, which have a high myoglobin content. In addition, they have a large number of mitochondria and capillaries and get their ATP mainly from oxidative phosphorylation. Fast-twitching fibers are referred to as type IIb fibers or fast glycolytic fibers. Because of the high density of actin and myosin proteins in them, they have the largest diameter of all the fibers. Because of their low myoglobin content, type IIb fibers—which have few mitochondria—are known as white fibers. These fibers have a high myosin ATPase activity, fast fatigue rates, and ATP obtained primarily from anaerobic glycolysis. Short-duration, high-intensity exercises like weightlifting and sprinting are the best fits for them.

3.2.2. Development

Most muscles originate from the mesoderm; in particular, the paraxial mesoderm gives rise to skeletal muscles. Myogenic cells, which are formed by mesodermal cells, go through mitosis to become postmitotic myoblasts. Actin and myosin are synthesized by these myoblasts, which then combine to form multinucleated myotubes. Actin, myosin, troponin, tropomyosin, and other muscle proteins are synthesized by myotubes. The muscle fibers, or myofibrils, are made up of all these proteins. The paraxial mesoderm first divides into segments, or somitomeres, in a craniocaudal manner before eventually forming the skeletal muscles.

The pharyngeal arches and the muscles of the head and neck are formed by seven somitomeres. For the trunk region, the remaining somitomeres combine to form 35 pairs of somites. Groups of epithelial cells are subsequently formed by the epithelialization of these somitomeres. The somite is the starting point for mesoderm, and the sclerotome, or bone-forming cells, are formed in the ventral region of each somite. Some clusters from the parietal mesoderm are divided into the primaxial and abaxial domains by the lateral somatic region. The notochord and neural tube send signals for differentiation to the primaxial domain, which is made up of somites surrounding the neural tube and forms the shoulder, back, and intercostal muscles. The lateral plate mesoderm sends signals to the abaxial domain, which then forms the limb, abdominal wall, and infrahyoid muscles.

3.2.3. Organ Systems Involved

Attached to the bones by tendons, skeletal muscle is distributed throughout the body. There is also skeletal muscle in the diaphragm, tongue, upper esophagus, and eye socket. Along with visceral and cardiac muscles, the human body has three different types of muscles: skeletal muscle. Skeletal muscle definition, anatomy, characteristics, uses, and kinds are covered in this lesson in an understandable and comprehensive way. Muscle tissue connected to the bones that is essential to the operation of various body parts is called skeletal muscle. Given that the body's nervous system is in charge of them, these muscles are also referred to as voluntary muscles.

The skeletal muscles have the following properties:

- Extensibility: It is the ability of the muscles to extend when it is stretched.
- Elasticity: It is the ability of the muscles to return to its original structure when released.
- Excitability: It is the ability of the muscle to respond to a stimulus.
- Contractility: It is the ability of a muscle to contract when in contact with a stimulus.

There are two types of skeletal muscles named as red and white muscles-

- Red Muscles: Red muscles are due to the red pigment called myoglobin, which is present in high amounts in the human body. These muscles are smaller in diameter and have a large number of mitochondria. Myoglobin stores the oxygen, which is used by the mitochondria for the synthesis of ATP. Red muscles have a large number of blood capillaries.
- White Muscles: In contrast to red muscles, white muscles are larger in diameter and contain a small amount of myoglobin. They also have fewer mitochondria.

3.2.4. Function

The primary functions include contracting to generate movement, maintaining body position and posture, regulating body temperature, storing nutrients, and stabilizing joints. Skeletal muscle's main job from a mechanical perspective is to transform chemical energy into mechanical energy, which produces force and power. From a metabolic perspective, skeletal muscle stores vital substrates like amino acids and carbohydrates and helps with basal energy metabolism. Additionally, skeletal muscle produces body heat. This heat is primarily wasted and is produced as a byproduct of muscular activity. Muscles are signaled to contract in order to produce heat as a homeostatic reaction to extreme cold.

The following are the important skeletal muscle functions:

1. The skeletal muscles are responsible for body movements such as typing, breathing, extending the arm, writing, etc., The muscles contract which pulls the tendons on the bones and causes movement.
2. The body posture is maintained by the skeletal muscles. The gluteal muscle is responsible for the erect posture of the body. The Sartorius muscles in thighs are responsible for body movement.
3. The skeletal muscles protect the internal organs and tissues from any injury and also provide support to these delicate organs and tissues.
4. These also support the entry and exit points of the body. The sphincter muscles are present around the anus, mouth and the urinary tract. These muscles contract which reduces the size of the openings and facilitates the swallowing of food, defecation, and urination.

5. The skeletal muscles also regulate body temperature. After strenuous exercise, the body feels hot. This is due to the contraction of skeletal muscles which converts energy into heat.

3.2.5. Mechanism

Employing excitation-contraction coupling, action potentials start a muscle contraction. Neural action potentials transition from cross-bridge cycling, or contraction, to excitation-contraction coupling. At the neuron terminus at the NMJ or motor endplate, the action potentials of the motor neuron trigger the release of ACh. Action potential transmission from the ACh to the muscle fiber is what depolarizes the NMJ. The signal is transferred to the interior of the muscle fiber by action potentials, which pass through the cell membrane and enter the T tubules. The dihydropyridine receptors of the T tubules undergo a conformational change upon depolarization, whether or not there is a calcium (Ca) release. The intracellular fluid (ICF) contains ten times more Ca due to the release of Ca from the sarcoplasmic reticulum's storage site as a result of this conformational shift, which also opens ryanodine receptors on the terminal cisternae of the sarcoplasmic reticulum. Troponin C is bound to the actin filament by the elevated ICF concentration of Ca, which alters the conformation of the troponin complex. The maximum number of Ca ions that each troponin C can bind is four, and the binding process is cooperative (much like the oxygen-binding hemoglobin). T Roponin C binding sites can thus be saturated with a slight variation in [Ca]. When tropomyosin is pulled out of the way by the conformational change of troponin C, the myosin-binding sites on actin are revealed, and the cross-bridge cycling that results in skeletal muscle contraction is initiated. In the terminal cisternae, the sarcoplasmic reticulum sequesters calcium from troponin C through a Ca-ATPase located in its membrane, a process known as SERCA, following the cessation of excitation and subsequent depolarization of the tubules. Actin's myosin-binding sites can be covered by tropomyosin when calcium is sequestered, which relaxes muscles.

Skeletal muscle contracts through a process called cross-bridge cycling. Actin and myosin are firmly bonded at the start of this cycle, a process known as rigor. This semi-permanent state is known as rigor mortis and occurs when basic physiologic energy is absent, as in death. In living tissue, this is a transient state because the myosin head's conformation changes in response to ATP binding, releasing the actin-myosin cross-link. Once the cross-link is broken and ATP is bound, it is hydrolyzed to produce inorganic phosphate and adenosine diphosphate (ADP), which causes the myosin head to "re-cock" and move in the direction of the positive end of actin, or nearer to the ends of the sarcomere. The myosin head and actin will form a cross-bridge as long as there is enough calcium present to maintain an uncovered actin-binding site. When ADP and inorganic phosphate are released, the myosin head moves toward the center of the sarcomere, or the negative end of actin, displacing the actin filament and shortening the sarcomere. This process is known as the power stroke. ADP is released to complete the cycle, and the sarcomere resumes its rigor. As long as calcium is bonded to troponin C, this cycle will continue. The total number of recruited motor units and the frequency at which those motor units receive action potentials add up to the force of contraction. A single motor neuron and all the muscle fibers it innervates are referred to as a motor unit, and multiple motor units can stimulate the same muscle. A motor unit's number of muscle fibers is determined by the muscle's intended use. Larger muscle groups will involve a significant number of muscle fibers, while muscles requiring fine motor control will involve fewer. Asynchronous recruitment of fibers occurs in muscles that work for extended periods of time, like the lower back muscles, distributing the fatigue of individual fibers over time and space.

The sum of the tensions in each muscle fiber causes tension in the muscles as a whole. When an action potential triggers the release of a specific quantity of calcium from the sarcoplasmic reticulum, resulting in a single muscle twitch and subsequent sequestration of calcium, muscle fiber recruitment occurs. More action potentials stimulate the muscle continuously, increasing calcium release and summation of twitches, which allows the muscle to contract further. When every Ca-binding site is occupied and every myosin-binding site is left unoccupied, a process known as tetany occurs, leading to maximal contraction. The energy required for the power stroke mechanism, which contracts skeletal muscle, and the reabsorption of calcium by the terminal cisternae is provided by the cleavage of ATP to ADP and inorganic phosphate. Muscle ATP stores quickly deplete, necessitating ATP regeneration. The process by which muscles produce ATP begins with the transfer of a phosphate group from creatine phosphate to ADP. When creatine phosphate stores are depleted, the electron transport chain and the citric acid cycle are used to produce ATP. When muscles actively contract, oxygen becomes the limiting factor along with glycolysis alone. Later, the primary source of ATP generation for muscles is the conversion of pyruvate to lactate. Skeletal muscle contains neuromuscular spindles, which are involved in proprioception. Extrafusal fibers are interspersed with intrafusal fibers, also known as neuromuscular spindles. The nuclear bag fiber and the nuclear chain fiber are the two distinct cells that make up intrafusal fibers. Due to the ability to contract, the entire fiber unit serves as a sensory receptor for contraction length, tension, and rate in addition to acting as a muscle. Primary afferent nerve fibers sense the length and rate of contraction of muscles. They have annulospiral endings around both the bag and chain fibers. Muscle length is sensed by secondary afferent fibers, which are mostly found on nuclear chain fibers and have flower spray endings.

3.2.6. Pathophysiology

3.2.6.1. Diseases Affecting the Neuromuscular Junction

- An autoimmune condition known as myasthenia gravis is brought on by antibodies to the neuromuscular junction's ACh receptors. By blocking ACh from binding, these antibodies lessen the depolarization that is transferred to the muscle cell. Lower concentrations of ACh released into the NMJ are unable to saturate the binding sites and cause an action potential in the muscle because repeated use depletes ACh stores. The patient experiences this as a fluctuating weakness that gets worse with use and gets better with rest. Extraocular muscles are frequently the first to be affected early in the course of the illness. Myasthenia gravis can be diagnosed with edrophonium, a short-acting acetylcholinesterase inhibitor. When edrophonium is injected, it delays the effects of ACh at the NMJ and temporarily avoids muscle fatigue.
- The NMJ condition known as Lambert-Eaton Myasthenic Syndrome (LEMS) is linked to small cell lung cancer (SCLC) in more than half of cases. It can manifest as a paraneoplastic phenomenon. Muscle weakness is the main

clinical symptom. The pathology results from antibodies being produced against voltage-gated calcium channels on presynaptic nerve terminals, which causes the neurotransmitter ACh to be reduced. LEMS patients may also exhibit oculobulbar weakness, autonomic dysfunction, dysphagia, and dysarthria in addition to muscle weakness. In the latter stages of LEMS, respiratory failure may sporadically happen. A phenomenon observed in LEMS that is linked to a reduction in muscle weakness after exertion is called post-exercise or post-activation facilitation. Increased Ca influx in the presynaptic membrane brought on by repeated muscle contractions makes it easier for ACh to be released by binding with multiple vesicles. This effect is only momentary because the extra calcium is eventually removed by the mitochondria.

- The NMJ's excitation-contraction coupling may also be impacted by toxins created by C. botulinum toxin. By blocking the presynaptic neuron at the NMJ's release of ACh, botulinum prevents the excitation of skeletal muscles and results in flaccid paralysis. One neurotoxin that C releases is tetanospasmin. Through blocking the release of inhibitory neurotransmitters by interneurons synapsing at the NMJ, tetani prevents relaxation and causes spastic paralysis.

3.2.6.1.1. Muscular Dystrophies

Muscular dystrophies include more than 30 inherited conditions that cause permanent muscle weakness. The two most common and well-known forms of muscular dystrophy include Duchenne muscular dystrophy (DMD) and Becker muscular dystrophy (BMD).

Mutations in the dystrophin gene result in Duchenne Muscular Dystrophy (DMD), an X-linked inherited neuromuscular disorder. The absence of dystrophin protein, which results in the degeneration of cardiac and skeletal muscle, is the cause of this disease's progressive muscle weakness and wasting. Around 1 in 3,600 male babies born worldwide are affected by DMD, and there are no clinical symptoms at birth. The age at which symptoms typically manifest and are diagnosed is approximately 4 years old. DMD is a rapidly progressing illness that causes patients to become wheelchair-dependent and develop severe cardiomyopathy by the time they are ten years old. Usually, cardiac and respiratory complications result in death.

With an incidence of 1 in 18,518 male births, Becker Muscular Dystrophy (BMD) is characterized as a milder form of DMD. Between the ages of 5 and 15, BMD usually manifests later than DMD and progresses more slowly in terms of clinical symptoms. Those with BMD typically experience symptoms after the age of 30, and they may continue to walk until they are 60 years old. Heart failure resulting from dilated cardiomyopathy is the most common cause of death and a common cause of morbidity in patients with BMD, despite milder involvement of the skeletal muscles.

3.2.6.2. Idiopathic Inflammatory Myopathies (Myositis)

Symmetric proximal muscle weakness that develops over weeks to months along with erythematous changes—which may occur before or after the myopathy—are the hallmarks of dermatomyositis (DM). A heliotropic rash, eyelid edema, Gottron papules at extensor surfaces, and subcutaneous calcifications are examples of erythematous changes. Although patients rarely experience myalgia, they may experience dysphagia, dysarthria, and interstitial lung disease. The prevalence of DM is higher in older and female patients.

The symptoms of polymyositis (PM) include a marked elevation of creatine kinase (CK) and a subacute onset of proximal muscular weakness, which is most noticeable in the shoulders and pelvic girdle. In certain instances, the neck extensors and flexors are also impacted. A biopsy that demonstrates cytotoxic CD8+ T cells and macrophage-rich cellular infiltrates separates PM from DM. With progressive, symmetrical weakness of the proximal muscles of the arms and legs, necrotizing myopathy (NM) is clinically identical to PM. Up to 80% of patients have myalgias, and in more severe cases, dysphagia and dysarthria may occur. With a mean age of onset in the fifth decade, NM exhibits a prevalence in males. The diagnosis of NM requires a biopsy, which reveals sporadic necrotic muscle fibers, sparse inflammatory cells surrounding the necrosis, a preponderance of macrophages, and a small number of lymphocytes (CD4+ and CD8+ T cells).

The most common acquired myopathy after age 50 is Inclusion Body Myositis (IBM). The slow-moving illness known as IBM usually affects knee extension and hand and finger flexion. Up to 80% of those affected have at least mild swallowing difficulties, and dysphagia is a common condition. Weakness in the arms and legs may come on before dysphagia. Although life expectancy is normal, patients eventually become dependent on wheelchairs. Myoglobin and other intracellular substances are released into the extracellular space as a result of a direct injury to the architecture of the skeletal muscle caused by rhabdomyolysis. Although too many to list here, some damages that can cause skeletal muscle injury include overuse (such as marathon running), compartment syndrome, and the use of illegal, prescription, and over-the-counter drugs. Large-scale ionized calcium release from the terminal cisternae, which triggers degradation processes, is the direct cause of the cellular damage. Damage to the skeletal muscle causes the release of breakdown products that impair kidney function and, in extreme situations, cause acute renal failure necessitating dialysis. These downstream effects of rhabdomyolysis can be systemic and potentially fatal. Many factors, such as chronic glucocorticoid use, malnourishment, systemic illness, disuse, and denervation, can cause atrophy of skeletal muscle. Atrophy is brought on by decreased protein synthesis, which lowers muscle mass by narrowing the diameter of individual muscle fibers, and increased proteolysis, which is mediated by the ubiquitin system. The pathways in each of these situations may be different (Gomes et al., 2002; Frontera & Ochala, 2015; Bordoni et al., 2023).

3.2.7. Clinical Significance

Humans can move and carry out daily tasks thanks to their skeletal muscles, which are also vital for breathing mechanics, maintaining balance and posture, and good posture. Skeletal muscle dysfunction can lead to many medical conditions. Myopathies, dysphagia, ataxia, weakness, tremors, ruptured tendons, and other conditions are among these illnesses. Clinically, patients may exhibit anything from skeletal muscle genetic abnormalities to muscular cramps. Understanding normal physiology serves as the foundation for understanding the pathology underlying skeletal muscle diseases. Notably, it's critical to advise patients to exercise to build muscle strength. Strengthening and preserving muscle is crucial for good posture, balance, flexibility, and bone health.

3.3. Anatomy of Skeletal Muscle

Skeletal muscles make up the majority of the muscles in your body. They comprise thirty to forty percent of your body's total mass. Tendons, which are strong bands of connective tissue, are responsible for joining skeletal muscle to bones all over your body. Skeletal muscles comprise your abdominal, hamstring, and shoulder muscles, among others. Flexible muscle fibers with a diameter ranging from less than half an inch to slightly over three inches make up skeletal muscles. Typically, these fibers run the entire length of the muscle. You can perform a wide range of movements because the muscles can move bones by contracting (tightening) the fibers. One of the main tissue/organ systems in the body is the musculoskeletal system. Skeletal, cardiac, and smooth muscle groups are the three primary categories of muscle tissue. All bodily movements are produced by the skeletal muscle and the tendons that connect it to the bone. The characteristic striated appearance of skeletal muscle is a result of the regular pattern of fine red and white lines crossing each other. As a result, another name for them is striated muscles.

3.3.1. Structure and Function

One of the human body's three major muscle tissues is skeletal muscle. Sheaths of connective tissue encase thousands of muscle fibers that make up each skeletal muscle. The skeletal muscle individual muscle fiber bundles are referred to as fasciculi. The term "epimysium" refers to the outermost sheath of connective tissue encircling the entire muscle. Perimysium is the connective tissue sheath that surrounds each fasciculus, and endomysium is the innermost sheath that encloses a single muscle fiber. Multiple myofibrils with multiple myofilaments make up each muscle fiber. Sarcomeres, the basic contractile unit of a skeletal muscle, are formed when all the myofibrils are bundled together in a distinctive striated pattern. Actin and myosin filaments, which are arranged differently to form different bands on the skeletal muscle, are the two most important types of myofilaments. Between the basement membrane and the sarcolemma, the cell membrane encircling the striated muscle fiber cell, are stem cells known as satellite cells that differentiate into mature muscle fibers. They differentiate and proliferate to create new muscle fiber cells when growth factors are applied. The intrinsic excitation-contraction coupling process of skeletal muscle is responsible for its main functions. Because the muscle and bone tendons are attached, when the muscle contracts, the bone moves, enabling the execution of particular movements. In addition to supporting structure, skeletal muscle aids in preserving the body's posture. A further function of skeletal muscle is to store amino acids that are needed by various body organs to synthesize proteins unique to those organs. A vital component in preserving homeostasis and serving as an energy source during famine is the skeletal muscle.

3.3.2. Conditions and Disorders that Affect Skeletal Muscles

A wide range of conditions can affect skeletal muscles, from mild injuries to serious or even life-threatening myopathies (diseases that affect skeletal muscles). A few are:

- *Muscular dystrophies:* This group of diseases causes progressive degeneration of skeletal muscle fibers. They're the result of having an abnormal gene and can be inherited (passed down through families). There are many different muscular dystrophies.
- *Myasthenia gravis (MG):* This autoimmune disease prevents muscles and nerves from communicating as they should. It

leads to severe muscle weakness and fatigue. MG can make it difficult to move, walk, speak, chew, see, hold your head up, or keep your eyelids open. It can even lead to severe breathing problems.

- *Rhabdomyolysis:* This life-threatening condition causes a breakdown of muscle tissue. The damaged muscles release proteins, electrolytes, and other substances into the blood. This can lead to serious organ damage. Traumatic injuries, heatstroke, or severe overexertion can cause rhabdomyolysis.
- *Sarcopenia:* We gradually lose skeletal muscle mass as we age. Sarcopenia begins around age 40. By 80, we lose about 50% of our muscle mass. Sarcopenia can lead to loss of function, mobility, balance problems, and falls. Obesity, hormonal changes, and other health conditions can accelerate muscle loss.
- *Strains:* Muscle strains, or pulled muscles, occur when you overstretch muscle fibers. These injuries are usually the result of overuse. Severe strains can lead to partial or complete muscle tears.
- *Tendonitis:* Tendons connect skeletal muscles to bones. Tendon inflammation can make it painful to use these muscles. Like strains, tendonitis is usually caused by overworking tendons.

3.3.3. Embryology

The differentiation of muscle fibers is regulated by distinct transcriptional mechanisms and particular gene regulatory activity. The para-axial mesoderm differentiates gradually during embryogenesis to produce muscle tissue. To create the somites, the para-axial mesoderm on either side of the neural tube begins to differentiate and segment. Myogenic regulatory factors facilitate the differentiation of somites into dermomyotome and sclerotome. The Wnt, Shh, and BMP4 proteins are some of these regulatory factors. Wnt proteins are primarily derived from the neural tube and surface ectoderm, Shh proteins (also known as Sonic Hedgehog) are sourced from the notochord, and BMP4 proteins are produced by the lateral mesoderm plate. As it migrates on the ventral side to form a distinct myotome beneath the dermatome, the lateral aspect of the dermomyotome experiences an epithelial-to-mesenchymal transition. The Sonic Hedgehog (Shh) signaling molecule from the notochord stimulates the myotome, which causes Myf5 expression and subsequent differentiation, resulting in the formation of the skeletal muscles in the body. Back muscles are produced when the dorsomedial aspect of the myotome differentiates into the epaxial myotome. The muscles of the body wall originate from the ventrolateral aspect, which differentiates into hypaxial myotome. This differentiation is brought about by several signaling molecules, including BMP and Wnt, as well as transcription factors, such as sine oculis homeobox. MyoD and Myf5 expression and their effects on various myoblasts are crucial for the development of skeletal muscles in the trunk and limbs. By uniting with other myoblasts in the fetus, these embryonic myoblasts undergo additional differentiation to form the primary muscle fibers and ultimately secondary myofibers. The continued growth and development of skeletal muscles is carried out by the satellite cells, which function as stem cells after birth.

3.3.4. Blood Supply and Lymphatics

Generally speaking, the longitudinal axis of the

muscle fiber and the main artery supplying blood to that specific skeletal muscle run parallel. The perimysium, the external connective tissue sheath surrounding the muscle fiber, is reached by feed arteries, which emerge from the main artery and run perpendicular to it. The feed artery splits into primary arterioles, which split into transverse arterioles, which split into terminal arterioles after two more orders of branching. The last vascular branches, known as terminal arterioles, run parallel to the muscle fiber's longitudinal axis and supply blood to the capillaries found inside the endomysium. A terminal arteriole is referred to as a microvascular unit, as are the capillaries it supplies. It is the tiniest skeletal muscle unit where blood flow regulation is possible. The microvascular unit in the endomysium close to the main capillary bed is where lymph capillaries begin in skeletal muscle, where they drain tissue fluid. While they drain the tissue fluid, these capillaries combine to form the lymphatic vessels. These lymphatic vessels connect to the larger lymphatic vessels after passing through the perimysium. Because there are no smooth muscles in the muscle wall, the lymph vessels within it cannot contract like blood vessels do. Instead, the lymph is drained out of the vessel by muscle movement and arteriolar pulsations.

3.3.5. Nerves

The neuronal innervation of a skeletal muscle normally consists of the neuromuscular junction, motor nerve fibers, and sensory nerve fibers. Both myelinated and non-myelinated nerve fibers make up the nerve fibers. Large, usually unbranched axons that travel to the target muscles for innervation originate from the cell bodies of the neurons. The axons split into several smaller branches close to the target muscle, innervating various muscle fibers. The motor nerve terminal is home to a large number of membrane-bound synaptic vesicles containing the neurotransmitter acetylcholine, as well as an endoplasmic reticulum. A sequence of events takes place when the action potential reaches the neuromuscular junction, leading to the union of the presynaptic and synaptic vesicle membranes and the subsequent release of the neurotransmitter into the synaptic cleft. Neurotransmitter (AChR) receptors are highly concentrated in the postsynaptic membrane of muscle fibers. These receptors are ligand-gated transmembrane ion channels. Muscle contraction results from a quick depolarization of the motor endplate brought on by the neurotransmitter's activation of these ion channels. This action potential causes the muscle fiber to contract.

3.3.6. Muscles

Numerous tissues make up each muscle, such as connective tissue sheaths, blood vessels, lymphatics, and contractile muscle fibers. The epimysium is the outermost sheath of connective tissue that envelops every muscle. Every muscle consists of fascicles, which are collections of muscle fibers encircled by a layer of connective tissue known as the perimysium. Each fascicle contains multiple units of individual muscle fibers encased in a connective tissue sheath called the endomysium. Actin and myosin are the two most important myofilaments that comprise the contractile components of the muscle fiber. The dark A band, the light I band, and the fundamental unit of contraction—also known as a sarcomere—are formed by their unique arrangement in a striated pattern. The thick myofilaments of myosin are attached to the central M line on either side of the sarcomere. This creates the shadowy A band. The Z-line, which partially overlaps the myosin filaments and acts as the origin of the thin actin myofilaments that project towards each other, borders the sarcomere. The myofilament sliding mechanism that results in contraction is largely dependent on the regulatory proteins, specifically troponin C, I, T, and tropomyosin. The other two main proteins that affect the mechanical characteristics of muscle are titin and nebulin. To improve coordination and consistent muscle contraction, a special T-tubule system is in place that conducts neuronal action potentials to the interior of muscle cells through sarcolemma releases.

3.3.7. Clinical Significance

Humans can move and carry out daily tasks thanks to their skeletal muscles. They support proper posture and balance as well as being vital to respiratory mechanics. They also shield the body's essential organs. Function abnormalities in the skeletal muscles lead to a variety of medical conditions. These illnesses include myopathy, paralysis, myasthenia gravis, ataxia, weakness, tremors, and incontinence of the bowels or urine. Nerve disorders can lead to neuropathy and interfere with the skeletal muscles' ability to function. Furthermore, skeletal muscle/tendon ruptures can happen suddenly in elite athletes or casual sports players, and they cause major disability in all patients, regardless of their level of activity (Gomes et al., 2002; Frontera & Ochala, 2015; Bordoni et al., 2023).

3.3.7.1. Muscle Cramps

An entire muscle group, a single muscle, or a subset of muscle fibers will contract continuously, involuntarily, painfully, and locally when they experience muscle cramps. If the cause of the cramp is idiopathic, known to occur in healthy subjects, or there is a disease present, it typically lasts minutes to a few seconds. A knot will be palpable in the cramped muscle area. The most common ailment requiring medical or therapeutic intervention during sports is exercise-induced muscle cramps. The precise cause of the cramps is unknown, and potential explanations vary depending on the physiological or pathological context in which they occur. It's important to know that a painful cramp in one spot doesn't always mean the cramp's source is close by. Under certain clinical conditions, the underlying cause may be chronic, spastic muscular contractions that have a major negative influence on human function. A common sign of this illness is pain in the sternocleidomastoid muscle. Clinically, this is identified in spasmodic or congenital torticollis.

Other relevant conditions in this realm include, but are not limited to the following:

- Exercise-induced and heat-related muscle cramping
- Piriformis syndrome
- Thoracic outlet syndrome (scalene muscle hypertrophy/spasticity)

3.3.7.2. Palsy/Compression Neuropathy

On the other end of the spectrum, a variety of muscle palsies can develop as a result of the long-term, downstream effects of different neuropathies and nerve conditions, which can lead to flaccid conditions (which can be either temporary or permanent).

These syndromes and conditions include but are not limited to the following:

- Bell's palsy
- Guyon canal syndrome
- AIN syndrome or PIN syndrome
- Carpal tunnel syndrome (secondary to compression neuropathy of the median nerve at the carpal tunnel)
- Supraspinatus and/or infraspinatus atrophy
- Klumpke palsy

3.4. Insulin Resistance and Skeletal Muscle

In terms of mass, the skeletal muscle is the largest organ in the body. In addition, it controls glucose homeostasis and accounts for 80% of the blood's postprandial glucose absorption. Because of its function in absorbing glucose and its significance concerning exercise and metabolic disorders, skeletal muscle is crucial for metabolism. Insulin resistance, a defining feature of type 2 diabetes and a risk factor for several metabolic diseases, is characterized by a decreased ability of target tissues, like skeletal muscle, to respond to the action of insulin. Insulin facilitates the uptake, utilization, and storage of glucose in skeletal muscle, which is essential for maintaining glucose homeostasis. When insulin binds to the insulin receptor on muscle cell plasma membranes, a series of intracellular events are set off, initiating insulin signaling. Translocation of glucose transporter type 4 (GLUT4) vesicles from intracellular compartments to the cell surface, which facilitates glucose transport into the cell, is one of the main mechanisms by which insulin increases glucose uptake in skeletal muscle. Nevertheless, this process is compromised in insulin resistance, which results in decreased GLUT4 translocation and decreased skeletal muscle cell uptake of glucose.

Skeletal muscle insulin resistance is caused by several molecular processes. Chronically high blood levels of free fatty acids can interfere with insulin signaling pathways, impairing intracellular insulin action. Obesity and metabolic syndrome are both associated with elevated free fatty acid levels. Insulin receptor substrate 1 (IRS-1) is phosphorylated on inhibitory serine residues by serine/threonine kinases like protein kinase C theta (PKCθ) and inhibitor of kappa B kinase (IKK), which are activated by increased intramuscular lipid accumulation, especially ceramides and diacylglycerols. This inhibits insulin receptor signaling. Furthermore, pro-inflammatory cytokines that are frequently elevated in obesity, such as interleukin-6 (IL-6) and tumor necrosis factor-alpha (TNF-α), can also induce IRS-1 serine phosphorylation, which exacerbates insulin resistance in skeletal muscle. Moreover, oxidative stress and modifications in mitochondrial function lead to insulin resistance in skeletal muscle. The pathophysiology of insulin resistance has been linked to impaired mitochondrial function, which is characterized by decreased oxidative capacity and increased production of reactive oxygen species (ROS). Mitochondria are essential for the metabolism of cellular energy. By obstructing insulin signaling pathways and triggering inflammatory reactions, ROS can cause insulin resistance. Furthermore, excessive lipid uptake and accumulation due to dysregulated lipid metabolism in skeletal muscle can harm mitochondrial function and worsen insulin resistance. Sedentary lifestyles and lack of exercise worsen insulin resistance in skeletal muscle by increasing intramuscular lipid accumulation, compromising mitochondrial function, and decreasing the ability to absorb glucose. On the other hand, consistent exercise increases skeletal muscle's sensitivity to insulin by enhancing mitochondrial biogenesis, enhancing glucose transport capability, and reducing inflammation. Insulin resistance is lessened by exercise-induced adaptations that improve skeletal muscle's insulin-stimulated glucose uptake, such as increased GLUT4 expression and translocation.

3.4.1. Links between Aging and Skeletal Muscle Insulin Resistance

When human skeletal muscle ages (after 40–50 years of age), it results in a progressive loss of muscle mass and mitochondrial function, a condition called sarcopenia. Along with a reduction in strength and muscle function, muscle mass loss is accompanied by a decrease in regenerative capacity. While sarcopenia's muscle dysfunction contributes to aging being a major risk factor for T2D, other hypothesized factors also play a role in the etiology of T2D. Secondary aging refers to the fact that T2D and other diseases can make this age-related muscle dysfunction worse. While it is currently impossible to stop aging, increased exercise or physical activity can prevent or postpone secondary aging. Sarcopenia, however, can make it more difficult to move, which can lead to a vicious cycle whereby sedentary behavior increases.

3.4.2. Combined effects of Aging and Obesity on Insulin Resistance

The three metabolic defects mentioned above—muscle atrophy/sarcopenia, obesity, and insulin resistance—occur and converge with one another as people age. The term "sarcopenic obesity" was actually coined to describe the toxic feedback loop between decreased skeletal muscle mass (sarcopenia) and increased fat mass (obesity), where one exacerbates the other. This is because these metabolic disorders are so intertwined. (Wolfe, 2006)

3.4.3. Links between Obesity/ Inflammation and Skeletal Muscle Insulin Resistance

Studies involving lean, non-diabetic individuals have traditionally shown a causal relationship between insulin resistance and weight. Obesity may raise the risk of insulin resistance because these people developed insulin resistance after receiving an overnutrition regimen. One major hypothesis for the pathophysiology of insulin resistance and type 2 diabetes is that obesity-related chronic inflammation plays a key role. Increased levels of pro-inflammatory cytokines in the blood, elevated blood glucose, and elevated free fatty acids—especially saturated ones—are commonly linked to type 2 diabetes (T2D), an illness that can cause insulin resistance. To illustrate, adipokines are released by adipose tissue and function as signaling molecules to promote tissue-to-tissue communication. The dysregulation of adipokines, particularly leptin, has been observed in patients with diabetes and obesity. Adipose tissue was recognized as an official endocrine organ after adipokines were discovered. The skeletal muscle can function as an endocrine organ by secreting substances known as "myokines," as has also been demonstrated over the past 20 years. Proteins called myokines are secreted by skeletal muscle and can communicate with other organs like the brain, adipose tissue, and bone. On the other hand, inflammation brought on by obesity can also target skeletal muscle. Table 3.1 indicates that specific cytokine hormones known as adipokines can be released from both tissues as a result of obesity-induced inflammation and insulin resistance. Interleukin-6 (IL-6), IL-8, IL-15, irisin, myonectin, and myostatin are among the substances that skeletal muscle can secrete. Unlike adipokines, muscle myokines are controlled by exercise and contraction. Obesity, inflammation, and insulin resistance can all change depending on the release of these circulating factors.

Table 3.1. *Summary of the Most Relevant Conclusions of Each Section (from 4 to 8)*

Authors and Year	Study Title	Aim of Study	Main Outcomes	Section
Tilg et al. (2006) [46]	Adipocytokines: Mediators Linking Adipose Tissue, Inflammation, and Immunity	Understand adipocyte-derived mediators.	Adipocytokines—mediators are mainly synthesized by adipocytes in white adipose tissue. Adiponectin and leptin are the two most abundant adipocytokines.	Adipokines and inflammation
Ohashi et al. (2014) [66]	Role of Anti-Inflammatory Adipokines in Obesity-Related Diseases.	Understand the role of the anti-inflammatory adipokines.	Adiponectin exerts beneficial actions on obesity complications.	
La Cava (2018) [59]	Leptin in inflammation and autoimmunity	Analyzes the known implications of leptin in multiple inflammatory conditions, including autoimmune diseases.	Leptin contributes to the generation and maintenance of low-grade inflammation.	
Mitsuhashi et al. (2007) [80]	Adiponectin Level and Left Ventricular Hypertrophy in Japanese Men	Analyze the relationship that might exist between the serum adiponectin level and electrocardiographically diagnosed left ventricular hypertrophy (ECG-LVH)	Adiponectin concentration was inversely and independently associated with ECG-LVH.	Adipokines and cardiovascular disease
Khafaji et al. (2012) [91]	Elevated Serum Leptin Levels in Patients with Acute Myocardial Infarction; Correlation with Coronary Angiographic and Echocardiographic Findings	Assess the relationship between serial serum leptin levels in patients with acute myocardial infarction (AMI)	There was a trend for an increase in the mean serum leptin levels with an increasing number of diseased vessels.	
Hassan-Ali et al. (2011) [121]	Serum Adiponectin and Leptin as Predictors of the Presence and Degree of Coronary Atherosclerosis	Determine the relationship between serum adiponectin and leptin with the presence and degree of coronary atherosclerosis.	Both serum adiponectin and leptin might play an important pathogenic role not only in the occurrence of coronary artery disease patients.	Adipokines and atherosclerosis

Satayesh et al. (2021) [135]	The Possible Mediatory Role of Adipokines in the Association between Low Carbohydrate Diet and Depressive Symptoms among Overweight and Obese Women	Explore the possible mediatory role of adipokines Galectin-3, transforming growth factor-beta (TGF-β), and endothelial plasminogen activator inhibitor (PAI-1) in the association between low carbohydrate diet (LCD) and depressive symptoms.	Higher adherence to Low Carbohydrate Diet is probably associated with a lower prevalence of depressive symptoms in obese adults through the mediatory role of adipokines.	Adipokines and mental disease
Yu et al. (2021) [323]	Gut Hormones, Adipokines, and pro- and Anti-Inflammatory Cytokines/Markers in Loss of Control Eating: A Scoping Review	Synthesize research that has investigated these biomarkers with loss of control eating.	The use of glucagon-like peptide 1 analog was able to decrease binge eating.	Adipokines and eating behaviors

Source: Clemente-Suárez VJ, Redondo-Flórez L, Beltrán-Velasco AI, Martín-Rodríguez A, Martínez-Guardado I, Navarro-Jiménez E, Laborde-Cárdenas CC, Tornero-Aguilera JF. The Role of Adipokines in Health and Disease. Biomedicines. 2023; 11(5):1290. https://doi.org/10.3390/biomedicines11051290

3.4.4. Mechanisms of Inflammation in Skeletal Muscle

Immune cells like T cells and macrophages can infiltrate skeletal muscle, and during obesity or type 2 diabetes in both human and rodent models, skeletal muscle can start to proliferate. The primary sources of pro-inflammatory immune cells are believed to be the intramuscular adipose tissue depots, which can make up to 10% of the total skeletal muscle mass and increase with obesity and type 2 diabetes. G. skeletal muscle (M1-like macrophages). In either the intramuscular or subcutaneous region, skeletal muscle contains two adipose-type depots. It is currently not technically possible to separate the distinct effects of these two depots. However, because of the change in myocyte metabolism brought about by inflammation, the interaction between skeletal muscle and adipose tissue promotes the proinflammatory phenotype in skeletal muscle and plays a significant role in the emergence of insulin resistance. The impact of signaling factors from adipose tissue, circulating immune cells, and the gastrointestinal tract on skeletal muscle metabolism is one area of tissue cross-talk in inflammation that is attracting increasing amounts of research interest. The technical difficulty of separating intramuscular adipose tissue from skeletal muscles in the in vivo disease models causes progress to be somewhat slow. According to recent research in mice, a high-fat diet causes endothelial cells to activate proinflammatory pathways, which in turn cause monocyte adhesion and transmigration. Infiltration of immune cells into muscle and other tissues is facilitated by this. After being exposed to saturated fatty acids, skeletal muscle cells draw monocytes and cause macrophage polarization to shift into an M1-like pro-inflammatory state. Insulin resistance may be brought on by these M1-like macrophages. Pro-inflammatory macrophages are elevated in the skeletal muscle of obese humans and mice fed high-fat diets. This increase has been connected to poor glucose tolerance and increased adiposity.

3.4.5. Mechanisms of Myokine Action

Myokines have been identified, proving that the skeletal muscle can function as an endocrine organ, in the same way that adipokines have established the adipose tissue as an endocrine organ. The bone, brain, and adipose tissue are among the organs with which myokines mediate cross-talk. Skeletal muscle has been found to produce and secrete more than 600 distinct peptides; efforts are currently underway to characterize the entire muscle secretome. Recent research has demonstrated that skeletal muscle contraction or exercise can cause the secretion of novel, previously unidentified myokines with anti-inflammatory properties. These are some of the most prominent and thoroughly researched myokines.

Interleukin-6 (IL-6)

Along with TNFα, skeletal muscle releases IL-6, a well-known pro-inflammatory cytokine that aids in the development of insulin resistance. Recent data, however, indicates that IL-6 may have anti-inflammatory properties as well; these effects are contingent upon the type of receptor binding and the signaling cascade. TNF activity coexists with pro-inflammatory NFκB signaling to induce IL-6 release in macrophages. On the other hand, a calcium-dependent MAPK signaling pathway rather than NFκB signaling is responsible for the release of IL-6 as a myokine in response to exercise. It is believed that this is controlled at the IL-6 receptor level. There are two varieties of IL-6 receptors: sIL-6R and IL-6R. Traditionally, IL-6 attaches to IL-6R, and this combination combines with widely expressed gp130 to activate the MAPK signaling pathway that inhibits apoptosis and reduces inflammation. However, only a small subset of lymphoid cells and hepatocytes express IL-6R. On the other hand, soluble IL-6R (sIL-6R) is expressed by a variety of cell types and induces IL-6 trans-signaling while having the same affinity for IL-6. Therefore, in cells lacking IL-6R, sIL-6R can trigger IL-6 signaling through gp130. Exercise duration and intensity in human skeletal muscle have been found to increase IL-6 release, which has been connected to lactate production. This release of IL-6 is dependent on the production of lactate brought on by exercise; lactate by itself, in the absence of exercise, mimics the release of IL-6 from skeletal muscle.

3.4.5.1. Myostatin

The first myokine to be identified was myostatin (growth differentiation factor 8), which was found in 1997. Following its discovery, multiple secretome analyses were conducted, which resulted in the identification of over 600 myokines. Myostatin, a highly conserved protein belonging to the TGF-β family, is primarily expressed in skeletal muscle, but it is also present in adipose and cardiac tissue. A "hypermuscle" phenotype, such as that of Belgian Blue cattle or whippets, is caused by the ablation or mutation of myostatin, a protein that negatively regulates muscle mass. Following resistance training, myostatin expression and protein abundance in humans decline, and there is a positive correlation between myostatin expression and IL-6 plasma levels. Myostatin suppresses the production of new proteins and myogenesis, which increases muscle mass. Myostatin has also been linked to muscle sarcopenia, and elevated serum levels are seen in female sarcopenic patients. Exploring the therapeutic potential of myostatin inhibition to counteract muscle atrophy is a topic of great interest to researchers. Numerous drugs, including follistatin and stamulumab (a myostatin antibody), have been tested as potential myostatin antagonists since the early 2000s. However, none of these drugs are clinically effective in improving muscle strength in patients with muscular dystrophy, and studies on these drugs have had to be stopped for safety concerns. There is evidence that myostatin inhibition through the ActRIIB agonist, also known as the activin receptor extracellular domain fusion protein (ACVR2B-Fc), can prevent cancer-induced cachexia in mice. Both myostatin and activin A, which are secreted factors belonging to the TGF-β family, affect skeletal muscle through the same pathway. Two type-I (ALK4 and ALK5) and two type-II (ActRIIA and ActRIIB) activin receptors form a multimeric receptor complex that myostatin binds to. ActRIIB has a greater affinity for myostatin and is more prevalent in skeletal muscle than ActRIIA. The Smad 2/3/4 complex is formed when the myostatin pathway is activated, the multimeric receptor complex forms, Smad2 and Smad3 are phosphorylated, and Smad4 is recruited. Muscle atrophy and cachexia result from the Smad complex's subsequent translocation into the nucleus, where it inhibits the genes responsible for skeletal muscle differentiation and proliferation. In actuality, myostatin levels are elevated in aging and cancer (diseases linked to muscle atrophy). AKT-mediated mTOR pathway, which is involved in muscle protein synthesis, can also be inhibited by myostatin signaling. When AKT is inhibited, autophagy is activated through the FoxO and ubiquitin-proteasome pathways, which are involved in protein degradation. In general, higher myostatin levels are linked to both increased muscle atrophy and decreased muscle growth.

Irisin

PGC1α stimulates the expression of irisin, also referred to as cleaved FNDC5, which is thought to mediate the positive effects of exercise by encouraging the browning of white adipose tissue. The uncoupling protein UCP1 is activated during this browning process, which leads to a partial brown adipose tissue phenotype in white adipose tissue. Elevated thermogenesis is linked to brown adipose tissue. In both human and rodent exercise models, it has been demonstrated that irisin transcript levels rise. This is believed to be due to an increase in mitochondrial number and oxygen consumption through elevated PGC1α expression. The difficulty in detecting irisin in the blood (due to low serum levels) is the main reason for the controversy surrounding the exercise-induced increase in serum irisin. Although measuring irisin levels has proven difficult, a recent study has demonstrated that exercise causes an increase in circulating irisin levels (as measured by tandem mass spectrometry). A mutant Fndc5 mouse model was developed to evaluate its capacity to mediate adipocyte "browning" and exercise. The mice did not exhibit any abnormalities in the development or function of their skeletal muscles, but they did exhibit decreased running ability, insulin sensitivity, and glucose uptake in response to running, which emphasizes the role that irisin plays in mediating the metabolic effects of exercise. Furthermore, PGC-1α and mitochondrial transcription factor A, which are both involved in increased mitochondrial content and function, are expressed more when irisin is applied to mouse myotubes. However, detrimental nutrients like palmitate can reduce the expression of irisin and, consequently, lessen the benefits of insulin sensitization. In particular, palmitate inhibits the expression of FNDC5 by driving Smad3 to bind to a Smad3 binding motif in the promoter of the FNDC5 gene. This demonstrates one possible mechanism by which the downregulation of insulin-sensitizing factors such as irisin results in insulin resistance in muscle.

3.4.5.2. Myonectin

Myonectin is a member of the CTRP family and is a myokine that is responsive to nutrients. It is similar in structure to adiponectin and is released during muscle contraction. Myonectin acts like insulin, promoting the uptake of fatty acids by increasing the expression of genes that transport fatty acids, such as CD36 and Fabp1/4, in response to physical activity. In mice, myonectin can prevent autophagy in the liver, but this effect is blocked when the PI3K/AKT pathway is inhibited. This pathway is crucial for muscle growth, and myonectin may help prevent muscle wasting through its interaction with this pathway. Myonectin also activates the AMPK pathway in muscle cells, which helps to increase the movement of the GLUT4 glucose transporter and glucose uptake. Additionally, myonectin is linked to mitochondrial DNA density, with levels increasing in response to insulin resistance. Myonectin levels vary depending on the type of muscle fibers, with slow-twitch fibers expressing higher levels than fast-twitch fibers.

3.4.5.3. Interleukin 15 (IL-15)

A potential therapeutic target to counteract the detrimental effects of obesity is IL-15, an exercise- and muscle contraction-regulated myokine that can reduce inflammation and obesity. Although the precise impact of exercise on IL-15 expression, protein, and secretion varies from study to study, it is believed to mediate the benefits of exercise. These studies vary in terms of exercise type and intensity (acute vs. instruction), in addition to IL-15 measurement techniques. People's serum levels of IL-15 are generally found to be positively impacted by moderate-intensity training. Myoblast differentiation is accompanied by an upregulation of IL-15, and IL-15 enrichment in cultured skeletal muscle can cause differentiation and boost muscle mass. Yet, a different group of researchers demonstrated that giving IL-15 to young rats causes them to lose muscle mass and increase apoptosis, indicating that the circumstances surrounding IL-15 administration may have an impact on the protein's function in skeletal muscle. In addition to raising adiponectin secretion and decreasing lipid accumulation in adipose tissue (much like exercise), IL-15 has been demonstrated to enhance fatty acid oxidation and glycogen synthesis in skeletal muscle. Similar to how exercise affects the STAT3 and AMPK pathways, IL-15 has also been demonstrated to enhance glucose uptake into rat skeletal muscle and cultured skeletal muscle cells. There is disagreement over the mechanism underlying IL-15 function as a myokine, which suggests that more research is necessary. Regarding this, a study has provided insight into the possible in vivo mechanism of IL-15 regulation.

3.4.5.4. Other Myokines

BDNF and Decorin are two other noteworthy myokines that are involved in muscle regeneration, differentiation, and fat metabolism. Furthermore, novel myokines that react to exercise have been discovered. Regarding the impact of exerkines on insulin resistance, further research is required to fully understand the role these exerkines play in insulin resistance before using them in therapeutic settings (Gomes et al., 2002; Frontera & Ochala, 2015; Bordoni et al., 2023).

A Closer Look

Muscle Mechanics

The biomechanics of skeletal muscle encompass a multitude of intricate processes that govern its function in generating force and facilitating movement. Central to this understanding is the principle of force generation, which is rooted in the molecular interactions occurring within muscle fibers during contraction. Within each muscle fiber, myosin heads interact with actin filaments, forming cross-bridges that cycle through attachment, force generation, and detachment, ultimately leading to the sliding of actin filaments past myosin filaments and muscle shortening.

Muscle architecture, referring to the arrangement of muscle fibers within a muscle, greatly influences its force-generating capabilities. Muscles can be classified based on their architecture into parallel, pennate, or fusiform types. Pennate muscles, characterized by obliquely oriented muscle fibers relative to the tendon, are particularly efficient in generating force due to their increased physiological cross-sectional area (PCSA), which allows for a greater number of muscle fibers to contribute to force production.

The length-tension relationship is a fundamental concept in muscle biomechanics, describing the relationship between muscle length and the force it can generate. At optimal lengths, muscles can generate maximal force due to optimal overlap between actin and myosin filaments. Deviation from this optimal length, either through excessive stretch or contraction, leads to diminished force production due to decreased cross-bridge formation and reduced overlap between filaments. This relationship is crucial in understanding muscle function during various activities, as muscles operate across a range of lengths during movement.

Pennation, the angle at which muscle fibers are oriented relative to the tendon, plays a significant role in muscle function by influencing the effective PCSA and force-generating capacity. Muscles with greater pennation angles have a larger PCSA and are thus capable of generating greater force per unit cross-sectional area. Additionally, pennation allows for a greater number of muscle fibers to be packed into a given volume, enhancing force transmission to the tendon and facilitating force generation along the muscle's line of action.

Summary

- Skeletal muscles (commonly referred to as muscles) are organs of the vertebrate muscular system and typically are attached by tendons to bones of a skeleton. The muscle cells of skeletal muscles are much longer than in the other types of muscle tissue and are often known as muscle fibers.
- Skeletal muscle comprises about 35% of the body of humans by weight. The functions of skeletal muscle include producing movement, maintaining body posture, controlling body temperature, and stabilizing joints.
- The skeletal muscles account for about half of a mammal's body weight, and as a result, they receive proportionately large amounts of administered doses of chemicals. Skeletal muscle is a target organ for a variety of chemicals and adverse or toxic effects can range from minor muscle weakness or slight pain to complete paralysis.
- Skeletal muscle tissue is made up of a collection of muscle fibers wrapped in connective tissue sheaths. There are three types of connective tissue sheaths named for their location. Endomysium surrounds individual muscle fibers.
- The sarcomere is the functional unit of a skeletal muscle cell. Each sarcomere is about 2.5 micrometers in length. It is made up of multiple myosin and actin filaments oriented in parallel. The actin and myosin filaments overlap in certain places creating several bands and zones.
- The thick and thin filaments in the myofibrils are supported by accessory proteins. These proteins maintain the speed and alignment of filaments during the contraction cycle.
- Skeletal muscle is innervated by α-motor neurons, which stimulate its muscle fibers to contract. The cell bodies of α-motor neurons are located in either the ventral horn of the spinal cord (for limbs and trunk muscles) or in the motor nuclei of the brainstem (for head and face muscles).
- Skeletal muscle contraction is triggered by an action potential arriving at the neuromuscular junction, causing the opening of voltage-gated calcium ion channels. The resulting increase in intracellular Ca^{2+} causes vesicles containing acetylcholine (ACh) to release their contents into the synaptic cleft.

References

1. Bordoni, B., Black, A. C., & Varacallo, M. (2023). Anatomy, tendons. In *StatPearls* [Internet]. StatPearls Publishing. Retrieved from: https://www.ncbi.nlm.nih.gov/books/NBK571433/ (accessed on 25 June 2024).
2. Bourne, M., Talkad, A., & Varacallo, M. (2023). Anatomy, bony pelvis and lower limb, foot fascia. In *StatPearls* [Internet]. StatPearls Publishing. Retrieved from: https://www.ncbi.nlm.nih.gov/books/NBK557493/ (accessed on 25 June 2024).
3. Buckingham, M., & Rigby, P. W. (2014). Gene regulatory networks and transcriptional mechanisms that control myogenesis. *Developmental Cell, 28*(3), 225–238. https://doi.org/10.1016/j.devcel.2014.01.020.

4. Calderón, J. C., Bolaños, P., & Caputo, C. (2014). The excitation-contraction coupling mechanism in skeletal muscle. *Biophysical Reviews, 6*(1), 133–160. https://doi.org/10.1007/s12551-013-0127-y.
5. Chang, A., Ly, N., & Varacallo, M. (2023). Piriformis injection. In *StatPearls* [Internet]. StatPearls Publishing. Retrieved from: https://www.ncbi.nlm.nih.gov/books/NBK567705/ (accessed on 25 June 2024).
6. Dean, S., McCracken, J., Kosmider, S., & Herath, D. (2018). Lambert-Eaton myasthenic syndrome developing post-diagnosis of small-cell lung cancer. *Internal Medicine Journal, 48*(12), 1541–1542. https://doi.org/10.1111/imj.14080.
7. Fitts, R. H. (2008). The cross-bridge cycle and skeletal muscle fatigue. *Journal of Applied Physiology (1985), 104*(2), 551–558. https://doi.org/10.1152/japplphysiol.01200.2007.
8. Frontera, W. R., & Ochala, J. (2015). Skeletal muscle: A brief review of structure and function. *Calcified Tissue International, 96*(3), 183–195. https://doi.org/10.1007/s00223-014-9915-y.
9. Gomes, A. V., Potter, J. D., & Szczesna-Cordary, D. (2002). The role of troponins in muscle contraction. *IUBMB Life, 54*(6), 323–333. https://doi.org/10.1080/15216540216035.
10. Goodman, C. A., Hornberger, T. A., & Robling, A. G. (2015). Bone and skeletal muscle: Key players in mechanotransduction and potential overlapping mechanisms. *Bone, 80*, 24–36. https://doi.org/10.1016/j.bone.2015.04.014.
11. Hernández-Hernández, J. M., García-González, E. G., Brun, C. E., & Rudnicki, M. A. (2017). The myogenic regulatory factors, determinants of muscle development, cell identity and regeneration. *Seminars in Cell & Developmental Biology, 72*, 10–18. https://doi.org/10.1016/j.semcdb.2017.11.011.
12. Hikida, R. S. (2011). Aging changes in satellite cells and their functions. *Current Aging Science, 4*(3), 279–297. https://doi.org/10.2174/1874609811104030279.
13. Hultman, E., & Greenhaff, P. L. (1991). Skeletal muscle energy metabolism and fatigue during intense exercise in man. *Science Progress, 75*(298 Pt 3–4), 361–370.
14. Jayam Trouth, A., Dabi, A., Solieman, N., Kurukumbi, M., & Kalyanam, J. (2012). Myasthenia gravis: A review. *Autoimmune Diseases, 2012*, 874680. https://doi.org/10.1155/2012/874680.
15. Lehman, W., Hatch, V., Korman, V., Rosol, M., Thomas, L., Maytum, R., Geeves, M. A., Van Eyk, J. E., Tobacman, L. S., & Craig, R. (2000). Tropomyosin and actin isoforms modulate the localization of tropomyosin strands on actin filaments. *Journal of Molecular Biology, 302*(3), 593–606. https://doi.org/10.1006/jmbi.2000.4071.
16. Periasamy, M., Herrera, J. L., & Reis, F. C. G. (2017). Skeletal muscle thermogenesis and its role in whole body energy metabolism. *Diabetes & Metabolism Journal, 41*(5), 327–336. https://doi.org/10.4093/dmj.2017.41.5.327.
17. Perreault, E. J., Day, S. J., Hulliger, M., Heckman, C. J., & Sandercock, T. G. (2003). Summation of forces from multiple motor units in the cat soleus muscle. *Journal of Neurophysiology, 89*(2), 738–744. https://doi.org/10.1152/jn.00682.2002.
18. Sellers, J. R. (2000). Myosins: A diverse superfamily. *Biochimica et Biophysica Acta (BBA)–Molecular Cell Research, 1496*(1), 3–22. https://doi.org/10.1016/s0167-4889(00)00017-1.
19. Shih, H. P., Gross, M. K., & Kioussi, C. (2008). Muscle development: Forming the head and trunk muscles. *Acta Histochemica, 110*(2), 97–108. https://doi.org/10.1016/j.acthis.2007.12.001.

20. Squire, J. M. (1997). Architecture and function in the muscle sarcomere. *Current Opinion in Structural Biology, 7*(2), 247–257. https://doi.org/10.1016/s0959-440x(97)80034-9.

21. Stone, W. L., Leavitt, L., & Varacallo, M. (2023). Physiology, growth factor. In *StatPearls* [Internet]. StatPearls Publishing. Retrieved from: https://www.ncbi.nlm.nih.gov/books/NBK565722/ (accessed on 25 June 2024).

22. Thornell, L. E., Carlsson, L., Eriksson, P. O., Liu, J. X., Österlund, C., Stål, P., & Pedrosa-Domellöf, F. (2015). Fiber typing of intrafusal fibers. *Journal of Anatomy, 227*(2), 136–156. https://doi.org/10.1111/joa.12348.

23. Wilke, J., Engeroff, T., Nürnberger, F., Vogt, L., & Banzer, W. (2016). Anatomical study of the morphological continuity between iliotibial tract and the fibularis longus fascia. *Surgical and Radiologic Anatomy, 38*(3), 349–352. https://doi.org/10.1007/s00276-015-1578-1.

24. Wolfe, R. R. (2006). The underappreciated role of muscle in health and disease. *The American Journal of Clinical Nutrition, 84*(3), 475–482. https://doi.org/10.1093/ajcn/84.3.475.

Chapter 4

SMOOTH MUSCLE

Contents

Introduction

Skeletal, cardiac, and smooth muscle tissue are the three primary types found in the human body. Smooth muscle is a non-striated muscle type that is frequently found in the walls of blood vessels and hollow organs. Though smooth muscle can be found all over the body, it is most frequently found in the walls of arteries, blood vessels, and the digestive tract, as well as surrounding other organs like the eyes. As previously mentioned, smooth muscle cells lack striations. This indicates that they lack the observable bands of contractile proteins that are present in skeletal muscles. Moreover, the contraction of these muscles occurs automatically without conscious thought because they are involuntary. Autonomic nerves and hormones such as vasopressin and adrenaline can send chemical or electrical signals to them, causing them to contract. Typically, smooth muscle tissues are positioned as sheets between connective tissue layers or as tubes and circular layers surrounding the intestines. Additionally, each cell in this type of muscle contains a single nucleus. Smooth muscle controls the vasculature system, which distributes blood throughout the body. Contracting smooth muscles helps control blood pressure and other cardiovascular functions. Peristalsis, the rhythmic, wave-like contraction of the muscles surrounding the digestive tract, is another way they help with food digestion.

Orientation and Directional Terms

Term	Definition	Illustration
Autonomic nerves	A network of nerves throughout your body that control unconscious processes. These are things that happen without you thinking about them, such as breathing and your heart beating.	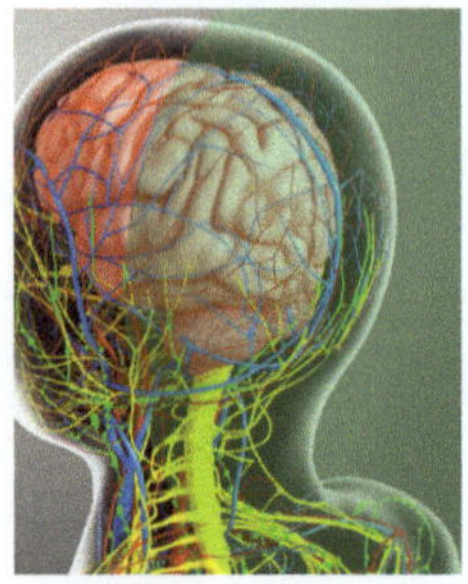
Atherosclerosis	Atherosclerosis is the buildup of fats, cholesterol and other substances in and on the artery walls. This buildup is called plaque. The plaque can cause arteries to narrow, blocking blood flow.	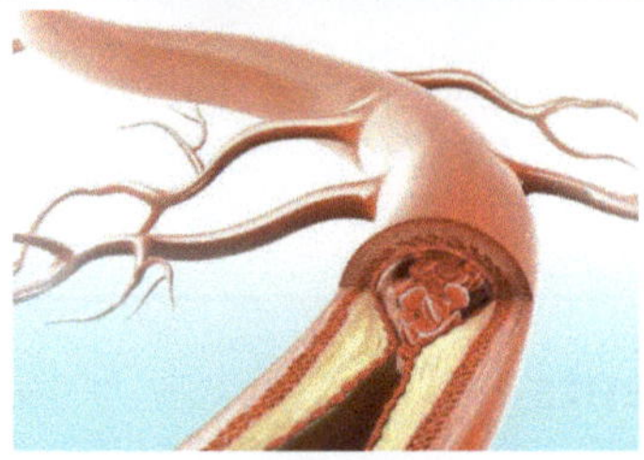
Cytoplasm	Cytoplasm is the gelatinous liquid that fills the inside of a cell. It is composed of water, salts, and various organic molecules. Some intracellular organelles, such the nucleus and mitochondria, are enclosed by membranes that separate them from the cytoplasm.	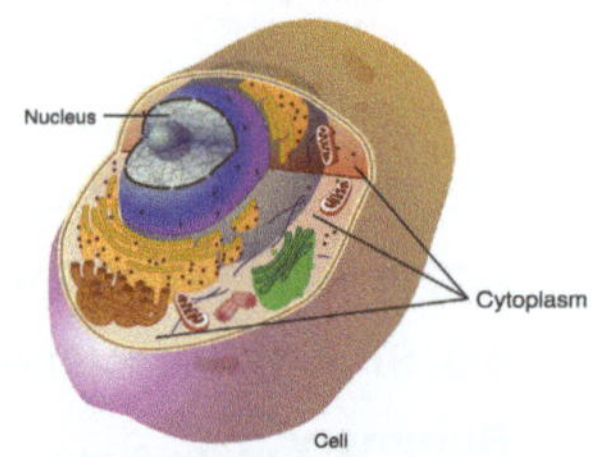
Electrolyte balance	An electrolyte imbalance means that the level of one or more electrolytes in your body is too low or too high.	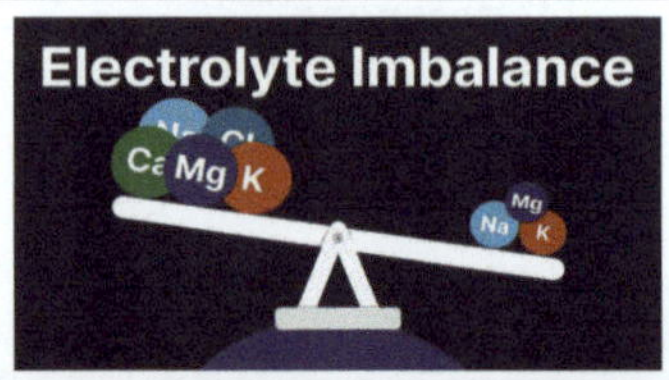
Neural crest	Neural crest cells are a temporary group of cells that arise from the embryonic ectoderm germ layer, and in turn give rise to a diverse cell lineage—including melanocytes, craniofacial cartilage and bone, smooth muscle, peripheral and enteric neurons and glia.	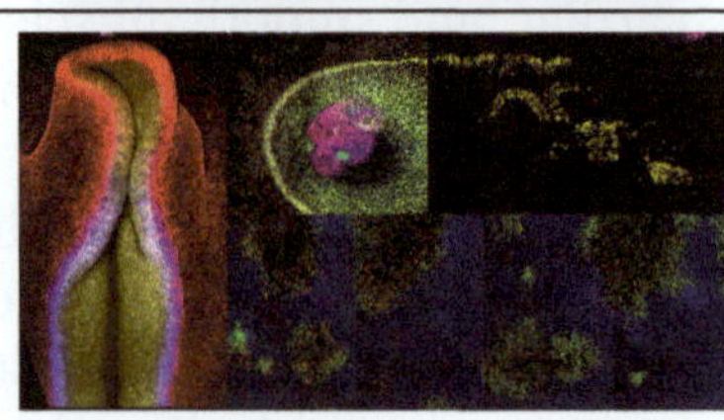

4.1. Anatomy of Smooth Muscle

Smooth muscle is distributed throughout the body and performs several roles. It aids in digestion and nutrient absorption in the stomach and intestines. It is present throughout the urinary system and aids in the body's detoxification as well as electrolyte balance. It is present in all veins and arteries, where it is essential for controlling tissue oxygenation and blood pressure. The body relies on essential functions for basic sustenance. Smooth muscle differs from skeletal muscle in various ways, with its ability for involuntary contraction being most notable. The nervous system can regulate body subsystems using smooth muscle without conscious effort. During exercise, blood pressure adjusts to oxygen demands without conscious awareness, as the nervous system naturally regulates smooth muscle using receptors, hormones, and neurotransmitters. Additionally, smooth muscle is crucial to the progression of disease throughout the body. For individuals with asthma, bronchodilators are a critical and potentially life-saving treatment because they relax the smooth muscle of the airways. Metoclopramide serves as an example of a medication that increases smooth muscle signaling to stimulate and enhance gastric emptying. When combined with ACEI, nitrates are utilized in the treatment of ischemic heart disease, a combination that has demonstrated a reduction in patient mortality. Understanding smooth muscle is essential for healthcare professionals due to its significant influence on various parts of the body. The fundamental mechanism of many treatments involves altering the signaling pathways that affect smooth muscle.

4.1.1. Structure and Function

Skeletal muscle and smooth muscle have different functions. Smooth muscle, in contrast to skeletal muscle, can contract without conscious thought and can sustain tone over time. Smooth muscle can be characterized as an involuntary, non-striated muscle at the cellular level. Smooth muscle has a non-striated pattern because its thick and thin filaments are not organized into sarcomeres. When viewed under a microscope, it will seem uniform. The cytoplasm of smooth muscle is highly concentrated in myosin and actin. The two primary proteins involved in muscle contraction are actin and myosin. Attached to dense bodies dispersed throughout the cell are actin filaments. Dense bodies appear dark when viewed under an electron microscope. The sarcoplasmic reticulum, which contains calcium and helps to maintain contraction, is another significant structure. Smooth muscle is characterized as fusiform, meaning that it is tapering at both ends and has a rounded center. Smooth muscle is more elastic than striated muscle, but it can still contract and relax. This is crucial for organ systems that depend on the preservation of contractile tone, such as the bladder. Within the smooth muscle cell, actin and myosin combine to form continuous chains that are secured at the dense bodies. The actin and myosin chains' intermediate and thin filaments can then extend to dense bodies on nearby smooth muscle cells, creating a mesh-like network that encircles a sizable number of smooth muscle cells. Adherens junctions, also known as connexins, allow smooth muscle cells to contract uniformly in a manner akin to a spiral corkscrew. One can extend the role of smooth muscle to include the organ systems that it assists in regulating on a much larger scale. The role of smooth muscle in each organ system is quite broad and goes beyond the scope of this article.

For simplicity, the basic functions of smooth muscle in the organ systems are listed below.

- Gastrointestinal tract: Propulsion of the food bolus
- Cardiovascular: Regulation of blood flow and pressure via vascular resistance
- Renal: Regulation of urine flow

- Genital: Contractions during pregnancy, propulsion of sperm
- Respiratory tract: Regulation of bronchiole diameter
- Integument: Raises hair with erector pili muscle
- Sensory: Dilation and constriction of the pupil as well as changing lens shape

4.1.2. Embryology

Neural crest and mesoderm cells are the sources of smooth muscle. The reason behind this is that smooth muscle plays a vital role in numerous bodily tissues. The migration of neural crest cells that takes place during embryonic development is one of its distinctive characteristics. Consequently, neural crest cells give rise to a wide variety of tissues found throughout the body. The development of smooth muscle in the body, particularly in the control of blood vessels, is significantly influenced by neural crest cells. Many sources give rise to vascular smooth muscle cells, which is important from a medical standpoint as it could influence how vascular diseases are localized at different sites. Examples of conditions that frequently manifest at particular vascular locations are atherosclerosis and aortic aneurysms. Hemodynamics and the underlying vessel structure were previously thought to be involved. The location and presentation of the disease, however, appear to be related to the smooth muscle cell embryonic lineage, according to mounting evidence. The development of the endothelium network is also partly dependent on smooth muscle cell development. A vital component of vascular development and stability are vascular smooth muscle cells, also known as mural cells. The regulation of blood flow, endothelial network growth, and vessel stability heavily depends on mural cells, which encircle larger vessels. The process of signaling that results in vessel development and their developmental origins, however, are not well understood. For vascular tissue engineering and therapeutic revascularization, the growth of vascular smooth muscle cells is a key objective.

4.1.3. Blood Supply and Lymphatics

The blood supply and lymphatic contributions differ by region because smooth muscles are widely distributed throughout the body. Nearly all of the body's arteries provide blood to smooth muscle, which can be either endothelial smooth muscle found inside the artery or smooth muscle found within an organ system, like the arteries of the gastrointestinal tract. The impact of smooth muscles on blood supply itself becomes increasingly significant. Smooth muscle, for instance, controls the diameter of the vessel within the cardiovascular system to help regulate blood flow. Vascular diseases of smooth muscle, as was previously mentioned, can have devastating consequences on the body and result in serious pathology. It was previously believed that atherosclerosis was solely related to hemodynamics and vessel structure, but more recent research has revealed a connection to smooth muscle development as well. Even the development of pulmonary hypertension has been linked to persistent activation of vascular smooth muscle, according to research. Asthma may arise from the pathologic activation of smooth muscle within the lungs. When the airway becomes obstructed due to smooth muscle constriction, asthma develops. According to recent research, the smooth muscle layer may thicken even before the onset of asthma, suggesting a potential genetic connection.

4.1.4. Nerves

The innervation of smooth muscle varies greatly depending on its function and location, much like the blood supply. The sympathetic nervous system is the main innervation of vascular smooth muscle. Vascular smooth muscle cells are contracted by alpha-1 and alpha-2 receptors, causing vasoconstriction and systemic hypertension. Although they also react to sympathetic stimulation, beta-2 receptors have a vasodilatory effect, which lowers blood pressure throughout the body. However, smooth muscle cell contraction is also significantly influenced by parasympathetic activation. Research on the subject as early as 1925 showed how the gastrointestinal tract is affected by parasympathetic innervation. Researchers have more recently demonstrated how the enteric, parasympathetic, and sympathetic nervous systems all function in unison to affect and contract smooth muscle. The spinal levels T1 through L2 of the spine contribute to the sympathetic stimulation of smooth muscle. All of these contributions end up in the sympathetic trunk, which is responsible for directing autonomic nerve impulses to various bodily tissues and organs. The cranial nerves, vagus nerve, and pelvic splanchnic nerves are the three components that make up the parasympathetic nervous system. The vagus nerve, for example, innervates the gastrointestinal tract from the esophagus to the proximal portion of the large intestines and branches out to the heart, larynx, trachea, bronchi, liver, and pancreas. Each parasympathetic nerve regulates a distinct area of the body. The autonomic nervous system is the combined name for the sympathetic and parasympathetic nervous systems. The intricate workings of the autonomic nervous system enable precise, unconscious regulation of many vital bodily processes, including blood pressure, heart rate, respiration rate, urination, and digestion.

In smooth muscle tissue, autonomic nervous system innervation ultimately results in the release of calcium. Intramuscular calcium is necessary for smooth muscle contraction. The smooth muscle cell increases its calcium content in two different ways. L-type channels found in the membrane's caveolae allow calcium to enter the cell in response to depolarization, hormones, or neurotransmitters. Through ryanodine receptors and IP3, intracellular calcium then triggers the release of calcium from the sarcoplasmic reticulum (SR); this process is known as calcium-induced calcium release. The sarcoplasmic reticulum's release of calcium into smooth muscle is not physically connected to the ryanodine receptor, in contrast to skeletal muscle. Activated calmodulin is created when calcium binds to calmodulin after it has entered the cell. Myosin light chain kinase (MLCK) is subsequently activated by calmodulin, and MLCK phosphorylates a regulatory light chain on myosin. Following phosphorylation, the myosin head undergoes a conformational shift that raises myosin ATPase activity and facilitates interaction between the myosin head and actin. After that, there is a cross-bridge cycling, which causes tension. The amount of tension produced is correlated with the cell's calcium concentration. Compared to skeletal muscle, smooth muscle exhibits substantially less ATPase activity. The much slower cycling speed of smooth muscle is caused by this factor. The longer contraction duration, however, may result in a smooth muscle contraction with a higher force. Connexins are utilized to further improve smooth muscle contraction. Connexins facilitate the passage of calcium and other molecules to nearby smooth muscle cells, enabling intercellular communication. This process enables quick cell-to-cell communication and a smooth contraction pattern.

The steps involved in smooth muscle cell contraction are as follows:

1. Depolarization of membrane or hormone/neurotransmitter activation
2. L-type voltage-gated calcium channels open
3. Calcium-induced calcium release from the SR

4. Increased intracellular calcium
5. Calmodulin binds calcium
6. Myosin light chain kinase activation
7. Phosphorylation of myosin light chain
8. Increase Myosin ATPase activity
9. Myosin-P binds Actin
10. Cross-bridge cycling leads to muscle tone

Dephosphorylation of myosin light chains terminates smooth muscle contraction. Unlike skeletal muscle, smooth muscle is phosphorylated during its activation. This creates a potential difficulty in that simply reducing calcium levels won't produce muscle relaxation. Myosin light chain phosphatase (MLCP) is instead responsible for dephosphorylation of the myosin light chains, ultimately leading to smooth muscle relaxation.

4.1.5. Muscles Tissues

Hollow organ walls contain smooth muscle, so-called because the cells lack visible striations (e.g., bladder), the lining of blood vessels, and the tissues inside the eyes (e.g., iris) and the skin (e.g., muscles- arrector pili). Smooth muscle exhibits involuntary control and is responsive to hormones, local stimuli, and neural stimulation from the autonomic nervous system.

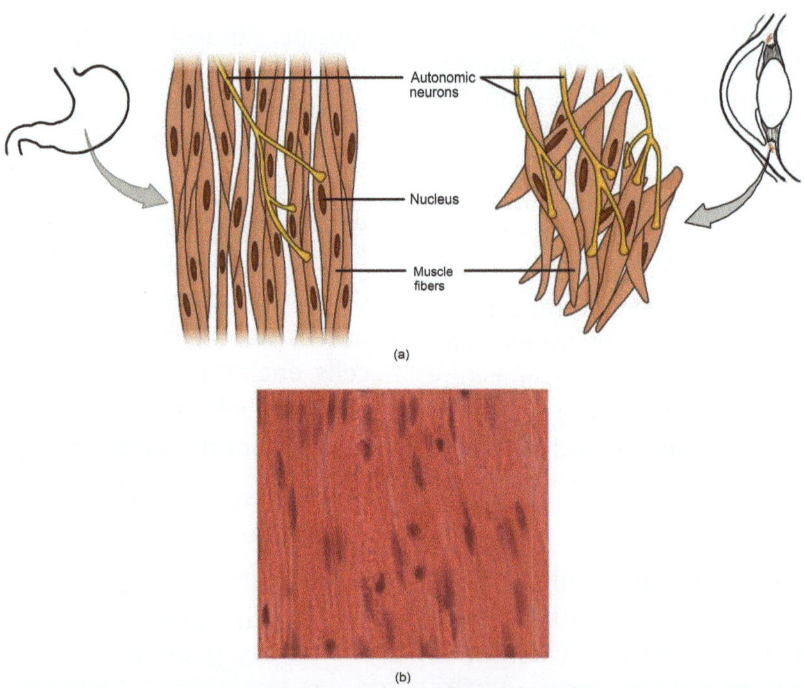

Figure 4.1. *Smooth muscle tissue: Smooth muscle tissue is found around organs in the digestive, respiratory, and reproductive tracts and the iris of the eye.*

Source: https://open.oregonstate.education/app/uploads/sites/157/2019/07/1021_Smooth_Muscle_new-768x652.jpg.

Stretching a muscle can cause it to contract in specific places, such as the walls of visceral organs. Individual smooth muscle cells range in size from 30 to 200 μm. Smooth muscle fibers are spindle-shaped and, in contrast to skeletal muscle fibers, have a single nucleus. Because gap junctions exist between the cells, smooth muscle fibers function in unison and are frequently observed forming sheets of tissue. Known as visceral or unitary smooth muscle, this kind of smooth muscle is the most prevalent kind found in the human body and forms the walls of hollow organs. Smooth muscle with a single unit contracts slowly and steadily to facilitate the passage of materials through the body, including food in the digestive tract. The second type of smooth muscle that has been observed is called multi-unit smooth muscle. It is made up of cells that are not electrically coupled because they hardly ever have gap junctions. As a result, contraction is limited to the cell that was initially stimulated rather than spreading to other cells. Large arteries, the arrector pili muscles connected to hair follicles, the lungs' large airways, and the internal eye muscles that control light entry and lens shape are examples of this kind of smooth muscle (Figure 4.1).

Actin and myosin, two contractile proteins found in smooth muscle fibers, work together to create tension even though smooth muscle cells lack striations. These fibers are attached to dense bodies that are dispersed throughout the cytoplasm and anchored to the sarcolemma rather than being organized into orderly sarcomeres, which explains why there are no striations. To give contractile proteins something to work against on the inside, a network of intermediate fibers runs between the dense bodies. Similar to the Z-discs of skeletal muscle, a dense body holds the thin filaments firmly in place. Our bodies get most of their calcium ions from the extracellular milieu. Although there are no T-tubules, the sarcolemma contains tiny indentations called caveoli that indicate areas with a high density of calcium channels that allow calcium entry. Although it is present in the fibers, the sarcoplasmic reticulum is not as developed as it is in skeletal muscle.

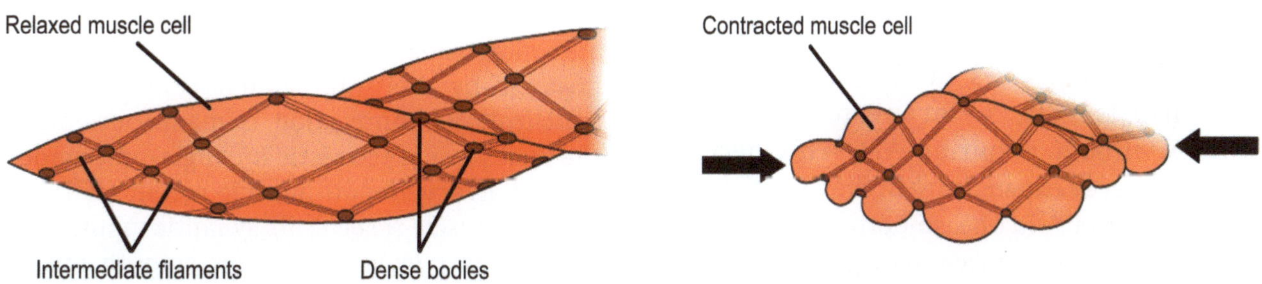

Figure 4.2. *Muscle Contraction: The dense bodies and intermediate filaments are networked through the sarcoplasm, which cause the muscle fiber to contract.*

Source: https://open.oregonstate.education/app/uploads/sites/157/2021/02/1028_Smooth_Muscle_Contraction-768x159.jpg.

Since smooth muscle cells lack troponin, the regulatory protein calmodulin controls cross-bridge formation rather than the troponin-tropomyosin complex. When a smooth muscle cell is stimulated, extra Ca^{++} is released by the sarcoplasmic reticulum and external Ca^{++} ions flow through open calcium channels in the sarcolemma. Myosin (light chain) kinase is activated when calcium binds to calmodulin in the cytoplasm, forming the Ca^{++}-calmodulin complex. ATP is converted to ADP and Pi by myosin light chain kinase, which then phosphorylates the myosin heads, causing the Pi to attach to the head. The thin filaments can then be pulled by the heads once they have attached to actin-binding sites. The dense bodies are pulled on by the thin filaments as they pass through the thick filaments, and the intermediate filament networks spread throughout the sarcoplasm are pulled on by the dense bodies. The entire muscle fiber contracts as a result of this configuration, pulling the ends toward the center and creating a corkscrew-shaped bulge in the middle (Figure 4.2).

The contraction of muscles persists until the active transport of Ca++ ions out of the cell or back into the sarcoplasmic reticulum by ATP-dependent calcium pumps. But to keep muscles toned, a small amount of calcium is still present in the sarcoplasm. The residual calcium maintains the muscle slightly contracted, which is critical for some processes like blood vessel pressure maintenance. Since most smooth muscles have to work for extended periods without rest, they produce relatively little power to use as little energy as possible. While myosin kinase is inactivated or dephosphorylated and Ca++ is eliminated, certain smooth muscles can continue to contract. This can occur when a subset of actin-myosin head cross-bridges, known as latch-bridges, maintain the thick and thin filaments connected for an extended amount of time without requiring ATP. This permits minimal energy expenditure in the maintenance of muscle "tone" in the smooth muscle lining arterioles and other visceral organs. The highly ordered neuromuscular junctions seen in skeletal muscle are not formed by the axons of autonomic nervous system neurons when they stimulate smooth muscle. Rather, a wide synaptic cleft is where neurotransmitters are released through a series of neurotransmitter-filled bulges known as varicosities that run along the axon of the neuron feeding the smooth muscle. Additionally, pacesetter cells are found in the visceral muscles of the hollow organ walls (apart from the heart). Muscle contractions and action potentials can be involuntarily triggered by a pacesetter cell.

Smooth muscle can be found in all the organ systems listed below:

- Gastrointestinal tract
- Cardiovascular: Blood vessels and lymphatic vessels
- Renal: Urinary bladder
- Genital: Male and female reproductive tracts
- Respiratory tract
- Integument: arrector pili of the skin
- Sensory: Ciliary muscle and iris of the eye

4.1.6. Physiologic Variants

Single-unit and multi-unit smooth muscle are the two types that exist. Multiple cells linked by connexins that can be stimulated synchronously by a single synaptic input comprise single-unit smooth muscle. Groups of smooth muscle cells that are single units can communicate with one another through connexins. Calcium waves are produced by the diffusion of ions and molecules between cells, which is made possible by this intercellular communication. Synchronous contraction is made possible by the special characteristic of single-unit smooth muscle. Every smooth muscle cell in multi-unit smooth muscle receives its synaptic input, which sets it apart from single-unit smooth muscle. This makes it possible for multi-unit smooth muscle to control much more precisely. Large arteries, the ciliary muscles in the eyes, and the airways of the lungs all contain multi-unit smooth muscle.

4.1.7. Surgical Considerations

Every surgery will be affected by the overall function of smooth muscle because of its regulatory effects on autonomic control. Keeping an eye on a patient's vital signs during surgery is essential for a successful procedure, and the autonomic nervous system—which controls smooth muscle contraction—can be greatly impacted by the stresses of the procedure. Even changing the way smooth muscle functions can be the goal of surgery, as in the case of a vagotomy. A vagotomy is a traditional surgical procedure used to treat peptic ulcer disease by excising the vagus nerve at the level of the stomach, thereby eliminating stimulation. Overstimulation of the vagus nerve has been suggested as a potential cause of the condition. Though recent improvements in medical therapy for peptic ulcer disease have made this procedure less popular, some patients may still benefit from it. An additional instance pertains to the management of specific neuroendocrine tumors, such as adrenal pheochromocytomas, which may result in cardiovascular issues during surgery due to the release of surplus catecholamines. Understanding how beta and alpha blockades impact smooth muscle and how those changes impact other body functions is essential for proper management. When planning and carrying out any surgery, having a thorough understanding of the role that smooth muscle contraction plays and how it affects various body systems becomes essential because of its regulatory control effects.

4.1.8. Clinical Significance

The estimated cost of asthma-related medical expenses in the United States in 2013 was $81.9 billion. It is astounding to learn that something as basic as smooth muscle contraction can cause asthma, given the massive burden on healthcare systems. Smooth muscle is an essential component of every organ system in the human body, serving a vital role in life. Smooth muscle has a variety of functions in the body, including maintaining blood pressure and flow in the cardiovascular system, opening and closing airways in the lungs, assisting in motility and nutrient collection in the gastrointestinal system, and being involved in nearly every other organ system. Medical professionals must possess a comprehensive understanding of smooth muscle anatomy, physiology, function, and disease applications due to the smooth muscle's widespread distribution throughout the body and numerous unique properties. From a functional perspective, each vital sign is preserved by smooth muscle physiology. Smooth muscle has probably contributed to the development of the illness, regardless of whether the patient presents with a chronic or acute emergent condition. Many life-saving treatments target smooth muscle directly in an acute setting. Health professionals can save lives in these situations if they have a solid foundation and understanding of smooth muscle. Clinicians will be able to improve their patients' quality of life if they have a deeper comprehension of smooth muscle. The psycho-social aspects of smooth muscle diseases are often disregarded in the context of the biopsychosocial model. For instance, a patient with neurogenic bladder disease may withdraw from society to minimize the stigma attached to their illness. When treating patients with smooth muscle dysfunction, medical professionals must recognize the various aspects that the illness will affect. Research on smooth muscle and its overall effects on disease will probably change in the future, as it does with all aspects of medicine. Future implications of the smooth muscle research, such as the potential to restore endothelial tissue and develop new strategies for promoting revascularization, appear promising. This small shift in understanding could have a massive effect on cardiovascular disease mortality and treatment in the future. Even though smooth muscle is still a very complex topic, medical professionals will be better equipped to provide better care both now and in the future if they have a firm grasp of how it affects healthcare, even at the most basic level.

4.1.9. Innervation

The innervation of the smooth musculature is complex. It lies under the influence of the visceral nervous system and works autonomously at the same time.

Furthermore, it is regulated by:

- Neurotransmitters: e.g., norepinephrine, acetylcholine;
- Hormones: e.g., estrogen, oxytocin;
- Tissue hormones: e.g., prostaglandins, histamine.

Regional alterations (e.g., extending) might be calming or stimulating. The smooth muscle is contracted automatically, in contrast to the skeletal muscle. Two types of single-unit and multi-unit systems are distinguished functionally. Gap junctions provide electrical connectivity between the single-unit type smooth muscle cells, which contract uniformly. Internal organs and blood vessel walls (visceral smooth musculature) contain these kinds of cells. To enable more precise muscle control, each of the multi-unit smooth cells must have its own innervation because they are not interdependent. Among the iris and hair arrector muscles are two places they can be found.

4.2. Physiology of Smooth Muscle

Smooth muscle is found all over the body and performs several tasks. It aids in digestion and nutrient absorption in the stomach and intestines. It is a component of the urinary system, which helps the body eliminate toxins and maintain electrolyte balance. It is found in all arteries and veins, where it is essential for controlling blood pressure and oxygenation of tissues. The body could not sustain even its most basic functions in the absence of these essential functions. There are several ways in which smooth muscle differs from skeletal muscle, but its capacity for involuntary contraction and control may be the most significant. Without conscious effort on the part of the user, the nervous system can use smooth muscle to tightly regulate many of the body's subsystems throughout life. When an individual engages in exercise, their blood pressure adjusts to the increased oxygen demands without their conscious awareness. Instead, the nervous system uses other receptors, hormones, and neurotransmitters to naturally regulate smooth muscle. Additionally crucial to the disease process throughout the body is smooth muscle. For asthmatics, bronchodilators are crucial and potentially life-saving as they relax the airway smooth muscle. Metoclopramide is a medication that enhances smooth muscle signaling to aid gastric emptying. The use of nitrates in treating ischemic heart disease is a well-known application of medical therapy for smooth muscle. Studies have demonstrated that nitrates can reduce patient mortality when combined with ACE inhibitors. Since many treatments fundamentally involve altering the signaling pathways that impact smooth muscle, medical professionals must comprehend the unique significance of smooth muscle throughout the body.

4.2.1. Cellular Level

Cellularly speaking, smooth muscle is an involuntary non-striated muscle. Smooth muscle has a non-striated pattern due to the presence of thick and thin filaments that do not group into sarcomeres. It looks homogeneous when viewed under a microscope. Actin and myosin are abundant in the cytoplasm of smooth muscle. Actin and myosin are the primary proteins involved in the contraction of muscles. Attached to dense bodies dispersed throughout the cell are actin filaments. When viewed through an electron microscope, dense bodies appear dark. The sarcoplasmic reticulum, another crucial structure that helps maintain contraction, contains calcium. Fusiform, or round in the middle and tapering at both ends, is the shape of smooth muscle. Compared to striated muscle, smooth muscle is more elastic and can tense and relax. This characteristic is crucial for organ systems that depend on the maintenance of contractile tone, such as the bladder.

4.2.2. Development

Mesoderm and neural crest cells are the sources of smooth muscle, which is responsible for supporting numerous bodily tissues. Neural crest cells are special because they migrate during the development of the embryo. For this reason, neural crest cells are the source of many tissues found throughout the body. In particular, neural crest cells are essential for the regulation of blood vessels and the development of smooth muscle throughout the body. Multiple vascular smooth muscle cell lineages can give rise to vascular diseases with potentially site-specific localization, making this a medically significant phenomenon. Aortic aneurysms and atherosclerosis, for instance, frequently manifest at particular vascular sites. This used to seem to be connected to the underlying vessel structure and hemodynamics. Nonetheless, there is mounting evidence that suggests the embryonic lineage of smooth muscle cells may influence the location and manifestation of certain diseases. The growth of the endothelium network is also significantly influenced by smooth muscle cell development. Mural cells, also known as vascular smooth muscle cells, are crucial for the growth and stability of arteries. Mural cells encircle larger vessels and have a major impact on blood flow regulation, endothelial network expansion, and vessel stability. On the other hand, little is understood about how their developmental beginnings or the signaling pathway leading to vessel development influence each other. A key goal for vascular tissue engineering and therapeutic revascularization is the development of vascular smooth muscle cells.

4.2.3. Organ Systems Involved

The smooth muscle cell ranges in length and thickness from 20 to 200 μm. Most myofilaments are found in the eosinophilic cytoplasm. During contraction, the nucleus at the center takes on a cigar shape. Similar to T-tubules in skeletal muscle, the cell membrane forms caveolae. A basal lamina connects smooth muscle cells to surrounding connective tissue. Smooth muscle fibers are grouped in branching bundles, creating a complex system rather than a strictly parallel structure like skeletal muscle. This results in greater contractile power. Actin and myosin filaments are positioned between dense bodies in the cytoplasm and attachment plaques at the cell membrane. Intermediate filaments like vimentin and desmin support the cell structure (Figure 4.3).

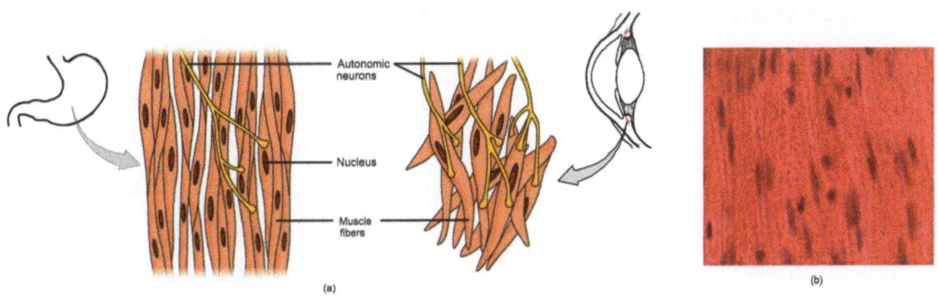

Figure 4.3. *Smooth muscle structure.*

Source: https://courses.lumenlearning.com/suny-ap1/chapter/smooth-muscle/.

Smooth muscle contraction is stopped by myosin light chain dephosphorylation. Smooth muscle is phosphorylated during activation, in contrast to skeletal muscle, which poses a potential challenge because lowering calcium levels alone won't cause muscle relaxation. On the other hand, smooth muscle relaxation is brought about by the dephosphorylation of the myosin light chains, which is the result of myosin light chain phosphatase (MLCP). The nitric oxide mechanism is a significant clinical aspect of smooth muscle relaxation. Nitric oxide synthase in endothelial cells produces nitric oxide, which diffuses from the endothelium into smooth muscle cells. The enzyme guanylyl cyclase is then bound to and activated by nitric oxide, which causes guanosine triphosphate (GTP) to be converted to cyclic guanosine monophosphate (cGMP). When cGMP levels in smooth muscle cells rise, cGMP-dependent protein kinase is stimulated. This, in turn, activates MLCP, which causes myosin light chain dephosphorylation and ultimately smooth muscle relaxation.

The membrane potential that starts or modifies contraction distinguishes smooth muscle action potentials from other types of potentials. Therefore, a variety of stimuli, such as local humoral factors, hormones in circulation, or mechanical stimulation such as stretching of the cells, can activate the graded membrane response. Smooth muscle action potentials can last nearly fifty times longer than skeletal action potentials, but they are slower. This feature seems to arise from the fact that smooth muscle cells' calcium channels open more slowly than those in skeletal muscle. This, in turn, causes the smooth muscle to repolarize slowly because potassium channels react slowly as well. The smooth muscle membrane may also contain sodium channels, which work by speeding up depolarization and assisting in the activation of calcium channels. Additionally, certain smooth muscle cells exhibit the capacity to generate a pacemaker current on their own. For example, the interstitial cells of Cajal maintain this pacemaker current in the intestines. The pacemaker current is an example of multiple-cycle, repetitive oscillations in the membrane potential. The intestines do not contract because of these slow waves of membrane potential fluctuation, which makes them special. Certain voltage-gated calcium channels appear to become active at resting membrane potential, and at some threshold, an influx of calcium will cause a slow wave to propagate. L-type calcium channels will open in response to a sufficiently high slow-wave amplitude, causing contraction. Sodium may contribute to the electrical activity oscillations. An influx of sodium results from the stimulation of Na-Ca exchange by calcium influx, which in turn raises the rate of the Na-K pump. Because the slow-wave activity and membrane potential oscillations occur independently of the central nervous system, this activity is still unique. As a result, the slow waves enable the smooth muscle to maintain its tonicity without requiring constant action potential firings.

Smooth muscle can contract without an action potential, according to research. Action potentials rarely occur in multi-unit smooth muscle. The smooth muscle in the iris of the eye serves as an illustration, wherein ACh and norepinephrine produce a depolarization known as a junctional potential. In these circumstances, the contraction is brought about by changes in the smooth muscle that are brought about by the neurotransmitters themselves. Eventually, an influx of calcium through L-type channels is triggered by the junctional potential. Certain G-proteins that are activated by neurotransmitters can then activate phospholipase C, which produces IP3, which can then cause the sarcoplasmic reticulum to release calcium. It might be necessary to use long-lasting smooth muscle contractions. If smooth muscle contractions happened similarly to skeletal muscle, the metabolic demand of a prolonged contraction would be far too expensive. As intracellular ATP supplies are exhausted, the muscle would probably tire. The process known as the latch state enables the smooth muscle to sustain high tension at low energy consumption. The tone of smooth muscle will not decrease even when phosphorylated myosin light chain kinase levels do.

4.2.4. Related Testing

Anti-smooth muscle antibodies (ASMA) are serum markers that can become elevated in some forms of autoimmune disease. They are typically associated with autoimmune hepatitis but may also increase in primary sclerosing cholangitis and systemic lupus erythematosus. The antibodies direct themselves against actin, troponin, and tropomyosin.

4.2.5. Pathophysiology

Below is a summary of how smooth muscle pathologies can impact various organ systems. A large portion of the content is also relevant to illnesses that aren't covered in this article. Being able to identify the moments in which smooth muscle may contribute to the course of a disease is increasingly crucial for clinicians. Smooth muscle is primarily responsible for motility in the gastrointestinal tract. Any harm to the intestinal smooth muscle could have disastrous consequences for the body. This loss of motility is known as gastroparesis. Numerous illnesses, such as nerve dysfunction, collagen disease, muscular dystrophies, amyloidosis, thyroid disease, diabetes mellitus, Chagas disease, neuropathy, and so forth, can affect stomach motility. These patients can have a wide range of illnesses; they could show up asymptomatic or in a crisis with a functional stomach blockage. Any time a stomach problem appears, one should always be suspicious of possible effects on smooth muscle physiology.

Within the renal system, vascular smooth muscle can be found in the bladder, ureters, and kidneys. Vascular smooth muscle dysfunction is linked to end-stage renal disease at the kidney level and is associated with chronic kidney disease.

Nephrolithiasis is one example of how damage to the ureters can also harm smooth muscle and compromise ureter function. Nearly all of the bladder's functions are dependent on the special qualities of smooth muscle. Damage to any of the bladder's regulatory systems that control smooth muscle can result in loss of tone and neurogenic bladder disease; the complexity of this condition increases when you take into account how much of an impact it has on a person's quality of life. Regarding its function in childbirth, smooth muscle in the genital system is frequently discussed. The uterus is lined with smooth muscle, which produces the contractile force during childbirth. There are numerous medications on the market designed expressly to improve smooth muscle contraction at birth. Even though this might not be a true pathology, it's important to understand that doctors can use their understanding of smooth muscle physiology to stop diseases from developing.

The smooth muscle contractions in the vas deferens and epididymis also contribute to fertility in males. Because there is a perceived dearth of knowledge regarding the potential pathologic connections between smooth muscle and infertility, it is crucial to understand that spermatozoa could never aid in fertilization without the contractile nature of smooth muscle. For example, several drugs commonly taken by men affect the contractility of smooth muscles, which may have an effect on fertility. The following are a few examples: nitrates, phosphodiesterase (PDE) inhibitors, nonsteroidal anti-inflammatory drugs, adrenergic receptor agonists and antagonists, psychotropic medications, anticholinergic medications, calcium antagonists, and ACE inhibitors.

4.3. Smooth Muscle: A Stiff Sculptor of Epithelial Shapes

The role of smooth muscle in mechanically shaping epithelia during embryonic development is becoming more widely acknowledged. The mesenchymal tissue known as smooth muscle envelops the epithelia of various organs, such as the intestines, blood vessels, lungs, bladder, ureter, uterus, oviduct, and epididymis. Because smooth muscle is more rigid than the surrounding epithelium, it frequently performs its morphogenetic role by physically preventing the proliferation of an epithelial layer. This restriction causes buckling, which results in mechanical instabilities and epithelial morphogenesis. It appears that smooth muscle cell shortening alone, in the absence of smooth muscle stiffness, is sufficient to drive epithelial morphogenesis. Finding out how smooth muscle develops is essential to comprehending the development of organs that use smooth muscle stiffness as a driver of morphogenesis. Differentiating smooth muscle-like tissues in vivo and in culture is a crucial step in this process. This calls for a thorough understanding of the genetic, anatomical, and functional markers that are used to differentiate similar cell types, such as myofibroblasts and myoepithelial cells, from the various subtypes of smooth muscle, such as vascular versus visceral.

It is now understood that smooth muscle plays a significant role in the morphogenesis of folded and branching organs. Because smooth muscle is a mesenchymal tissue, it can engage in reciprocal signaling with the epithelium to produce intricate patterns of epithelial folds. Additionally, smooth muscle can physically shape epithelia by exerting mechanical forces. Physical mechanisms using smooth muscle can affect changes over longer length scales than morphogen diffusion and may require simpler regulatory schemes than biochemical mechanisms that rely on intricate morphogen gradients. Physical mechanisms can directly induce epithelial folding through mechanical instabilities. For instance, a single buckling event can produce branches throughout an epithelium, starting from a uniform, unbranched tube, by uniformly adjusting the epithelium's proliferation rate with the nearby smooth muscle. However, to specify the location of each branch through local changes in cell shape or proliferation, multiple short-range foci of high morphogen concentration would be needed to create this architecture through diffusion.

Experiments and modeling have been used to study the physical contributions of smooth muscle to tissue morphogenesis in developing organisms, such as the small intestine, esophagus, lung, oviduct, and epididymis. Smooth muscle also appears to support the physical structure of developing organs, as evidenced by the development of aneurysms or dilated epithelial or endothelial tubes in developing blood vessels and ureters when smooth muscle is absent. While the primary function of smooth muscle is contraction, it appears that the morphogenetic effects of smooth muscle are not dependent on smooth muscle cell shortening. Instead, it has been suggested by computational models that a stiff, static smooth muscle layer surrounding the growing epithelium may be the driving force behind epithelial folding. Thus, the characteristic of smooth muscle that appears to be most important for controlling the morphogenesis of epithelial cells is its high mechanical stiffness in comparison to the surrounding epithelium. Building a comprehensive picture of the morphogenetic events requires an understanding of the intricate interplay between physical and biochemical mechanisms in smooth muscle-induced physical mechanisms of morphogenesis. To learn more about how the differentiation of smooth muscle is regulated, a combination of in vivo and cell and tissue culture assays will be needed to further explore these phenomena. The interpretation of these assays is largely dependent on the ability to differentiate between the various smooth muscle-like tissues.

4.3.1. Properties of Smooth Muscle

From the intestines to blood vessels and hair follicles, smooth muscle is an involuntary contractile tissue present in nearly every part of the body. Since at least Galen's time in the second century, people have known that the intestines can move independently. However, Fallopius did not describe the muscle fibers that cause this motion until the sixteenth century, when he grossly dissected the intestines from the stomach. In the early 1700s, Reisseisen discovered muscle fibers in the lung, demonstrating that similar tissues were still being found by gross dissection. Still, until the research of Henle and von Kölliker, there was a great deal of disagreement over whether arteries had a muscle sheath. The histopathologist Henle noticed that the layer of muscle surrounding the arteries lacked the striations characteristic of voluntary muscles. To prove that smooth muscle is comprised of these tissues, Von Kölliker separated the spindle-shaped muscle cells found in the vasculature from those that formed the involuntary muscles of other organs.

Nowadays, tissue expressing α-smooth muscle actin (α-SMA) is classified as smooth muscle. To differentiate between distinct smooth muscle subtypes (vascular versus visceral) or related cell types (myofibroblasts and myoepithelial cells), more precise markers are employed. Certain proteins, contractile function, and histological characteristics like appearance and anatomical location are examples of these markers. Involuntary contraction is the main physiological function of smooth muscle cells. Smooth muscle tissues are made up of multiple cells that contract to cause a variety of movements, such as the peristalsis of food particles moving through the digestive tract or the piloerection of body hair. All cell types can contract in some way using actomyosin, but smooth muscle cells have a unique contractile apparatus made up of actin and myosin isoforms specific to smooth muscle. This apparatus is typically activated by calcium influx, but it does so in a different way than it does for skeletal muscle because calcium influx triggers a signaling cascade that phosphorylates myosin light chain, which in turn activates cross-bridge cycling of myosin heads on actin.

Actomyosin contractility and cytoskeleton rearrangements, such as actin repolymerization, allow smooth muscle cells to contract with both increased and decreased stiffness. A smooth muscle cell's intermediate filament cytoskeleton, which consists of vimentin and desmin, as well as its contractile network of actin fibers and myosin, are what give it its stiffness (figure 4.4). The muscular layer is less stiff than the epithelium, according to atomic force microscopy (AFM) studies on relaxed, dissected embryonic chicken gut sections. However, even when muscle cells are not physically able to shorten, individual smooth muscle cells can become at least twice as stiff as epithelial cells following contractile stimulation. Because individual cells, tissue sections, and short length-scale AFM measurements cannot account for the cellular and matrix organization of native smooth muscle tissue, these measurements most likely underestimate the tissue-scale stiffness of smooth muscle. Stretching smooth muscle tissues does not increase or decrease their force-generating capacity, in contrast to striated muscle. In contrast to skeletal muscle, where the extremely regular configurations of actin and myosin prevent interaction if the cell is stretched or compressed too much, the contractile apparatus's fiber meshwork allows myosin heads to interact with nearby actin filaments regardless of how stretched the cell is. Smooth muscle cells are particularly well-positioned to control epithelial morphogenesis due to their highly developed cytoskeletal network and capacity to maintain stiffness over a range of cell lengths.

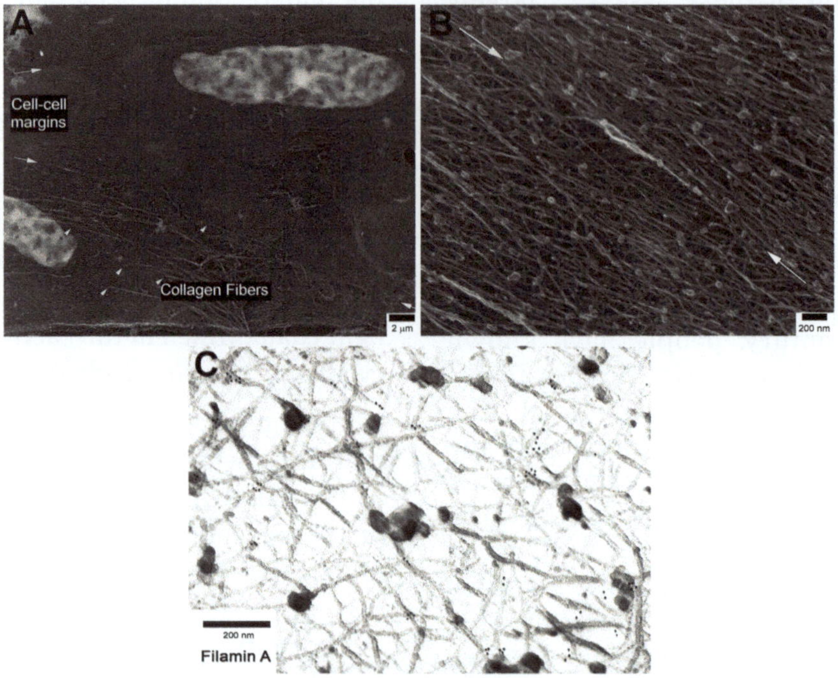

Figure 4.4. *The structure of a smooth muscle cell.*

The contractile apparatus of smooth muscle consists of a meshwork of actin and myosin fibers that undergo cross-bridge cycling upon activation of the cell. This meshwork is interconnected with the cytoskeletal network including intermediate filaments, cell-matrix, and cell-cell adhesions.

Source: Suphamungmee W, Lehman W, Morgan KG. Functional Remodeling of the Contractile Smooth Muscle Cell Cortex, a Provocative Concept, Supported by Direct Visualization of Cortical Remodeling. Biology. 2022; 11(5):662. https://doi.org/10.3390/biology11050662––.

Geometric anisotropy, or the tendency of muscle fibers to orient in one direction within a tissue, is another characteristic of smooth muscle that may help promote morphogenesis. Although it is not evident whether smooth muscle tissues are actually stiffer in that direction, they do shorten predominantly in the direction of their fibers. Significant changes in stiffness anisotropy occur after contraction. Research on the stiffness of individual smooth muscle cells and entire smooth muscle tissues in various organisms has produced contradictory results, with some reporting higher stiffness along the short axis and others reporting stiffer tissues along the long axis of the cells. In terms of embryonic smooth muscle, this is even less well-researched. Multiple smooth muscle layers are found in many organs that contain smooth muscle. These layers are frequently oriented longitudinally and circumferentially, and this may be especially significant in tissues where the different layers differentiate at different times. These characteristics make smooth muscle an efficient tool for reshaping embryonic epithelial tissues, as more research has been done on the physical mechanisms of morphogenesis. The gastrointestinal tract, the lungs, and the reproductive systems of both sexes are where this is most noticeable.

4.3.2. Gastrointestinal System

a) Intestine

The mucosa and its epithelium fold into thousands of projections called villi, increasing the amount of surface area that the gut can absorb nutrients. The mucosa is encircled by two primary smooth muscle layers, an outer longitudinal layer and an inner circular layer, both of which support the motility of the digestive system. The muscularis mucosa, a thin layer of smooth muscle that lies between the mucosa and the submucosa and has less obvious functional significance in adults, is also present (figure 4.5a,b). Although some observers distinguish between distinct inner and outer circular layers in the chicken's circular smooth muscle, this anatomy is similar to that of the mammalian gut. Furthermore, the chicken small intestine lacks the submucosal folds (plicae circulares) found in the human gut, and the chicken submucosal connective tissue is far thinner than the mammalian submucosa (and absent in some parts of the intestine).

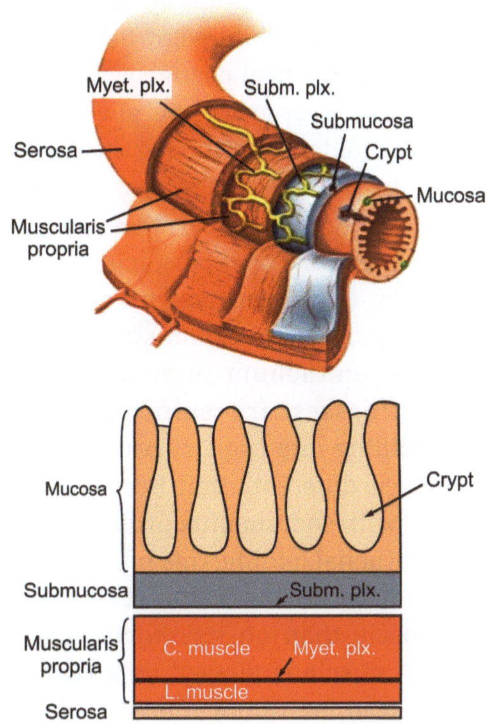

Figure 4.5. *The layered structure of the large intestine.*

Subm. plx. = submucosal plexus; Myet. plx. = myenteric plexus; C. muscle = circular muscle layer; L. muscle = longitudinal muscle layer. Adapted from [44] with permission. Fiber.

Source: Siri S, Zhao Y, Maier F, Pierce DM, Feng B. The Macro- and Micro-Mechanics of the Colon and Rectum I: Experimental Evidence. Bioengineering. 2020; 7(4):130. https://doi.org/10.3390/bioengineering7040130.

The three muscle layers in a White Leghorn chicken embryo develop for a few days. The circular layer forms at embryonic day 8 (E8), the longitudinal layer forms at E13, and the muscularis mucosa forms at E16. Each of these layers is accompanied by morphological changes in the epithelium and, following the appearance of the last muscle layer, the formation of villi. Different chicken breeds have reported different times for these events to occur. Inhibiting smooth muscle differentiation after each differentiation event eliminates the epithelial morphological change. Dissecting the smooth muscle layer from the gut epithelium eliminates the folds, and encasing the epithelium in a silk tube preserves the folded epithelial phenotype, suggesting that this interaction is purely mechanical. This conclusion is supported by computational modeling using finite elements, which demonstrates that the proliferating epithelium and muscle layers' varying stiffnesses are sufficient to cause epithelial folding into the structures seen after smooth muscle differentiation. Because reducing gut motility with sodium nitroprusside does not abrogate epithelial folding, this process appears to depend more on the static stiffness of the smooth muscle than on its shortening. When the smooth muscle is viewed as a rigid, static tissue, the computational model consistently produces epithelial folds. The mechanical model encounters multiple local energy minima en route to the final configuration, despite eventually recapitulating the observed geometry. To prevent these local minima in vivo, the system might need to be disturbed, and smooth muscle contraction might be able to perform this role. Notably, the model is run in stages where the epithelium is subjected to a longitudinal constraint after a circumferential constraint, matching each muscle layer as it differentiates. Smooth muscle plays a crucial role in the morphogenesis of the chicken gut and might also play a role in other organisms. In mice, on the other hand, it appears to have a secondary function to cellular migration in response to a morphogen pattern.

b) Eesophagus

The small intestine and the mammalian esophagus share a similar structure, with the exception that the esophagus lacks villi and has a much thicker epithelial layer. The muscle lining of the esophagus is composed of skeletal muscle in the proximal region, which changes to smooth muscle in the distal region. Each species has a different location for this transition along the esophagus. The mucosa of the esophagus in humans, cattle, and pigs is folded longitudinally in a pattern resembling the initial stages of a chick's gut folding. Numerous studies have looked into longitudinal folding in the esophagus as a straightforward, approachable model for the longitudinal folding of biological tubes generally. Longitudinal folding is a common structural motif throughout the body.

The longitudinal folds of the esophagus remain after death, and they vanish when the mucosa and submucosa are separated from the surrounding musculature. When considered collectively, these findings imply that the surrounding muscle passively contracts the soft mucosa and submucosa, causing mucosal folding. The esophageal folding pattern can be replicated through mechanical modeling, which views the mucosa and submucosa as hyperelastic solids subjected to an external pressure exerted by the smooth muscle. On the other hand, the mucosa is probably multiplying and expanding during development. By representing the mucosa as a tube that grows radially and circumferentially and is bounded by a static muscle layer without constriction from smooth muscle, other models have more accurately simulated the developmental case. In this instance, the number of folds can be computationally adjusted by varying the model's total mucosal and submucosal layer thickness. When the model's mucosal and submucosal thicknesses are matched to those of the bovine esophagus, the number of folds in the esophagus is accurately predicted by the model. According to these studies, the esophageal mucosa can develop longitudinal folds by constraining the proliferating mucosal epithelium inside a stiff, static layer of smooth muscle during development.

4.3.3. Respiratory System

The airway epithelium in the adult mouse lung is surrounded by smooth muscle, which progressively thins and sparsely bundles around the small conducting airways and bronchi. The gut tube buds off the trachea at E9.5, and two bronchial buds soon branch off of the growing trachea during development. Currently, an epithelial tube encircled by mesenchyme surrounds each side of the developing lung. By repeatedly using two branching motifs, terminal bifurcation—where the end of an epithelial tube splits into two new tubes—and domain branching, which occurs when one epithelial tube buds off of the side of another—the epithelium forms the architecture of the mature lung. When the growing branch wraps around the tube, cells in the mesenchyme next to its leading edge differentiate into smooth muscle. For this reason, smooth muscle appears to differentiate along the branch, consistently trailing the tip of the epithelium by a small amount. Before the epithelial tip flattens and eventually forms a cleft at bifurcating branches, smooth muscle cells differentiate. In the process, the epithelium fully bifurcates into two daughter branches. More smooth muscle cells differentiate and form a continuous layer that surrounds the cleft site and extends around the original branch. When the proliferating epithelium is genetically or pharmacologically inhibited from differentiating into smooth muscle, it buckles into intricate, uncontrollable shapes. Epithelial bifurcation is eliminated when smooth muscle fully envelops the bud through enhanced smooth muscle differentiation. Since the smooth muscle causes the bifurcating epithelium to revert to an unbifurcated geometry when it is separated from it, interactions between the epithelium and smooth muscle are most likely primarily mechanical. Isolating the effects of smooth muscle contraction from tissue stiffness is challenging because blocking calcium channels while inhibiting smooth muscle contraction also inhibits smooth muscle differentiation in this system. Considering that airway smooth muscle in adults lacks a defined physiological purpose, its fundamental role in shaping the lung is especially noteworthy (Figure 4.6).

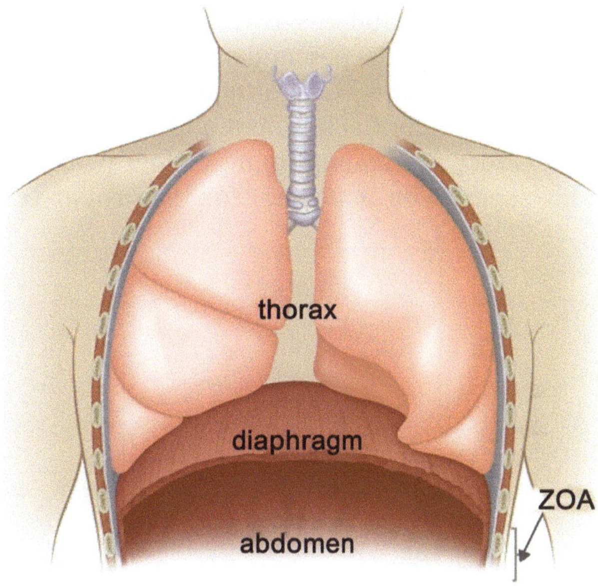

Figure 4.6. *The lung.*

Source: Hu J, Guo R, Li H, Wen H, Wang Y. Perioperative diaphragm dysfunction. Journal of clinical medicine. *2024; 13(2):519. https://doi.org/10.3390/jcm13020519---.*

There is evidence to suggest that domain branching can also be influenced by smooth muscle. Smooth muscle appears to reorganize to make room for new buds to form when they form in an epithelial region that is already covered in it. Future research is necessary to ascertain whether mechanics plays a part in this process, as it is still unknown how smooth muscle in this system influences branching. Lastly, the longitudinal folds of the adult respiratory mucosa resemble those of the adult esophagus. Research on the instabilities caused by smooth muscle that cause esophageal folding has suggested that airway folding could be a part of this mechanism as well.

4.3.4. Reproductive System

a) Oviduct

The passageway that connects the ovary to the uterus is called the mouse oviduct, sometimes referred to as the fallopian tube or uterine tube (figure 4.7). Though experimental and computational evidence indicates that the longitudinal folds in both organs arise through a common mechanism—mechanical instabilities in a proliferating epithelium constrained by a static sheath of smooth muscle—it has deeper and more complex longitudinal folds than the esophagus. The oviduct's structure is quite straightforward: a circular and a longitudinal smooth muscle layer directly encircles a folded epithelium and a thin layer of mucosal connective tissue. Since ciliated cells of the oviduct are mainly found at fold peaks and fold loss is linked to infertility in humans, these folds seem to be important for the proper transport of eggs and sperm along the oviduct.

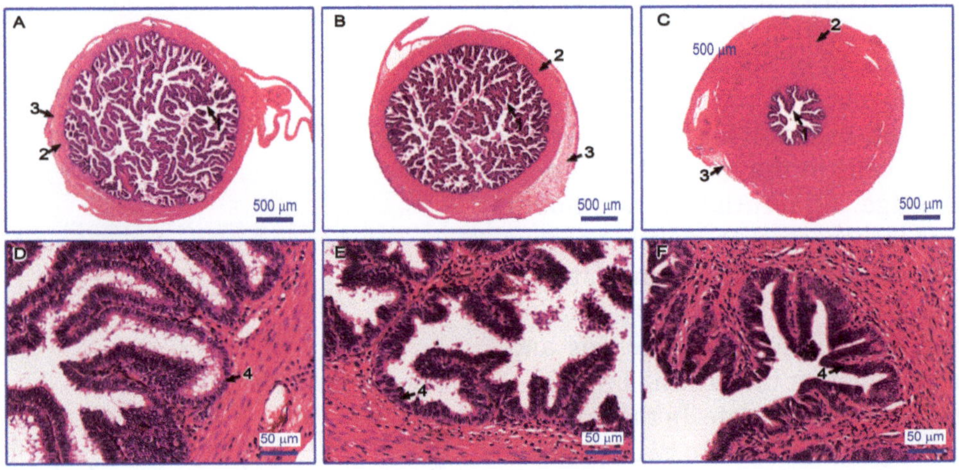

Figure 4.7. *Representative sections of porcine oviducts stained with hematoxylin and eosin. (A) the infundibulum, (B) the ampulla, (C) the isthmus, (D–F) epithelium lining the mucosal folds, in the infundibulum, the ampulla and the isthmus, respectively. Arrows: 1: mucosal folds, 2: muscle layer, 3: serosa, and 4: simple columnar ciliated epithelium.*

Source: Budna-Tukan J, Świątły-Błaszkiewicz A, Celichowski P, Kałużna S, Konwerska A, Sujka-Kordowska P, Jankowski M, Kulus M, Jeseta M, Piotrowska-Kempisty H, et al. "Biological Adhesion" is a Significantly Regulated Molecular Process during Long-Term Primary In Vitro Culture of Oviductal Epithelial Cells (Oecs): A Transcriptomic and Proteomic Study. International Journal of Molecular Sciences. 2019; 20(14):3387. https://doi.org/10.3390/ijms20143387.

The shape and folding pattern of the adult mouse oviduct are altered during ovulation. Since the smooth muscle layer does not fold with the epithelium, it is possible that the surrounding smooth muscle caused the epithelial folds to form through a buckling mechanism because the epithelium's circumferential length is longer than that of the smooth muscle. Deletions in the planar cell polarity gene Celsr1 cause disordered epithelial cell alignment, disordered longitudinal folding, and the formation of some circumferential folds. The epithelium in these mutants has a longer longitudinal length than the surrounding smooth muscle, whereas in wild-type mice, the lengths of the two tissues are almost equal. These findings suggest that the epithelium's circumferential and longitudinal constriction by smooth muscle may have contributed to the oviduct's morphology. The epithelial folding pattern seen in wild-type oviducts could be replicated using a mathematical model that treated the thin epithelium as a grid of springs inside a stiff smooth muscle cylinder. By lengthening the epithelium's longitudinal axis with its constraining cylinder, this model may also replicate the folding pattern observed in Celsr1-knockout mice. Furthermore, supporting this mechanical perspective, laser ablation experiments verified that the mutant epithelium retracts less than the wild-type epithelium in the longitudinal direction, suggesting that the mutant is under lower longitudinal tension. This is expected if the complex folds of the knockout were caused by the epithelium being compressed longitudinally. Through adjustments to the epithelium's circumference and length with respect to its constraining cylinder, this basic model can further reproduce a variety of intricate folding patterns. It is unclear whether smooth muscle contraction is required for oviduct folding in this system because the mechanical investigations treat the muscle as a stiff boundary constraint once more.

b) *Epididymis*

Sperm travel via the muscular tube known as the epididymis from the testis's efferent ductules to the ductus deferens, also known as the vas deferens. It is made up of smooth muscle that is tightly encircled by a layer of pseudostratified epithelial cells. The lumen of the epididymis does not have folds, in contrast to the uterine and gut tubes. The tube is extremely convoluted, with multiple loops and waves forming. However, this morphology also appears to be the consequence of the growing epithelium being restricted by smooth muscle. The epididymis of a mouse begins at E15.5 as a straight tube. Beginning at the head, the epididymis starts to fold into its twisted pattern, eventually twisting the entire tube by E18.5. Along the length of the epididymis, smooth muscle differentiates during this same time frame. Epithelial uncoiling occurs when the mesenchyme is separated from certain sections of the convoluted epithelium. In addition, the epithelial tube spreads out when the mesenchyme is severed, acting as a spring that is freed from a confining box. According to these findings, the mesenchyme may be mechanically restricting the growing epithelium's longitudinal growth, which would explain epididymal epithelial coiling. The fact that no circumferentially biased pattern of proliferation could explain the coiling and that the head of the epididymis, which folds first, proliferates more quickly than the body or tail lends more credence to this mechanism.

The epididymal epithelium is modeled as a chain of spheres embedded in a viscous mesenchyme in a mechanical model. The growth of the epididymal epithelium is simulated by adding new spheres to the chain at random. This model simulates what happens when growth is limited to the head region, with the head region folding first in the temporal pattern. The wavelength of the epididymal folds in the embryo is widened by blocking smooth muscle differentiation. In other words, the model indicates that smooth muscle contributes mechanically to epididymal folding by raising the effective viscosity of the mesenchyme. Reduction of the mesenchyme's viscosity causes a corresponding increase in wavelength. In this system, the smooth muscle was not specifically modeled as a static tissue; however, it appears to contribute to the development of epididymal structures by passively increasing stiffness instead of actively contracting on the epithelium.

4.3.5. Urinary and Vascular Systems

Even in systems where the mechanical morphogenetic effects of smooth muscle have not been directly investigated, some experimental evidence hints at a possible mechanical role for smooth muscle in determining epithelial architecture.

(a) Urinary system

Urine is transported from the kidneys to the bladder through the ureter, an epithelial tube encircled by thick layers of smooth muscle. Many research endeavors examining the routes preceding the ureter's smooth muscle development have resulted in ureteric smooth muscle knockouts in rodents. While some of these models lack smooth muscle only proximally, others do not develop smooth muscle throughout the entire ureter. These ultimately cause the ureter as a whole or just the proximal ureter to dilate. It is believed that this dilatation occurs when there is no smooth muscle to support peristalsis. However, considering smooth muscle's structural function in other tissues, it's plausible that smooth muscle keeps the ureter from dilating in wild-type mice by providing physical support.

(b) Vascular system

A layer of smooth muscle that lines the vascular endothelium controls blood pressure and blood flow. Medium-sized arteries have more pronounced smooth muscle coats, whereas larger blood vessels, like the aorta, have walls made of elastic and smooth muscle tissue. The thin layers of smooth muscle found in vein walls serve to control the fluid capacitance of the veins. Pericytes, which are sparsely wrapped around the thin endothelia in capillaries, seem to have similar purposes to those of the smooth muscle cells found in larger blood vessels. The vascular smooth muscle cells originate from a variety of developmental processes. For instance, the smooth muscle cells lining the aortic arch originate from neural crest cells that migrate from the folding neural tube, in contrast to the smooth muscle cells of the abdominal aorta, which originate directly from the local mesenchyme. Smooth muscle in adults has a mechanical role in shaping blood vessels: contraction of smooth muscle can support blood vessels against buckling into twisted patterns, which is the opposite of its function in the developing epididymis, and constriction of smooth muscle causes the vascular endothelium to fold similarly to the esophagus. Transgenic mice with reduced vascular smooth muscle recruitment or differentiation have been produced for numerous studies on vascular development. According to these models, smooth muscle mechanically shapes the structure of blood vessels by supporting the walls against dilation under blood pressure. The blood vessels also develop tortuously, and aneurysms and hemorrhages appear diffusely in the embryo. Aneurysms form in the body's microcirculation in models of aberrant pericyte development, indicating that the capillary analog of smooth muscle performs a similar mechanical function.

4.3.6. Smooth Muscle Differentiation

Selecting a particular smooth muscle tissue of interest from histological sections, whole-mount organs, or cultured explants is necessary for additional research on smooth muscle in these systems. These studies represent an important next step toward understanding how smooth muscle directs epithelial architecture downstream of instructions or toward identifying other organs that are mechanically shaped by similar muscle. The smooth muscle in the lung, for instance, differentiates in a specific pattern that propels epithelial bifurcation. However, one crucial aspect of lung morphogenesis remains unclear: how this pattern is established. Here, we provide an overview of markers and assays that are frequently used to differentiate between tissues related to smooth muscle in vivo and in culture, to facilitate these investigations. Typically, smooth muscle is seen on histology as a sheet of elongated, interconnected cells within connective tissue. Due to the absence of the distinctive striations seen in histological sections of cardiac and skeletal muscle, this muscle type is referred to as "smooth." This is because smooth muscle lacks the highly regular, regimented arrangement of skeletal and cardiac muscle sarcomeres, and instead has a contractile apparatus made up of a meshwork of contracting actin and myosin filaments. The adult's smooth muscle tissues are well-known, so identifying smooth muscle in anatomical areas known to contain it—like the wall of the bladder or the area surrounding the epithelium of the airway—usually only requires observing a sheet of cells expressing α-SMA. Some additional distinct markers have been found, though, to help differentiate smooth muscle cells from other related cell types, particularly in differentiation or cell sorting experiments or early in embryonic development when the final tissue architecture is still developing. Serum response factor (SRF) is one of the signaling molecules or transcription factors that are associated with the cytoskeleton or contractile machinery, whereas the majority of smooth muscle markers are proteins like α-SMA, smooth muscle myosin heavy chain (smMHC), transgelin, calponin, or meta-vinculin.

However, other cell types, such as myofibroblasts and myoepithelial cells, express the traditional smooth muscle markers. Like fibroblasts, myofibroblasts are found in the stroma of numerous organs and produce extracellular matrix. Myofibroblasts, in contrast to fibroblasts, multiply and produce matrix when epithelia are damaged. They also use their contractile qualities to pull on the damaged site, reducing its area. Myofibroblasts are involved in the development of organs as well. For example, they lay down a matrix that directs the growth of pulmonary alveoli. Whereas smooth muscle typically forms larger tissues of many cells in the stroma, myofibroblasts are typically found within stromal tissue as single cells. Myoepithelial cells are a component of the epithelium in glands that secrete secretions, like the mammary and salivary glands. They express both smooth muscle and epithelial markers there, living between the basement membrane, which divides the epithelium from the underlying stroma, and the secretory epithelial layer. They aid in expelling the gland's exocrine products by contracting. Because they are located above the epithelial basement membrane and express E-cadherin and other epithelial markers, these cells can be distinguished from smooth muscle.

Even within the smooth muscle itself, there is a great deal of variation: visceral smooth muscle, which lines internal organs like the gut, is not the same as vascular smooth muscle, which lines blood vessels. Even vascular smooth muscle from various vascular beds, such as the aorta, pulmonary artery, and coronary arteries, exhibits distinct phenotypic variations. Furthermore, because of its extensive research into the pathophysiology of asthma, the smooth muscle that envelops the epithelium of the lung's larger airways—known as airway smooth muscle, or ASM—is treated differently from visceral smooth muscle. Several markers have been found to differentiate between these cell types in light of this heterogeneity. For instance, smoothelin, which has two isoforms, A and B, is only expressed in smooth muscle cells and not in myofibroblasts. The longer isoform, smoothelin B, is found in vascular smooth muscle, whereas the shorter isoform, smoothelin A, is found in visceral smooth muscle and ASM. Furthermore, vascular smooth muscle expresses hairy/enhancer-of-split related with YRPW motif-like protein (HEYL), whereas ASM expresses noggin. These genes' reporters have been used to identify between these tissues as the lungs develop. These markers are used to identify cells that have differentiated into smooth muscle during embryonic development, along with information on cellular morphology, tissue structure, and contractile function (Tablle 4.1).

Table 4.1. *Table Representing the Expression of Different Integrin Subunits, Their Implication in Smooth Muscle Cell (SMC) Function and Disease Conditions Such as Atherosclerosis and Neointimal Hyperplasia, and Integrin-Directed Drugs Used in Clinics. Collagen, Col; Laminin, LN; Fibronectin, Fn; Vascular Cell Adhesion Molecule, VCAM; Osteopontin, OPN; Tenascin, TN; Vitronectin, VN; Fibrinogen, Fib; EDA, Extra Domain A*

Integrin	ECM	SMC Expression	SMC Function	Implication in Atherosclerosis/ Restenosis	Integrin-Targeting Agents in Clinics
α1β1	Col 1-IV, LN	High expression in resting SMCs. Downregulated in culture conditions and during neointimal hyperplasia	Promotes SMC adhesion and contractile phenotype	$\alpha_1\beta_1$ deletion induces a stable plaque phenotype	SAN-300
α2β1	Col 1 and IV, LN	Undetectable levels in normal human SMCs, and high expression in cultured SMCs	promote chemotaxis of arterial SMCs	$\alpha_2\beta_1$ deletion had no effect on atherosclerosis	Vatelizu-mab
α3β1	Col 1, Fn, and LN	Detectable levels in normal human SMCs, and high expression in cultured SMCs	No conclusive reports		
α4β1	Cellular-Fn, VCAM, OPN	Undetectable levels in normal human SMCs, expressed in SMCs in culture and in intimal atherosclerotic thickening	Induction of SMC differentiation	blocking $\alpha_4\beta_1$ prevents neointimal hyperplasia	Natalizu-mab AJM300
α5β1	Fn and LN	Low levels in normal human SMCs, and high expression in cultured SMCs and during neointimal hyperplasia	Promote SMC proliferation and migration	Mediates early atherosclerosis	Volocixi-mab ATN61
α7β1	LN	High levels in normal SMCs, and low expression in synthetic SMC	Promotes contractile SMC phenotype	α7 deletion promotes neointimal hyperplasia	No conclusive reports

α8β1	Fn, TN, VN	Overexpressed in SMCs that display a contractile phenotype low expression in synthetic SMC phenotype and during neointimal hyperplasia	Promotes contractile SMC phenotype. Prevents SMC proliferation and migration	α8 deletion aggravates intimal thickening	No conclusive reports
α9β1	Fn-EDA, TN, VCAM	Expression increases in synthetic SMC phenotype	Promotes SMC proliferation, migration, and synthetic phenotype.	α9 deletion prevents NH	ASP5094
αvβ1	VN, Fn	Weakly expressed in normal SMCs, and upregulated in SMCs cultured on fibronectin	Inhibits contractility in SMC exposed to serum	No conclusive reports	PLN-74809 PLN-1474
αvβ3	VN, OPN, Fn	Weakly expressed in normal SMCs, and upregulated in SMCs cultured on fibronectin and during neointimal hyperplasia	Promotes SMC adhesion, proliferation and migration	Promotes neointimal hyperplasia	LM609, Abcixi-mab (c7E3Fab; ReoPro), Vitaxin, Intetumu-mab, Cillengitide
αvβ5	Fib, Fn, OPN VN	highly abundant in cultured SMCs, upregulated upon vascular injury	Promotes SMC adhesion and migration	Promotes neointimal hyperplasia	LM609 Intetumu-mab

Source: Jain M, Chauhan AK. Role of Integrins in Modulating Smooth Muscle Cell Plasticity and Vascular Remodeling: From Expression to Therapeutic Implications. Cells. *2022; 11(4):646. https://doi.org/10.3390/cells11040646*

A Closer Look

Muscle Fatigue

Muscle fatigue is a complex phenomenon characterized by a decline in muscle performance during sustained or repeated contractions. Understanding the mechanisms underlying muscle fatigue involves exploring both central and peripheral factors that contribute to this phenomenon.

Peripheral fatigue refers to processes occurring within the muscle itself, while central fatigue involves changes in the central nervous system's ability to drive muscle contraction.

One key peripheral factor contributing to muscle fatigue is the depletion of energy stores, particularly adenosine triphosphate (ATP), phosphocreatine (PCr), and glycogen. ATP is the primary energy source for muscle contraction, and its availability is crucial for sustaining muscle activity. During prolonged or intense exercise, ATP and PCr levels can become depleted, leading to impaired muscle function and fatigue. Similarly, glycogen depletion in muscle fibers can limit the availability of glucose for energy production, further contributing to fatigue.

Additionally, the accumulation of metabolites such as lactate, hydrogen ions (H+), and inorganic phosphate (Pi) can interfere with muscle function and contribute to fatigue. Lactate, produced during anaerobic metabolism, can lower intracellular pH, impairing enzyme function and muscle contractility. Elevated levels of H+ ions can also inhibit key enzymes involved in ATP hydrolysis and calcium release, leading to impaired muscle function. Furthermore, the accumulation of Pi can interfere with cross-bridge cycling and reduce the force-generating capacity of muscle fibers.

Central fatigue involves changes in the central nervous system (CNS) that impair the ability to voluntarily activate motor units and generate force. This can occur due to alterations in neurotransmitter release, neuromuscular junction function, or the excitability of motor neurons. During prolonged exercise, the CNS may perceive fatigue based on sensory feedback from muscle receptors, such as muscle spindles and Golgi tendon organs, as well as from metabolic and hormonal changes circulating in the bloodstream. As a result, there may be a reduction in the neural drive to the muscles, leading to decreased muscle activation and force production.

Summary

- The human body contains three main types of muscular tissue: skeletal, cardiac, and smooth. Smooth muscle is a type of non-striated muscle that is common in the walls of hollow organs and blood vessels.
- Smooth muscle is present all over the body, serving various functions. In the stomach and intestines, it aids in digestion and nutrient absorption. It can be found in the urinary system, where it helps eliminate toxins and maintains electrolyte balance.
- Smooth muscle differs from skeletal muscle in function. Unlike skeletal muscle, smooth muscle is capable of maintaining tone for extended periods and often contracts involuntarily. At a cellular level, smooth muscle can be described as an involuntary, non-striated muscle.
- Smooth muscle is derived from both mesoderm and neural crest cells. This is because smooth muscle contributes to many different tissues throughout the body. One unique feature of neural crest cells is their migration that occurs during embryological development.
- Smooth muscle, so-named because the cells do not have visible striations, is present in the walls of hollow organs (e.g., urinary bladder), lining the blood vessels, and in the eye (e.g., iris) and skin (e.g., arrector pili muscle).
- A dense body is analogous to the Z-discs of skeletal muscle, anchoring the thin filaments in position. Calcium ions are supplied primarily from the extracellular environment.
- Muscle contraction continues until ATP-dependent calcium pumps actively transport Ca^{++} ions out of the cell or back into the sarcoplasmic reticulum. However, a low concentration of calcium remains in the sarcoplasm to maintain muscle tone.
- Smooth muscle consists of two types: single-unit and multi-unit. Single-unit smooth muscle consists of multiple cells connected through connexins that can be stimulated in a synchronous pattern from only one synaptic input.
- Smooth muscle is present throughout the body, where it serves a variety of functions. It is in the stomach and intestines, where it helps with digestion and nutrient collection. It exists throughout the urinary system, where it functions to help rid the body of toxins and works in electrolyte balance.

References

1. Bargehr, J., Low, L., Cheung, C., Bernard, W. G., Iyer, D., Bennett, M. R., Gambardella, L., & Sinha, S. (2016). Embryological origin of human smooth muscle cells influences their ability to support endothelial network formation. *Stem Cells Translational Medicine, 5*(7), 946–959. https://doi.org/10.5966/sctm.2015-0316.
2. Bolton, T. B., & Large, W. A. (1986). Are junction potentials essential? Dual mechanism of smooth muscle cell activation by transmitter released from autonomic nerves. *Quarterly Journal of Experimental Physiology, 71*(1), 1–28.

3. Fernandes, D. J., McConville, J. F., Stewart, A. G., Kalinichenko, V., & Solway, J. (2004). Can we differentiate between airway and vascular smooth muscle? *Clinical and Experimental Pharmacology and Physiology, 31*(11), 805–810. https://doi.org/10.1111/j.1440-1681.2004.04084.x.

4. GISSI-3: Effects of lisinopril and transdermal glyceryl trinitrate singly and together on 6-week mortality and ventricular function after acute myocardial infarction. Gruppo Italiano per lo Studio della Sopravvivenza nell'infarto Miocardico. (1994). *Lancet, 343*(8906), 1115–1122.

5. Giuseppe, C., Paul, J., & Hans-Ulrich, I. (2015). Use of nitrates in ischemic heart disease. *Expert Opinion on Pharmacotherapy, 16*(11), 1567–1572. https://doi.org/10.1517/14656566.2015.1052807.

6. Goss, C. M. (1968). On movement of muscles by Galen of Pergamon. *The American Journal of Anatomy, 123*(1), 1–26. https://doi.org/10.1002/aja.1001230102.

7. Hellstrom, M., Kalen, M., Lindahl, P., Abramsson, A., & Betsholtz, C. (1999). Role of PDGF-B and PDGFR-beta in recruitment of vascular smooth muscle cells and pericytes during embryonic blood vessel formation in the mouse. *Development, 126*(13), 3047–3055.

8. Hirashima, T. (2014). Pattern formation of an epithelial tubule by mechanical instability during epididymal development. *Cell Reports, 9*(2), 866–873. https://doi.org/10.1016/j.celrep.2014.09.041.

9. Hrousis, C. A., Wiggs, B. J., Drazen, J. M., Parks, D. M., & Kamm, R. D. (2002). Mucosal folding in biologic vessels. *Journal of Biomechanical Engineering, 124*(3), 334–341. https://doi.org/10.1115/1.1489450.

10. Jackson, W. F., & Boerman, E. M. (2018). Voltage-gated Ca^{2+} channel activity modulates smooth muscle cell calcium waves in hamster cremaster arterioles. *American Journal of Physiology. Heart and Circulatory Physiology, 315*(4), H871–H878. https://doi.org/10.1152/ajpheart.00292.2018

11. Kim, H. Y., Pang, M. F., Varner, V. D., Kojima, L., Miller, E., Radisky, D. C., & Nelson, C. M. (2015). Localized smooth muscle differentiation is essential for epithelial bifurcation during branching morphogenesis of the mammalian lung. *Developmental Cell, 34*(6), 719–726. https://doi.org/10.1016/j.devcel.2015.08.012.

12. Kim, H. Y., Varner, V. D., & Nelson, C. M. (2013). Apical constriction initiates new bud formation during monopodial branching of the embryonic chicken lung. *Development, 140*(15), 3146–3155. https://doi.org/10.1242/dev.093682.

13. Koyama, H., Shi, D., Suzuki, M., Ueno, N., Uemura, T., & Fujimori, T. (2016). Mechanical regulation of three-dimensional epithelial fold pattern formation in the mouse oviduct. *Biophysical Journal, 111*(3), 650–665. https://doi.org/10.1016/j.bpj.2016.06.032.

14. Li, B., Cao, Y. P., & Feng, X. Q. (2011). Growth and surface folding of esophageal mucosa: A biomechanical model. *Journal of Biomechanics, 44*(1), 182–188. https://doi.org/10.1016/j.jbiomech.2010.09.007.

15. Pogoda, K., Kameritsch, P., Mannell, H., & Pohl, U. (2019). Connexins in the control of vasomotor function. *Acta Physiologica, 225*(1), e13108. https://doi.org/10.1111/apha.13108.

16. Shyer, A. E., Tallinen, T., Nerurkar, N. L., Wei, Z., Gil, E. S., Kaplan, D. L., Tabin, C. J., & Mahadevan, L. (2013). Vilification: How the gut gets its villi. *Science, 342*(6155), 212–218. https://doi.org/10.1126/science.1238842.

17. Sinha, S., Iyer, D., & Granata, A. (2014). Embryonic origins of human vascular smooth muscle cells: Implications for in vitro modeling and clinical application. *Cellular and Molecular Life Sciences, 71*(12), 2271–2288. https://doi.org/10.1007/s00018-013-1520-8.

18. Varner, V. D., Gleghorn, J. P., Miller, E., Radisky, D. C., & Nelson, C. M. (2015). Mechanically patterning the embryonic airway epithelium. *Proceedings of the National Academy of Sciences of the United States of America, 112*(30), 9230–9235. https://doi.org/10.1073/pnas.1504102112.

19. Volckaert, T., & De Langhe, S. (2014). Lung epithelial stem cells and their niches: Fgf10 takes center stage. *Fibrogenesis & Tissue Repair, 7*(8). https://doi.org/10.1186/1755-1536-7-8.

20. Wenzel, S. E., & Balzar, S. (2006). Myofibroblast or smooth muscle: Do in vitro systems adequately replicate tissue smooth muscle? *American Journal of Respiratory and Critical Care Medicine, 174*(3), 364–365. https://doi.org/10.1164/rccm.200606-755ED.

21. Williams, D. M., & Rubin, B. K. (2018). Clinical pharmacology of bronchodilator medications. *Respiratory Care, 63*(6), 641–654.

22. Yan, J., Zhang, L., Xu, J., Sultana, N., Hu, J., Cai, X., Li, J., Xu, P. X., & Cai, C. L. (2014). Smad4 regulates ureteral smooth muscle cell differentiation during mouse embryogenesis. *PLOS ONE, 9*(8), e104503. https://doi.org/10.1371/journal.pone.0104503.

Chapter 5

CARDIAC MUSCLE

Contents

Introduction

Within vertebrates, cardiac muscle is one of the three main muscle types that are exclusive to the heart. Sarcomeres, which are contractile units, are a feature that sets cardiac muscle apart from smooth muscle, the third major muscle type, but it also unites cardiac muscle with skeletal muscle, another major muscle type. Unlike skeletal muscle, cardiac muscle is not controlled voluntarily and exhibits rhythmic contractions. As the heart's pacemaker, the sinoatrial node controls the heart's rhythmic contraction of cardiac muscle. Myocardium, or cardiac muscle cells, make up the majority of the heart. The heart's contractility, which underpins its pumping action, and the rhythmicity of its contractions are what make its action so remarkable. To meet the metabolic needs of peripheral tissues, including the skeletal muscles, kidneys, brain, skin, liver, heart, and gastrointestinal tract, the heart pumps different amounts of blood per minute or cardiac output. The contractile force produced by the cardiac muscle cells and their frequency of activation (rhythmicity) determine the cardiac output. The heart's ability to pump blood normally and adapt to variations in demand is largely dependent on the parameters influencing the frequency and force of heart muscle contraction.

The heart's highly branched cellular network is made up of cardiac muscle cells. The heart's chambers are encircled by layers of myocardial tissue, which are arranged and linked end to end by intercalated disks. The contraction of individual cardiac muscle cells results in force and shortening of these muscle bands, which in turn causes the heart chamber size to decrease and blood to be ejected into the pulmonary and systemic vessels. The longitudinal sarcoplasmic reticulum and terminal cisternae, the mitochondria, and the plasma membrane in alignment with the Z lines are crucial elements of every cardiac muscle cell involved in excitation and metabolic recovery processes. Sarcomeres extend from Z line to Z line and are arranged into contractile units with thick (myosin) and thin (actin, troponin, and tropomyosin) protein filaments. These units have a distinctive cross-striated pattern resembling that of skeletal muscle. Heart contraction rate and the coordination of atrial and ventricular contraction needed for effective blood pumping are determined by the electrical characteristics of cardiac muscle cells and the flow of electrical signals throughout the heart. The muscle's activation, or action potential, is separated into five stages. The permeability of the plasma membrane to potassium (K^+), sodium (Na^+), and calcium (Ca^{2+}) ions varies with time, resulting in the formation of each phase of the action potential.

Orientation and Directional Terms:

Term	**Definition**	**Illustration**
Cardiac cells	Cardiac cells are striated and consist of sarcomeres just like the skeletal muscle. Unlike skeletal muscle, cardiac fibres branch and interdigitate.	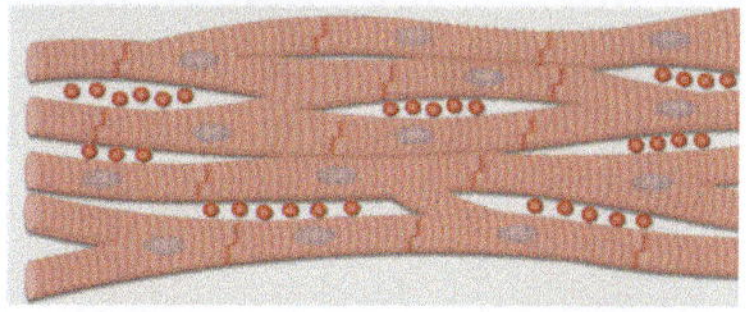
Cardiomyocyte	Cardiomyocytes contain many more mitochondria than skeletal muscle cells reflecting the dependence of cardiac muscle cell on aerobic metabolism.	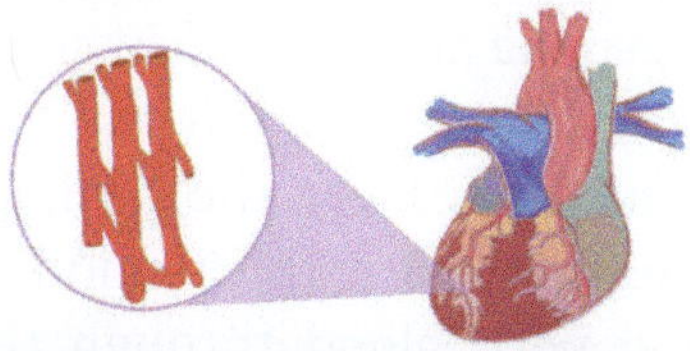
Central nuclei	The central nucleus of the amygdala is a roughly spherical cell group located in the rostral and dorsomedial aspect of the amygdaloid complex.	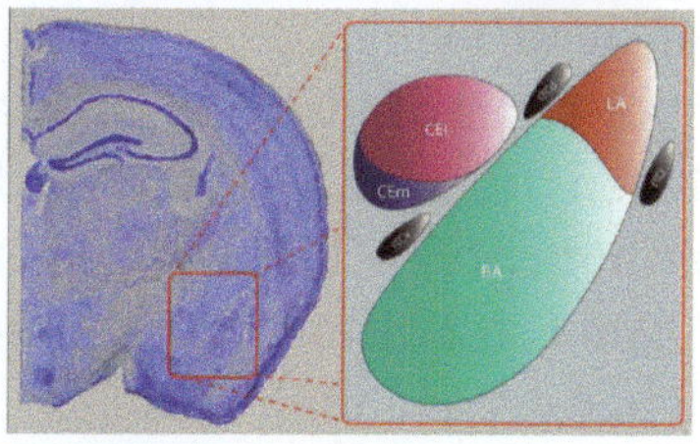
Coronary veins	Coronary veins return deoxygenated blood back to the heart. Smaller veins fuse to become a large, thin-walled vein, coronary sinus, on the posterior surface of the heart emptying directly into the right atrium.	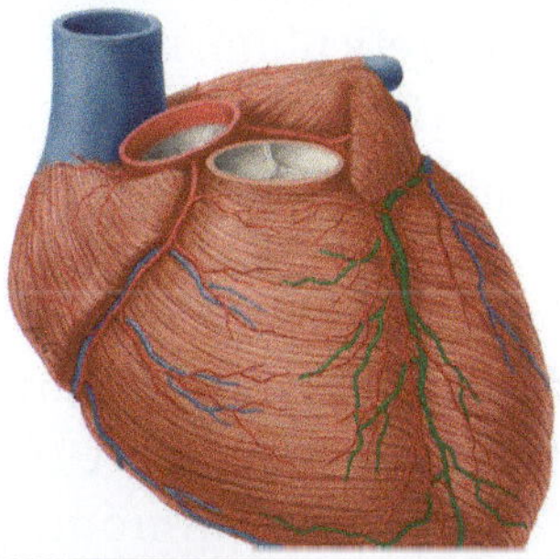
Myocardium	Myocarditis is inflammation of the heart muscle, called the myocardium. The condition can reduce the heart's ability to pump blood.	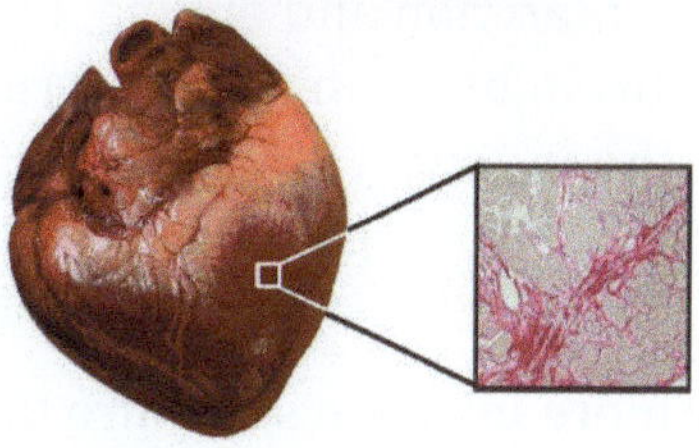

5.1. Basics of Cardiac Muscle

Two other types of vertebrate muscle tissues are smooth muscle and skeletal muscle. Cardiac muscle is also referred to as heart muscle or myocardium. The primary tissue of the heart wall is made up of this striated, involuntary muscle.

Between the pericardium, which is the outer layer of the heart wall, and the endocardium, which is the inner layer, the cardiac muscle, or myocardium, forms a thick middle layer that is supplied with blood through the coronary circulation. It is made up of separate cardiac muscle cells connected by intercalated discs, with collagen fibers and other extracellular matrix components encasing the cells. Although there are some significant distinctions, the way that cardiac and skeletal muscles contract is similar. The internal calcium store of the cell, the sarcoplasmic reticulum, releases calcium in response to electrical stimulation, specifically a cardiac action potential. The cell's myofilaments slide past one another as a result of an increase in calcium, a phenomenon known as excitation-contraction coupling. Cardiomyopathies—diseases affecting the heart muscle—are extremely significant. Among them are myocardial infarction and angina, two ischemic disorders brought on by a constricted blood supply to the muscle.

5.1.1. Structure

With a far more intricate structure than skeletal muscle, cardiac muscle is very different from the latter. While skeletal muscles can only contract, cardiac muscles can also relax. Consequently, compared to skeletal muscles, cardiac tissue will have a far more irregular morphology. The sarcoplasmic reticulum, which houses the calcium ions required for cell contraction, is connected to cardiac muscle cells via T tubules. Encircling and safeguarding the heart and its related structures is the myocardium, a thin but resilient membrane. An epicardium, myocardium, and endocardium make up the three layers of the heart wall. All four heart chambers and the heart valves are lined with tissue called the endocardium. In addition to covering any gaps in this layer, the epicardium forms a thin layer on top of the heart's exterior surface.

5.1.1.1. Gross Anatomy

The majority of the heart is made up of cardiac muscle, or myocardium. With a thick layer of myocardium positioned between the inner endocardium and the outer epicardium (also referred to as the visceral pericardium), the heart wall is a three-layered structure. Along with lining the cardiac chambers and covering the cardiac valves, the inner endocardium also connects to the endothelium that lines the blood vessels that supply the heart. The epicardium is located on the outside of the myocardium and is a component of the pericardial sac, which envelops, shields, and lubricates the heart. Cardiomyocytes, or cardiac muscle cells, are found in multiple sheets within the myocardium. In relation to the epicardium, the muscle sheets that encircle the left ventricle closest to the endocardium are oriented perpendicularly. To squeeze the most blood out of the heart with each heartbeat, the ventricle can squeeze in three directions at once when these sheets contract in unison: longitudinally (becoming shorter from apex to base), radially (becoming narrower from side to side), and twistingly (like wringing out a damp cloth).

Heart muscle requires a steady flow of blood to supply oxygen and nutrients because it expends a lot of energy during contraction. The coronary arteries supply blood to the myocardium. The aortic root is the source of these, which are located on the heart's exterior, or epicardial surface. The right atrium then receives blood flow from the coronary veins (Figure 5.1).

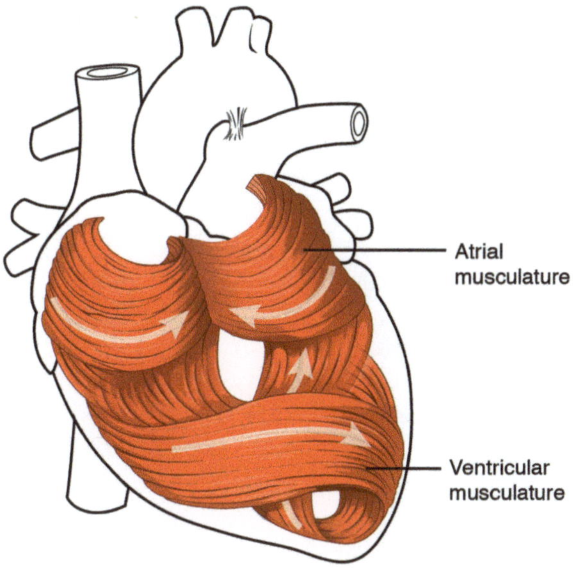

Figure 5.1. *Differently oriented cardiac muscle fibers.*

Source: https://upload.wikimedia.org/wikipedia/commons/thumb/0/0e/2006_Heart_Musculature.jpg/800px-2006_Heart_Musculature.jpg.

5.1.1.2. Microanatomy

The contractile myocytes of the heart muscle are known as cardiomyocytes or cardiac muscle cells. The extracellular matrix that surrounds the cells is made by the fibroblast cells that support them. The pacemaker cells are specialized modified cardiomyocytes that regulate the heart's contractions. Without sarcomeres, the pacemaker cells are only weakly contractile. Instead, they are connected to nearby contractile cells by gap junctions. The primary pacemaker, the sinoatrial node, is situated close to the superior vena cava entrance on the right atrium wall. The atrioventricular node contains additional pacemaker cells (secondary pacemaker). The impulses that cause the heart to beat are carried by pacemaker cells. They perform many tasks and are dispersed throughout the heart. They are in charge of their ability to produce and release electrical impulses on their own. They also need to be capable of picking up on and reacting to brain electrical impulses. The ability to transmit electrical impulses from one cell to another is the last requirement. Smaller and conduct at a slower rate between the cells are the pacemaker cells found in the atrioventricular and sinoatrial nodes. The Purkinje fibers and the specialized conductive cells in the bundle of His have a bigger diameter and conduct signals more quickly. Purkinje fibers can swiftly conduct electrical signals; veins and a capillary network remove waste products; coronary arteries supply muscle cells with nutrients.

The heart's pumping action is facilitated by the contraction of cardiac muscle cells. For the heart to pump blood effectively, each cardiomyocyte must contract in unison with the cells nearby, forming a functional syncytium. If this unison is disrupted, the heart may not contract at all, as might happen in irregular heart rhythms like ventricular fibrillation. Heart muscle cells are approximately rectangular in shape when viewed under a microscope, measuring between 100 and 150 μm by 30 and 40 μm. Long fibers are created by intercalated discs connecting individual cardiac muscle cells at their ends. Myofibrils are specific actin and myosin protein contractile fibers that slide past one another in every cell. Sarcomeres are the basic contractile units of muscle cells, and these are arranged into groups. Under a microscope, the striated or striped appearance of cardiac muscle cells is similar to that of skeletal muscle due to the regular organization of myofibrils into sarcomeres. The lighter actin-based I bands and the darker myosin-based A bands are what cause these striations. T-tubules, which are membrane-bound sacs that extend from the surface of cardiomyocytes to their interior, aid in enhancing the contraction's efficiency. These cells are not like skeletal muscle cells, which have many nuclei; most of them have just one nucleus (some may have two central nuclei). The numerous mitochondria found in cardiac muscle cells give the cell the adenosine triphosphate (ATP) energy it needs to function, which helps the cells withstand fatigue (Figure 5.2).

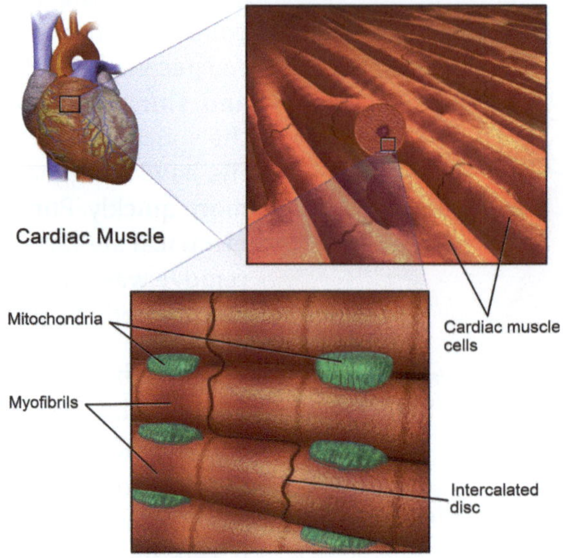

Figure 5.2. *Cardiac muscle.*

Source: https://upload.wikimedia.org/wikipedia/commons/thumb/7/73/Cardiac_Muscle.png/800px-Cardiac_Muscle.png.

5.1.1.3. T-tubules

T-tubules are tiny tubes that extend from the cell's surface to its interior. They share the same phospholipid bilayer, are continuous with the cell membrane, and are exposed to the extracellular fluid that envelops the cell at its surface. Compared to skeletal muscle, cardiac muscle has fewer, larger, and more numerous T-tubules.

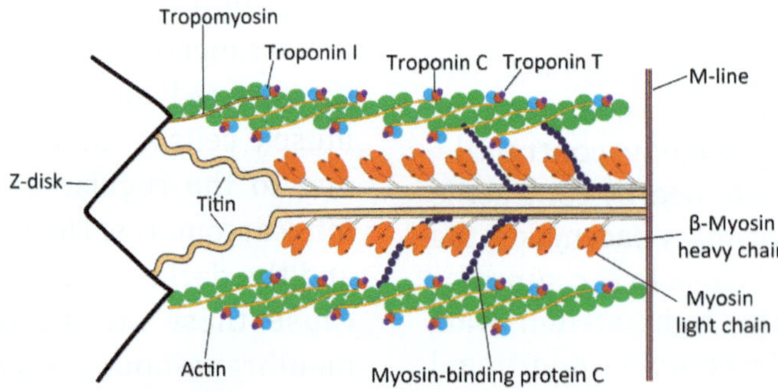

Figure 5.3. *Cardiac sarcomere structure.*

Source: https://upload.wikimedia.org/wikipedia/commons/thumb/7/7f/Cardiac_sarcomere_structure.png/1280px-Cardiac_sarcomere_structure.png.

They unite at the cell's center and form a transverse-axial network that runs into and through the cell. They are located close to the sarcoplasmic reticulum, the cell's internal calcium store. In this instance, a single tubule forms a diad with a terminal cisterna, a portion of the sarcoplasmic reticulum. T-tubules perform a variety of tasks for cells, such as quickly transmitting electrical impulses from the cell surface to the interior known as action potentials and assisting in the excitation-contraction coupling process, which controls the amount of calcium present in the cell. As demonstrated by cell contraction-induced T-tubular content exchange (advection-assisted diffusion), which was validated by confocal and 3D electron tomography observations, they are also involved in mechano-electric feedback (Figure 5.3).

5.1.1.4. Intercalated Discs

To facilitate the quick transmission of electrical impulses throughout the network and allow the cardiac syncytium to act in a coordinated contraction of the myocardium, the cardiomyocytes are arranged in a network connected by intercalated discs. The heart's connection fibers link the two syncytia, the atrial and ventricular. Ion diffusion is made possible by the extremely low electrical resistance across intercalated discs. Since ions move so easily along the axes of cardiac muscle fibers, action potentials can pass through cardiac muscle cells with very little resistance. The law of all or none is followed by every syncytium (Figure 5.4).

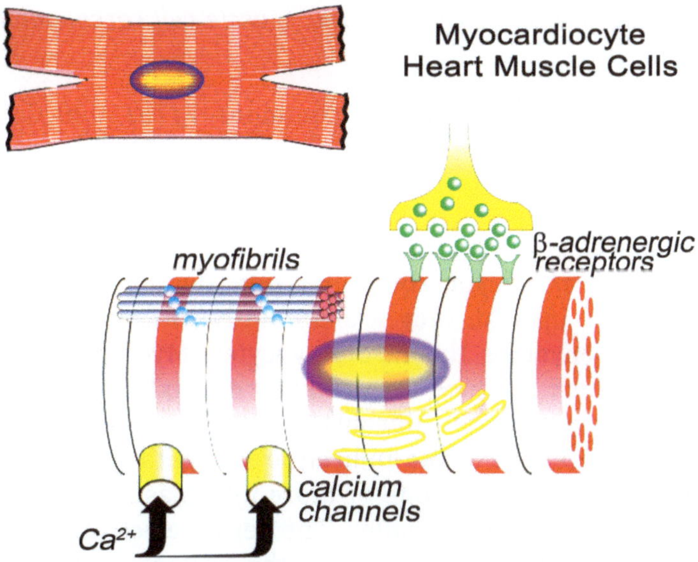

Figure 5.4. *Illustration of a cardiac muscle cell.*

Source: https://upload.wikimedia.org/wikipedia/commons/c/c6/Myocardiocyte.png.

Unlike skeletal muscle, which develops into a multicellular syncytium during embryonic development, intercalated discs are intricate adhering structures that link individual cardiomyocytes to an electrochemical syncytium. The primary mechanism for transmitting force during muscle contraction is the discs. The actin filament anchoring fascia adherens junctions, the intermediate filament anchoring desmosomes, and gap junctions are the three types of cell-cell junctions that make up intercalated discs. They cause the heart muscle to depolarize and allow ions to move between cardiac cells, which in turn allows action potentials to propagate amongst them. Together, the three different types of junctions form a single area composita. Intercalated discs are thin, dark-staining lines that appear to divide adjacent cardiac muscle cells under light microscopy. The direction of the intercalated discs is opposite to that of the muscle fibers. An intercalated disc's path appears more complicated when viewed under an electron microscope. This could show up as a tangled electron-dense structure covering the location of the hidden Z-line at low magnification. With both longitudinal and transverse areas appearing in the longitudinal section, the intercalated disc's path appears even more twisted when magnified at a high magnification (Figure 5.5).

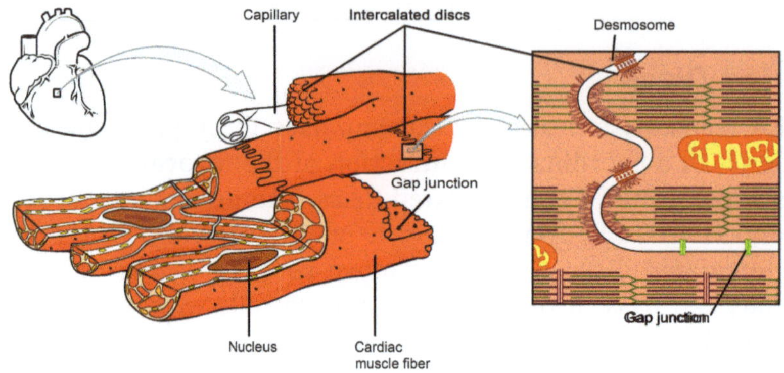

Figure 5.5. *Intercalated discs are part of the cardiac muscle cell sarcolemma and they contain gap junctions and desmosomes.*

Source: https://upload.wikimedia.org/wikipedia/commons/7/7e/1020_Cardiac_Muscle.jpg.

5.1.1.5. Fibroblasts

Heart fibroblasts are essential cells that provide support to the heart muscle. Fibroblasts are essential in the response to injury, such as a myocardial infarction, because they cannot contract with the same force as cardiomyocytes. Instead, they are primarily in charge of forming and preserving the extracellular matrix that envelops the cardiomyocytes. Myofibroblasts, which behave like a cross between fibroblasts (which produce extracellular matrix) and smooth muscle cells (which can contract), can develop from activated fibroblasts after an injury. By producing collagen and slowly contracting to bring the edges of the injured area together, fibroblasts can heal an injury in this way. Cardiomyocytes can only hold one or more fibroblasts at a time. Fibroblasts are more numerous than cardiomyocytes but are smaller. The term "electrically coupled" refers to their ability to modify the electrical currents that cross the surface membrane of a cardiomyocyte. This phenomenon was first demonstrated in vitro in the 1960s and, with the aid of optogenetic techniques, was ultimately verified in native cardiac tissue. Fibroblasts may also play a role in the electrical insulation of the heart conduction system and in cell transformation into adipocytes and cardiomyocytes, among other cell types.

5.1.1.6. Extracellular Matrix

The fibroblasts and cardiomyocytes are surrounded by extracellular matrix (ECM). The extracellular matrix (ECM) is made up of polysaccharides, or sugar chains, called glycosaminoglycans, and proteins like collagen and elastin. When combined, these compounds provide cardiac muscle with elasticity, strengthen and support the muscle cells, and bind water molecules to the muscle cells to keep them hydrated. Type IV collagen and laminin make up the majority of the basement membrane, which is the matrix that comes into direct contact with the muscle cells. Cardiomyocytes and the basement membrane are connected by integrins, which are specialized glycoproteins.

5.1.2. Development

Cardiomyocytes, or heart muscle cells, are present in all humans at birth and grow larger as the heart expands during childhood development. Less than half of the cardiomyocytes present at birth are replaced during a normal lifespan, despite evidence suggesting that cardiomyocytes are slowly turned over during aging. Individual cardiomyocytes grow not only during normal heart development but also in response to heart disease, excessive exercise (atherosclerosis), and damage to the heart muscle, such as myocardial infarction. A normal adult cardiomyocyte is round, measuring between 10 and 25 μm in diameter and about 100 μm in length. Sarcomerogenesis, or the cellular production of new sarcomere units, is the process that leads to cardiomyocyte hypertrophy. Cardiomyocytes grow through eccentric hypertrophy during heart volume overload. Ventricular dilatation results from the lengthwise extension of cardiomyocytes with constant diameter. The process of concentric hypertrophy is how cardiomyocytes enlarge during heart pressure overload. The heart wall thickens as a consequence of the cardiomyocytes growing in diameter but staying the same length.

5.1.3. Physiology

There are numerous similarities between the physiology of skeletal and cardiac muscle. Both muscle types' main job is to contract, and in both situations, the action potential—a distinctive flow of ions across the cell membrane—marks the start of a contraction. By raising the calcium concentration in the cytosol, the cardiac action potential then causes muscle contraction. The fundamental morphology and function of cardiac muscle are strikingly similar to those of skeletal muscle, and the two muscles are highly organized. For example, individual muscle fibers, which comprise multiple, alternating thick and thin contractile filaments, give each type of muscle its characteristic striated appearance. This is true for both types of muscle. Skeletal and cardiac muscle, however, differ significantly from one another despite their many similarities, which makes each specially adapted to carry out its intended function.

5.1.3.1. Cardiac Cycle

The human heart's activity from the start of one heartbeat to the start of the next is known as the cardiac cycle. It is divided into two phases: the diastole, when the heart muscle refills with blood and relaxes, and the systole when the heart muscle contracts forcefully and pumps blood. The heart immediately expands and relaxes after emptying to take in fresh blood returning from the lungs and other bodily systems. It then contracts once more to pump blood to the lungs and those systems. It is thought that the rest phase is polarized. The ions like calcium, potassium, and sodium are separated by the resting potential at this point in the beat. The ability for automatic or spontaneous depolarization exists in cardiac cells. This is directly related to a membrane that permits sodium ions to gradually enter the cell up until the point at which depolarization is achieved. The depolarization is then followed and extended even further by calcium ions. Repolarization is caused by potassium ions slowly moving out once calcium stops moving inward. The extended refractory period is caused by the CMC membrane's extremely slow repolarization. However, the process by which the cytosolic calcium concentrations increase varies in cardiac and skeletal muscle. The action potential in cardiac muscle is made up of an inward flow of calcium and sodium ions. While the flow of calcium is sustained and provides the plateau phase that is typical of cardiac muscle action potentials, the flow of sodium ions is fast but very brief. A phenomenon called calcium-induced calcium release occurs when a relatively small amount of calcium flows through L-type calcium channels and causes a much larger release of calcium from the sarcoplasmic reticulum. The sarcoplasmic reticulum in skeletal muscle cells is directly coupled to the surface membrane, whereas during an action potential, very little calcium enters the cell. The finding that skeletal muscle fibers can contract without extracellular calcium whereas cardiac muscle fibers need calcium to be present in the solution surrounding the cell to do so serves as an example of this distinction.

According to the sliding filament theory, long protein myofilaments oriented along a cardiac muscle cell's length slide over one another during contraction. Actin, troponin, and tropomyosin are the proteins that make up thin filaments, whereas myosin is the protein that makes up thick filaments. The cell gets shorter and fatter as the thick and thin filaments slide past one another. The protein troponin and tropomyosin bind to calcium ions through a process called cross-bridge cycling, which subsequently reveals important binding sites on actin. Actin can then bind to myosin in the thick filament, causing the thick filaments to pull along the thin filaments. Troponin and tropomyosin cover the actin-binding sites once more when the cell's calcium concentration drops, which relaxes the cell.

5.1.3.2. Regeneration

Heart muscle cells were generally thought to be non-regenerative. That being said, a 2009 report provided evidence to the contrary. At the Karolinska Institute in Stockholm, samples of heart muscle from people born before 1955 were examined by Olaf Bergmann and his colleagues. These individuals had very little cardiac muscle surrounding their hearts, and many of them displayed disabilities as a result of this abnormality. The researchers calculated that a 4-year-old renews roughly 20% of heart muscle cells annually and that approximately 69% of a 50-year-old's heart muscle cells were created after birth using DNA samples from numerous hearts. The identification of adult endogenous cardiac stem cells was announced in the 2000s, and research findings suggested that different stem cell lineages, such as bone marrow stem cells, could differentiate into cardiomyocytes and could be employed as a treatment for heart failure. Other teams were unable to confirm these results, though, and a number of the initial studies were eventually withdrawn due to accusations of scientific fraud.

5.1.3.3. Differences Between Atria and Ventricles

The cardiac ventricles and atria are formed by cardiac muscle. There are some variations even though the muscle tissue in the cardiac chambers is remarkably similar. While the myocardium in the atria is significantly thinner, the myocardium in the ventricles is thicker and can withstand strong contractions. The individual myocytes of the myocardium vary depending on the cardiac chamber. Ventricular cardiomyocytes have a denser T-tubule network and are wider and longer. While atrial myocytes and ventricular cardiomyocytes share similar basic mechanisms for handling calcium, atrial myocytes have a smaller and faster-decaying calcium transient, which leads to an increase in their capacity to buffer calcium. Because each chamber has a different complement of ion channels, the ventricles have longer action potential durations and effective refractory periods. Since atrial cardiomyocytes are the only cells that produce some ion currents, like IK(UR), these cells may be the target of atrial fibrillation treatments.

5.1.4. Clinical Significance

Cardiomyopathies, or diseases affecting the heart muscle, are the main cause of death in industrialized nations. The most prevalent ailment is coronary artery disease, which results in a diminished blood supply to the heart. The development of atherosclerotic plaques narrows the coronary arteries. The angina pectoris syndrome may develop if these narrowings worsen to the point where blood flow is only partially restricted. Usually, this results in chest pain during activity that goes away when you rest. A myocardial infarction or heart attack happens when a coronary artery abruptly narrows or blocks completely, stopping or drastically reducing blood flow through the vessel. If the blockage is not removed as soon as possible through medication, surgery, or percutaneous coronary intervention, a section of the heart muscle may sustain permanent damage and scarring. An abnormally thick (hypertrophic cardiomyopathy), abnormally large (dilated cardiomyopathy), or abnormally stiff (restrictive cardiomyopathy) heart muscle can result from a particular cardiomyopathy. Certain illnesses can be inherited and are brought on by genetic mutations. Even with a regular blood supply, heart muscle can sustain damage. Myocarditis is a condition where the heart muscle becomes inflamed; it is typically caused by a viral infection, but it can also occasionally be caused by the body's immune system. Drugs like alcohol, chronic hypertension or high blood pressure, and irregular heartbeats can also cause damage to the heart muscle. If the damage is severe enough, many of these conditions can impair the heart's ability to pump blood. Heart failure occurs when the heart can no longer pump enough blood to meet the body's requirements. Myocytolysis is the term used to describe severe injury to cardiac muscle cells. It is classified as a coagulative or colliquative form of cellular necrosis (Rehman et al., 2023).

5.2. Anatomy of Thorax – Cardiac Muscle

The heart's thick middle layer is made up of cardiac muscle, also known as the myocardium. Together with skeletal and smooth muscle, it is one of the three different kinds of muscle in the body. An inner endocardium and a thin outer layer known as the epicardium (also known as the visceral pericardium) encircle the myocardium. Cardiac veins remove blood from the heart muscle, while coronary arteries supply it. The individual cells that comprise the cardiac muscle are called cardiomyocytes. The main job of cardiomyocytes is to contract; this produces the pressure required to move blood through the circulatory system. One of the three types of muscles in the human body, the cardiac muscle is located in the heart's walls. Cardiomyocytes are specialized cells that comprise cardiac muscle. Because they resemble fibrils in shape and are long and cylindrical, these cells are also referred to as contractile myofibrils because they contract regularly to maintain blood flow through the heart. The sarcomere is the contractile functional unit of the myofibril. The cells that make up the atria and ventricles of muscles are called cardiomyocytes. Because cardiomyocytes are a type of muscle cell that depends on myosin and actin for contraction, their structure is crucial. Cardiomyocytes can also produce an electrical signal known as an action potential to contract because a membrane containing salt ions surrounds them. The numerous mitochondria in cardiac muscle provide the energy necessary for the muscle's proper operation. Furthermore, unlike skeletal muscles, cardiac muscle fibers lack cross-bands, or T-tubules, which prevents them from storing or releasing calcium ions.

5.2.1. Structure and Function

The heart muscle must contract and relax quickly and involuntarily in order to pump blood throughout the circulatory system. The unique characteristics of cardiac muscle's structure enable it to contract in a coordinated manner and withstand fatigue to achieve this. A cardiac muscle cell, also known as a cardiomyocyte, is a tubular structure made up of chains of rod-like cell components called myofibrils. Sarcomeres, the basic contractile units of muscle cells, are repeated in sections to form myofibrils. Long proteins called myofilaments, which can form both thick and thin filaments, make up sarcomeres. Actin is found in thin myofilaments, while myosin is found in thick myofilaments. When the muscle contracts and relaxes, the myofilaments glide past one another. In a process known as excitation-contraction coupling, this mechanism is triggered by the release of calcium from the sarcoplasmic reticulum (SR) when an action potential is applied to the muscle. Actin and myosin slide past one another to form "cross-bridges," which result in the heart contracting and force being produced. Rectangular, branching cells with a single, centrally located nucleus are known as cardiomyocytes. Skeletal muscle cells, on the other hand, typically have a large number of nuclei. In order to generate large amounts of adenosine triphosphate (ATP) and myoglobin, which stores oxygen to meet the demands of muscle contraction, cardiomyocytes have a large number of mitochondria. When examined under a microscope, the arrangement of thin and thick myofilaments overlapping within the cell's sarcomere gives the impression of being striated, similar to skeletal muscle. Thick, dark A-bands (mostly myosin) with a bright center H-zone and lighter colored I-bands (primarily actin) with a dark center Z line (also called Z disc) connecting the actin filaments give this appearance its distinctive look.

The sarcolemma, a plasma membrane that serves as a partition between the extracellular and intracellular contents, envelops the outside of the cardiomyocyte. T-tubules are the extensions of the sarcolemma into the cardiomyocyte's cytoplasm. They are made up of many proteins, including beta-adrenergic receptors, sodium-calcium exchangers, calcium ATPases, and L-type calcium channels, which enable ion exchange with the extracellular fluid that surrounds the cell. T-tubules run alongside enlarged sections of the sarcoplasmic reticulum known as the terminal cisternae at the Z-line of the cardiomyocyte. This combination of a single T-tubule and one terminal cisterna is known as a diad. In contrast, skeletal muscle forms "triads," which emerge at the A-I junction, by combining two terminal cisternae and one T-tubule. A syncytium of cardiac cells is formed when adjacent cardiomyocytes are connected at their ends by intercalated discs. There are three distinct kinds of cell junctions found in the intercalated disc: gap junctions, desmosomes, and fascia adherens. Using desmosome connections and fascia adherens, the transverse side of the intercalated discs, which runs perpendicular to the muscle fibers at the Z lines, contributes a structural element. Gap junctions on the lateral side of the discs enable intercellular communication by transferring ions from one cardiomyocyte to another without first needing to be expelled into the extracellular space. Due to the low resistance of gap junctions, depolarization can spread quickly throughout the syncytium, facilitating the quick transmission of action potentials that cause the cardiomyocytes to contract in unison in synchrony.

The fact that cardiac muscle fibers have their own autorhythmicity is another unique characteristic. In contrast to skeletal or smooth muscle, which contract only with brain activity, cardiac fibers possess their own pacemaker cells, such as the sinoatrial (SA) node, which depolarizes on its own. These depolarizations happen at a steady rate, but the autonomic nervous system can also send signals to the pacemaker cells that alter the heart rate in response to the body's needs. Phase 0 is characterized by rapid depolarization, which is followed by initial partial repolarization in Phase 1, a plateau period in Phase 2, rapid repolarization in Phase 3, and stabilization at the resting potential in Phase 4. These five steps make up the myocardial action potential. A distinct characteristic of the myocardial action potential that is absent in skeletal muscle is the phase 2 plateau. It is brought on by a calcium influx via voltage-gated L-type calcium channels (also known as dihydropyridine receptors) on the cell surface, which counteracts the effects of potassium efflux from the cell. This calcium inflow is comparatively small and insufficient to initiate contraction on its own. Nevertheless, it sets off a process known as calcium-triggered calcium release, which causes the sarcoplasmic reticulum to release its calcium reserves into the myocyte's myoplasm. The process of myocyte contraction, which is visible with every heartbeat, can then start when the calcium binds to troponin on the thin filament.

5.2.2. Embryology

Among the first organs to develop in utero is the heart. The cardiac muscle develops from the visceral splanchnic mesoderm that envelops the heart tube. After gastrulation, mesodermal cells intercalate between the primitive streak's ectoderm and endoderm germ layers, where signals from the surrounding tissue encourage the growth of cardiac progenitor cells in the lateral plate mesoderm. Between the second and seventh weeks of pregnancy is when the heart develops.

5.2.3. Blood Supply and Lymphatics

Heart muscle needs a steady flow of nutrients and oxygen to meet its energy needs during contraction and relaxation. The coronary arteries, which are the aortic root's initial branches, supply blood to the myocardium. The cardiac veins empty blood into the right atrium via the coronary sinus. Left and right coronary arteries exist. The right ventricle and the bundle of His are supplied by the right coronary artery (RCA), which emerges from the right aortic sinus. The posterior descending artery (PDA), which supplies the AV node, posteromedial papillary muscle, posterior part of the interventricular septum, and the ventricles, arises in 85% of individuals (right dominance). The left aortic sinus gives rise to the left main coronary artery. It divides to form the left anterior descending artery (LAD) and the left circumflex coronary artery (LCX). The LCX supplies the anterolateral portion of the papillary muscle, the SA and AV nodes, and the lateral and posterior walls of the left ventricle. The anterior surface of the left ventricle and the anterior portion of the interventricular septum are supplied by the LAD. A myocardial plexus, which is housed inside the myocardium, is where lymph drains. The myocardial plexus empties into a subepicardial plexus, which gives rise to the left and right coronary trunks, in addition to a subendocardial plexus that receives lymphatics from the ventricles. The brachiocephalic lymph nodes and the thoracic duct are the next stops for lymph that leaves the right side of the heart through the right coronary trunk. The inferior tracheobronchial lymph nodes receive lymph from the left side of the heart's left coronary trunk, which then moves on to the right lymphatic duct.

5.2.4. Nerves

An important regulator of contractility, heart rate, stroke volume, and cardiac output is the autonomic nervous system (ANS). The vagus nerves on the left and right sides supply parasympathetic innervation (CN X). The sympathetic trunk fibers that emerge from the upper segments of the thoracic spinal cord are responsible for sympathetic innervation. Afferent nerves also transmit pain from the heart to the central nervous system and provide feedback on blood chemistry and blood pressure.

5.2.5. Muscles

Cardiac muscle makes up the thick middle

layer of the heart and is surrounded by a thin outer layer called the epicardium or visceral pericardium and an inner endocardium.

5.2.6. Physiological Variants

In the past 20 years, research has identified a large number of genes that cause cardiomyopathies, or diseases of the heart muscle. These genes include those that encode proteins that are involved in the development of sarcomeres in hypertrophic cardiomyopathy (HCM), cell-cell junctions in arrhythmogenic cardiomyopathy (AVC), cytoskeletal and sarcomeres in dilated cardiomyopathy (DCM), and sarcomeres or Z-disks in restrictive cardiomyopathy (RCM).

5.2.7. Surgical Considerations

Cardiopulmonary bypass is a technique used in heart surgery to stop the heart muscle from contracting while keeping the body's tissues and organs supplied with blood and oxygen. The cardiac surgeon is currently attempting to employ less intrusive methods. For instance, a lateral or inferior mini-thoracotomy could be used in place of the median sternotomy. The phrenic nerve (left and right), which runs beneath the pericardium, may sustain iatrogenic injury following cardiac surgery as a result of induced hypothermia. Only a small proportion of patients will experience permanent damage from these lesions, which are characterized by an over-elevation of the diaphragmatic portion, particularly on the left.

5.2.8. Clinical Significance

Heart muscle disorders have a significant global health impact, with ischemic heart disease being the world's leading cause of morbidity and mortality (measured in disability-adjusted life-years, or DALYs). An imbalance between the supply and demand of oxygenated blood for cardiac tissue is a hallmark of irreversible heart disease. This disease usually arises from reduced blood flow to the heart tissue, as in the case of coronary artery atherosclerosis, in which the lumen of a major epicardial artery is blocked by an atherosclerotic plaque, possibly with a superimposed thrombosis. Angina pectoris, acute myocardial infarction, and sudden cardiac death are examples of ischemic syndromes. Ischemia-induced myocardial damage results in an irreversible loss of cardiac function. When there is an adequate blood supply, damage to the heart muscle can also happen. An example of this is myocarditis, or inflammation of the heart muscle, which is primarily caused by a viral infection but can also have a bacterial infection etiology, as well as certain drugs, poisons, or autoimmune disorders. Cardiomyopathies are the collective term for primary heart muscle disorders. These include hypertrophic cardiomyopathy, which has abnormally thick heart walls, restrictive cardiomyopathy, which has abnormally stiff heart walls from conditions like amyloid deposition, and dilated cardiomyopathy, which is characterized by an abnormally large heart. Due to the limited capacity of cardiac muscle cells to regenerate, any damage or injury to these cells can have serious repercussions. However, there is still work to be done in the field of using stem cells to grow cardiac muscle (Rehman et al., 2023).

5.3. Physiology of Cardiac Muscle

Along with smooth muscle and skeletal muscle, the human body consists of three main types of muscles: cardiac muscle, also known as the myocardium. Similar to skeletal muscle, cardiac muscle is composed of sarcomeres, which enable contractility. Nevertheless, cardiac muscle is not under voluntary control like skeletal muscle is. The myocardium, endocardium, and pericardium are the three layers that make up the heart. The endocardium, which forms the inner lining of the heart chambers and valves, is made up of simple squamous epithelial cells and is not the same as cardiac muscle. The epicardium, pericardial space, parietal pericardium, and fibrous pericardium make up the fibrous sac that surrounds the heart. The heart's pumping action and contractility are attributed to the heart's cardiac muscle. The heart needs to pump enough blood and exert enough force during a contraction to meet the body's total metabolic needs. This idea, known as cardiac output, is calculated by multiplying the heart rate by the stroke volume. It is based on the frequency and contractile forces of the heart muscle. The heart's contractility varies in tandem with changes in metabolic demand.

5.3.1. Cellular Level

Cardiomyocytes, or cardiac muscle cells, are branched, striated, packed with mitochondria, and controlled involuntarily. Every myocyte has a single, central nucleus that is encircled by the sarcolemma, a type of cell membrane. Voltage-gated calcium channels are specialized ion channels that are absent from skeletal muscle and are present in the sarcolemma of cardiac muscle cells. Branching fibers linked by intercalated discs containing desmosomes and gap junctions are found in cardiac muscle cells. The heart can function as a pump because of these connections, which enable the cardiomyocytes to contract simultaneously. Electrical coupling is the process by which coordinated action potentials can move from one cardiomyocyte to the next via gap junctions between adjacent cardiomyocytes. Cardiac desmosomes are intercellular structures that serve as anchors for cardiac muscle fibers and are essential for preserving the heart's structural integrity. The sarcomere, which is made up of thick (myosin) and thin (actin) filaments, is the functional unit of cardiomyocyte contraction. The sliding filament theory is based on these interactions. The cardiomyocyte plasma membrane with transverse tubules (t-tubules) is called the sarcolemma. These highly branched releases of the cardiomyocyte sarcolemma, known as t-tubules, are involved in signal transduction, action potential initiation and regulation, excitation-contraction coupling (ECC), and maintaining the resting membrane potential. By concentrating voltage-gated L-type calcium channels and placing them close to calcium sense and release channels, or ryanodine receptors (RyRs), at the sarcoplasmic reticulum's junctional membrane, T-tubules control the cardiac extracellular calcium gradient (ECC).

5.3.2. Development

There are different phases in the heart's development. The beginning of gastrulation is marked by the formation of the primitive streak during embryogenesis, which comes after the invagination of epiblast cells. The embryonic plate, which was initially composed of two layers between the yolk sac and the amniotic cavity, is divided into three germ layers—the ecto-, meso-, and endoderm—by gastrulation. Between the ectoderm and endoderm layers, the mesoderm spreads laterally and cranially during development to form a variety of structures, most notably the heart. In the dorsal mesocardium, the myocardium starts to develop during the second week of pregnancy. Three weeks after conception, the primitive heart starts to form as a straight tube that gradually changes shape. This involves the tube folding, resulting in bulges that resemble the adult heart: the sinus venosus develops into the right atrium (sinus venarum) and coronary sinus; the truncus arteriosus becomes the aorta and pulmonary artery; the bulbus cordis becomes the smooth left and right ventricles; the primitive ventricle becomes the trabeculated LV/RV; and the primitive atrium becomes the trabeculated atria. The heart goes through a cardiac looping process that determines its left-sided orientation around the fourth week of development. A protein called dynein and cilia, a motile structure, work together to accomplish this. The condition known as dextrocardia, in which the heart is positioned on the right side of the chest, will arise if these elements stop working properly. Primary ciliary dyskinesia (PCD) and Kartagener syndrome are common conditions associated with this cardiac defect. As the heart takes on its correct shape, more developmental changes take place. The heart has one chamber at first, but as different septa grow, it divides into four distinct chambers. The membranous septum forms soon after the muscular ventricular septum, which joins the aortic-pulmonary septum as it twists and fuses together at the bottom of the ventricle. At this point, the endocardial cushions also emerge, dividing the left and right ventricles and atria. Birth defects or structural alterations in these processes may result in congenital cardiac disorders.

5.3.3. Function

The main job of cardiac muscle is to generate enough force to pump blood into circulation. Each coordinated contraction is powered by electrical impulses in the cardiac muscle. The heart needs ATP for its contractile activities, and it can be produced by the body using a variety of substrates, such as fatty acids, proteins, carbohydrates, and ketones. The core utilization process is aerobic production, though the heart can occasionally employ anaerobic processes. The cells that make up the cardiac muscle are specialized for pumping and contraction. To pump blood through the heart and into the rest of the body, they contract periodically. A unique type of cell found in cardiac muscles is known as a Purkinje fiber, and it plays a crucial role in the heart's ability to pump electrical impulses to and from the muscle cells.

5.3.4. Mechanism

The cardiac action potential lasts approximately 200 ms and is divided into 5 phases: (4) resting, (0) upstroke, (1) early repolarization, (2) plateau, and (3) final repolarization.

Approximate resting membrane potential (RMP): -90 mV

- Phase 4 – RMP due to activity of the Na/K ATPase pump. The exchange of three sodium ions out for two potassium ions maintains the negative intracellular potential.
- Phase 0 – depolarization to approximately +52 mV due to sodium influx via fast sodium channels
- Phase 1 – partial repolarization due to the closure of fast sodium channels and efflux of potassium and chloride
- Phase 2 – plateau phase maintained by the influx of calcium. Potassium efflux also occurs.
- Phase 3 – repolarization back to RMP due to potassium efflux and closure of sodium and calcium channels

The process of excitation-contraction coupling (ECC) is responsible for the involuntary generation of a cardiac action potential. To depolarize the membrane, action potentials move into the t-tubules via the sarcolemma. During the action potential's plateau phase (phase 2), calcium can enter the cell through L-type (long-lasting) calcium channels thanks to voltage-sensitive dihydropyridine (DHP) receptors on t-tubules. The sarcoplasmic reticulum releases more calcium through the ryanodine receptor in response to an increase in intracellular calcium concentration. This process is referred to as calcium-induced calcium release. When troponin C binds to the released calcium, tropomyosin separates from the actin myosin-binding sites. After myosin and actin create a cross-bridge, contraction takes place. Cross bridges persist as long as troponin is bound to calcium. The word "lusitropy" refers to the myocardium's relaxation after excitation-contraction coupling (ECC). The sarcoplasmic reticulum calcium-ATPase pump, or SERCA pump, is responsible for mediating lusitropy. It works by removing calcium from troponin-C and reestablishing the relaxed state of the myocardium by sequestering calcium into the sarcoplasmic reticulum.

Since phases 1 and 2 are missing, the action potential of pacemaker cells is divided into three phases rather than five, as is the case with cardiac muscle cells. The nodes that make up pacemaker cells are the atrioventricular (AV) and sinoatrial (SA) nodes. These nodes are known to fire on their own initiative, sending electrical activity throughout the heart without the need for stimulation. Funny current channels, which permit sodium ions to continuously leak into the cell (Phase 4), gradually raise the membrane potential until a certain threshold is reached, causing the cell to depolarize, are the cause of this autorhythmicity. The membrane potential is subsequently raised by opening calcium channels, which allows calcium ions to enter the cell (Phase 0). Potassium channels open in response to a positive membrane potential, which causes ions to flow outward and brings the membrane potential back to rest (Phase 3).

5.3.5. Related Testing

Many clinical tests are utilized to evaluate the function of the cardiac muscle. This list discusses high-yield clinical testing and is not meant to be exhaustive.

Echocardiogram: a routine cardiac ultrasound used to detect abnormalities in the heart. Valvular abnormalities, masses, pericardial disease, congenital abnormalities, and pulmonary hypertension can all be evaluated with an echocardiogram. Echocardiography is also frequently used to evaluate the function of the heart muscle and is helpful in the diagnosis of cardiomyopathies and congestive heart failure. Transthoracic echocardiograms (TTEs) and transesophageal echocardiograms (TEEs) are two different types of echocardiograms.

- TTE: a non-invasive test that utilizes an echocardiography probe placed on the chest wall.
- TEE: a specialized probe with an ultrasound transducer at the tip passed into the patient's esophagus, allowing for a posterior view of the heart.

Echocardiogram reports are detailed and offer essential information regarding the heart's function. Echo reports typically include:

- Rate and rhythm
- Chamber size
- Indications of hypertrophy
- Right ventricular function
- Left ventricular systolic function and ejection fraction
- Left ventricular diastolic function
- Valvular pathology (if any)
- Evidence of mass or thrombus
- Congenital abnormalities
- Pericardial anomalies
- Incidental findings

Electrocardiogram (ECG or EKG): an EKG is a non-invasive test that utilizes electrodes placed on the body's surface to record the heart's electrical rhythms. These electrical rhythms cause depolarization of the heart, which, in turn, leads to the contraction of the myocardium. With this knowledge, one can understand that the EKG indirectly indicates the heart's contraction.

Cardiac biomarkers: blood tests may be performed to identify enzymes and proteins that can indicate heart disease or cardiac damage.

- Troponin: measures the levels of cardiac proteins troponin T and troponin I. These proteins are found in cardiac muscle and are released upon damage to cardiac muscle, with troponin I being the more sensitive and specific marker of cardiac injury.

- Creatine kinase (CK): This enzyme is released from cardiac and skeletal muscle following damage. The isozyme CK-MB is more sensitive in diagnosing heart damage after a heart attack, with CK-MB levels rising 4 to 6 hours after a heart attack, peaking at 24 hours, and returning to baseline in 48 to 72 hours.
- Brain natriuretic peptide (BNP): a hormone secreted by the ventricular myocardium in response to ventricular wall stress (i.e., pressure overload or volume expansion). The gold standard in diagnosing heart failure is the measurement of BNP levels, with an elevated level indicating heart failure.

(Rehman et al., 2023)

5.3.6. Pathophysiology

The pathophysiology of cardiac muscle is based on damage to cardiac muscle cells, leading to inappropriate contractility.

Cardiomyopathy: Cardiomyopathies are disorders of the myocardium that are either acquired or genetically based and are linked to heart failure. Distinctive non-ischemic cardiomyopathies include dilated cardiomyopathy (DCM), hypertrophic cardiomyopathy (HCM), restrictive cardiomyopathy (RCM), arrhythmogenic right ventricular cardiomyopathy (ARVC), and unclassified cardiomyopathies, as per the World Health Organization.

- **Dilated cardiomyopathy (DCM):** This condition is characterized by dilation and impaired contraction of one or both ventricles, and it is not attributable to hypertension, valvular disease, or coronary artery disease. Patients with DCM exhibit heart failure symptoms as well as decreased systolic contraction. At least forty distinct genes have been found to have mutations in inherited forms of DCM, many of which encode structural elements of the sarcomere and desmosome. Nongenetic causes of DCM can arise, primarily from viral infections that cause myocardial inflammation. DCM can also result from systemic autoimmune diseases, toxins or allergies, or specific medications.
- **Hypertrophic cardiomyopathy (HCM):** A mutation in the sarcomere protein genes causes this autosomal dominant disease, which results in a thicker (hypertrophied) left ventricle and abnormal heart contraction. The conditions that result from this hypertrophied left ventricle include diastolic dysfunction, mitral regurgitation, myocardial ischemia, and outflow obstruction. Severe circumstances may result in abrupt cardiac death.
- **Restrictive cardiomyopathy (RCM):** This condition results in impaired ventricular filling in the setting of nondilated ventricles. RCM is typically characterized by nondilated nonhypertrophied ventricles, with biatrial enlargement secondary to increased atrial pressures. Diseases in which RCM may be seen include

sarcoidosis, amyloidosis, and hemochromatosis.

- **Arrhythmogenic right ventricular cardiomyopathy (ARVC):** This is the replacement of the myocardium with fibrofatty tissue leading to an increased predisposition to ventricular tachycardia and sudden cardiac death, especially in young adults and athletes. The release of exercise-induced catecholamines provokes ventricular arrhythmias in predisposed individuals. ARVC typically affects the right ventricle.
- **Unclassified cardiomyopathies:**
- *Stress-induced cardiomyopathy (Takotsubo cardiomyopathy):* A condition known as "broken heart syndrome" presents as a reversible transient ballooning of the apex of the left ventricle leading to wall motion abnormalities brought on by severe emotional or physical stress.
- *Cirrhotic cardiomyopathy:* This is a condition of diastolic and systolic dysfunction, impaired cardiac response to stress, and ECG abnormalities (QT prolongation) in patients with cirrhosis. Cardiac function is typically altered only under stressful conditions.
- **Ischemic cardiomyopathy (ICM)** is a form of dilated cardiomyopathy related to coronary artery disease (CAD). ICM is the decreased ability of the heart to properly pump blood throughout the body due to myocardial damage from cardiac ischemia. The lack of blood supply to the cardiomyocytes leads to cell death, cardiac fibrosis, and left ventricular enlargement and dilation. Globally, ischemic heart disease (IHD) is the leading cause of death, with approximately 7.2 million deaths yearly.

Heart Failure: impairment of blood systolic ejection and ventricular filling caused by anatomical and functional defects in the myocardium. In the particular evaluation of heart failure, the left ventricular ejection fraction (LVEF) is essential. Heart failure with preserved ejection fraction (HFpEF) is the diagnosis given to a patient with heart failure whose ejection fraction (EF) is 50% or higher. Heart failure with reduced ejection fraction (HFrEF) is defined as having an ejection fraction of less than or equal to 40%, while heart failure with mid-range ejection fraction (HFmrEF) is defined as having an ejection fraction of 41 to 49%. Clinical significance lies in differentiating between these three forms of heart failure because they require different therapies and drugs.

Myocarditis: an inflammatory disease of the myocardium most commonly caused by acute rheumatic fever or viral infections (Coxsackie virus, parvovirus B19). The long-term outcome of untreated myocarditis is dilated cardiomyopathy with heart failure.

5.3.7. Clinical Significance

In the US and around the world, heart disease is the leading cause of death for both men and women. Myocardial function assessment and the use of interventions to enhance cardiac muscle function and avoid myocardial maladaptations form the foundation of clinical care for patients with heart disease. Individual patients will receive different treatment modalities based on the previously mentioned pathophysiology. Since heart failure is commonplace worldwide, clinicians need to be knowledgeable about the physiology and treatment of this condition. The usual treatments for symptomatic heart failure include digoxin, vasodilators, diuretics, and positive inotropes. A diuretic and a vasodilator, such as an ACE inhibitor or hydralazine plus isosorbide dinitrate, would be the optimal treatment regimen. Digoxin may or may not be used in conjunction with this therapy, depending on how the patient presents. Every patient needs to hear from clinicians about the significance of cardiovascular health. In other words, cardiac muscles become more efficient the stronger they are. Frequent aerobic exercise helps strengthen muscle tissue and improves cardiac muscle health overall, reducing the risk of heart attack and stroke. Running, walking, swimming, cycling, dancing, and stair climbing are examples of aerobic exercise.

5.3.8. Cardiomyopathy

Cardiomyopathy is one of the main conditions that can affect your cardiac muscle tissue. It's a disease that makes it harder for your heart to pump blood.

There are several different types of cardiomyopathy:

- Hypertrophic cardiomyopathy. The cardiac muscles enlarge and thicken for no apparent reason. It's usually found in the lower chambers of the heart, called the ventricles.
- Dilated cardiomyopathy. The ventricles become larger and weaker. This makes it hard for them to pump, which makes the rest of your heart work harder to pump blood.
- Restrictive cardiomyopathy. The ventricles become stiff, which prevents them from filling to their full volume.
- Arrhythmogenic right ventricular dysplasia. The cardiac muscle tissue of your right ventricle is replaced with fatty or fiber-rich tissue. This can lead to arrhythmia, which refers to an abnormal heart rate or rhythm.

Not all cases of cardiomyopathy produce symptoms. However, it can sometimes cause:

- trouble breathing, especially when exercising
- fatigue
- swollen ankles, feet, legs, abdomen, or neck veins

It's usually hard to pinpoint the cause of cardiomyopathy. But several things can increase your risk of developing it, including:

- a family history of cardiomyopathy or heart failure
- high blood pressure
- obesity
- heavy alcohol consumption
- use of certain recreational drugs
- past heart attacks or heart infections

5.3.9. How Does Exercise Impact Cardiac Muscle Tissue?

Exercise can strengthen your cardiac muscle, just like it can many other muscles in your body. In addition to improving heart function, exercise can lower your chance of developing cardiomyopathy. 150 minutes or more of moderate exercise per week is advised by the American Heart Association. Aim for five days a week of roughly 30 minutes of exercise to meet this goal. Regarding exercise style, cardio workouts get their name from the advantages they provide for the heart muscle. Frequent aerobic exercise helps improve the efficiency of your heart's pumping action, lower blood pressure, and lower heart rate. Cardio exercises that are frequently done include swimming, biking, walking, and running. Try these 14 different kinds of aerobic exercise as well. Consult your doctor before beginning any kind of exercise program if you already have a cardiac condition. To prevent overstressing your heart, you may need to take certain precautions (Towbin et al., 2014).

A Closer Look

Cardiomyopathies and Inherited Heart Disorders

Cardiomyopathies encompass a diverse group of heart muscle disorders characterized by abnormalities in cardiac structure and function, often leading to impaired pump function and increased risk of arrhythmias and heart failure. Among the cardiomyopathies, hypertrophic cardiomyopathy (HCM), dilated cardiomyopathy (DCM), arrhythmogenic right ventricular cardiomyopathy (ARVC), and familial cardiomyopathies stand out as significant contributors to cardiovascular morbidity and mortality.

Hypertrophic cardiomyopathy is primarily a genetic disorder characterized by abnormal thickening (hypertrophy) of the heart muscle, typically affecting the left ventricle. Mutations in genes encoding sarcomere proteins, such as beta-myosin heavy chain (MYH7) and cardiac myosin-binding protein C (MYBPC3), underlie the pathogenesis of HCM. The hallmark feature of HCM is asymmetric hypertrophy of the myocardium, leading to dynamic left ventricular outflow tract obstruction, diastolic dysfunction, and increased risk of sudden cardiac death. Clinical manifestations range from asymptomatic individuals to exertional dyspnea, chest pain, syncope, and arrhythmias. Management strategies focus on symptom relief, risk stratification for sudden cardiac death, and prevention of adverse outcomes through lifestyle modifications, pharmacotherapy, and implantable cardioverter-defibrillator (ICD) placement in high-risk individuals.

Dilated cardiomyopathy is characterized by dilatation and impaired contractility of the left ventricle, resulting in systolic dysfunction and heart failure. DCM can be caused by genetic mutations affecting structural proteins (e.g., titin, dystrophin) or sarcomere proteins, as well as non-genetic factors such as viral infections, toxins, and autoimmune diseases. The pathophysiology involves myocyte loss, fibrosis, and chamber enlargement, leading to decreased cardiac output and increased ventricular filling pressures. Clinical manifestations include dyspnea, fatigue, peripheral edema, and arrhythmias. Management strategies focus on optimizing heart failure treatment with medications, cardiac resynchronization therapy (CRT), left ventricular assist devices (LVADs), and heart transplantation in severe cases.

Arrhythmogenic right ventricular cardiomyopathy is an inherited disorder characterized by the progressive replacement of the myocardium with fibrofatty tissue, predominantly affecting the right ventricle. Mutations in desmosomal genes, such as plakophilin-2 (PKP2) and desmoplakin (DSP), disrupt cell-cell adhesion, leading to myocyte detachment and fibrofatty infiltration. The pathophysiology involves electrical instability, arrhythmias, and sudden cardiac death, particularly in young individuals. Clinical manifestations include palpitations, syncope, ventricular tachycardia, and right ventricular dysfunction. Management strategies focus on arrhythmia suppression with antiarrhythmic drugs, catheter ablation, and ICD placement, along with lifestyle modifications and genetic counseling. Familial cardiomyopathies encompass a spectrum of inherited heart disorders with diverse genetic etiologies, including familial DCM, HCM, ARVC, and restrictive cardiomyopathy (RCM). These conditions often exhibit autosomal dominant inheritance patterns, with variable penetrance and expressivity. Genetic testing and counseling are essential for identifying at-risk family members, facilitating early diagnosis, and implementing appropriate management strategies tailored to individual risk profiles.

Summary

- The heart consists mostly of cardiac muscle cells (or myocardium). The outstanding characteristics of the action of the heart are its contractility, which is the basis for its pumping action, and the rhythmicity of the contraction.
- Cardiac muscle, in vertebrates, is one of three major muscle types, found only in the heart. Cardiac muscle is similar to skeletal muscle.
- Electrical stimulation in the form of a cardiac action potential triggers the release of calcium from the cell's internal calcium store, the sarcoplasmic reticulum. The rise in calcium causes the cell's myofilaments to slide past each other in a process called excitation-contraction coupling.
- Cardiac muscle is able to contract and relax, unlike skeletal muscles which only contract. This means that cardiac tissue will have far more irregular shapes than skeletal muscles. Cardiac muscle cells contain T tubules that connect to the sarcoplasmic reticulum which stores the calcium ions needed for the contraction of the cell.
- Pacemaker cells carry the impulses that are responsible for the beating of the heart. They are distributed throughout the heart and are responsible for several functions. First, they are responsible for being able to spontaneously generate and send out electrical impulses.
- T-tubules are microscopic tubes that run from the cell surface to deep within the cell. They are continuous with the cell membrane, are composed of the same phospholipid bilayer, and are open at the cell surface to the extracellular fluid that surrounds the cell.
- The cardiac syncytium is a network of cardiomyocytes connected by intercalated discs that enable the rapid transmission of electrical impulses through the network, enabling the syncytium to act in a coordinated contraction of the myocardium.
- Under light microscopy, intercalated discs appear as thin, typically dark-staining lines dividing adjacent cardiac muscle cells. The intercalated discs run perpendicular to the direction of muscle fibers. Under electron microscopy, an intercalated disc's path appears more complex.
- Cardiac fibroblasts are vital supporting cells within cardiac muscle. They are unable to provide forceful contractions like cardiomyocytes, but instead are largely responsible for creating and maintaining the extracellular matrix which surrounds the cardiomyocytes. Fibroblasts play a crucial role in responding to injury, such as a myocardial infarction.
- The extracellular matrix (ECM) surrounds the cardiomyocyte and fibroblasts. The ECM is composed of proteins including collagen and elastin along with polysaccharides (sugar chains) known as glycosaminoglycans.

References

1. Brakenhielm, E., & Alitalo, K. (2019). Cardiac lymphatics in health and disease. *Nature Reviews Cardiology, 16*(1), 56–68. https://doi.org/10.1038/s41569-018-0106-x.
2. Di Maio, A., Karko, K., Snopko, R. M., Mejía-Alvarez, R., & Franzini-Armstrong, C. (2007). T-tubule formation in cardiac myocytes: Two possible mechanisms? *Journal of Muscle Research and Cell Motility, 28*(4–5), 231–241. https://doi.org/10.1007/s10974-007-9115-9.
3. Forleo, C., Carmosino, M., Resta, N., Rampazzo, A., Valecce, R., Sorrentino, S., Iacoviello, M., Pisani, F., Procino, G., Gerbino, A., Scardapane, A., Simone, C., Calore, M., Torretta, S., Svelto, M., & Favale, S. (2015). Clinical and functional characterization of a novel mutation in lamin A/C gene in a multigenerational family with arrhythmogenic cardiac laminopathy. *PLoS One, 10*(4), e0121723. https://doi.org/10.1371/journal.pone.0121723.
4. Frontera, W. R., & Ochala, J. (2015). Skeletal muscle: A brief review of structure and function. *Calcified Tissue International, 96*(3), 183–195. https://doi.org/10.1007/s00223-014-9915-y.
5. GBD 2016 DALYs and HALE Collaborators. (2017). Global, regional, and national disability-adjusted life-years (DALYs) for 333 diseases and injuries and healthy life expectancy (HALE) for 195 countries and territories, 1990–2016: A systematic analysis for the Global Burden of Disease Study 2016. *The Lancet, 390*(10100), 1260–1344. https://doi.org/10.1016/S0140-6736(17)32130-X.
6. Giacomelli, E., Mummery, C. L., & Bellin, M. (2017). Human heart disease: Lessons from human pluripotent stem cell-derived cardiomyocytes. *Cellular and Molecular Life Sciences, 74*(20), 3711–3739. https://doi.org/10.1007/s00018-017-2576-0.
7. Hong, T., & Shaw, R. M. (2017). Cardiac T-Tubule microanatomy and function. *Physiological Reviews, 97*(1), 227–252. https://doi.org/10.1152/physrev.00037.2015.
8. Huang, W. A., Boyle, N. G., & Vaseghi, M. (2017). Cardiac innervation and the autonomic nervous system in sudden cardiac death. *Cardiac Electrophysiology Clinics, 9*(4), 665–679. https://doi.org/10.1016/j.ccep.2017.07.007.
9. Kanno, S., & Saffitz, J. E. (2001). The role of myocardial gap junctions in electrical conduction and arrhythmogenesis. *Cardiovascular Pathology, 10*(4), 169–177. https://doi.org/10.1016/S1054-8807(01)00096-4.
10. Kolwicz, S. C., Purohit, S., & Tian, R. (2013). Cardiac metabolism and its interactions with contraction, growth, and survival of cardiomyocytes. *Circulation Research, 113*(5), 603–616. https://doi.org/10.1161/CIRCRESAHA.113.302095.
11. Kruithof, B. P., van den Hoff, M. J., Wessels, A., & Moorman, A. F. (2003). Cardiac muscle cell formation after development of the linear heart tube. *Developmental Dynamics, 227*(1), 1–13. https://doi.org/10.1002/dvdy.10291.
12. Mollova, M., Bersell, K., Walsh, S., Savla, J., Das, L. T., Park, S. Y., Silberstein, L. E., Dos Remedios, C. G., Graham, D., Colan, S., & Kühn, B. (2013). Cardiomyocyte proliferation contributes to heart growth in young humans. *Proceedings of the National Academy of Sciences of the United States of America, 110*(4), 1446–1451. https://doi.org/10.1073/pnas.1214608110.
13. Moorman, A., Webb, S., Brown, N. A., Lamers, W., & Anderson, R. H. (2003). Development of the heart: (1) formation of the cardiac chambers and arterial trunks. *Heart, 89*(7), 806–814. https://doi.org/10.1136/heart.89.7.806.

14. Nair, R., & Muthukuru, S. R. (2022). Dextrocardia. In *StatPearls* [Internet]. StatPearls Publishing. Retrieved from: https://www.statpearls.com/ArticleLibrary/viewarticle/25357 (accessed on 25 June 2024).

15. Papakonstantinou, N. A., Sykaras, A. G., Vourlakou, C., Goudevenos, J., Papadopoulos, G., & Apostolakis, E. (2020). Cardioplegic storage solution: Is it the guardian of saphenous vein graft endothelium? *Journal of Cardiac Surgery, 35*(5), 996–1003. https://doi.org/10.1111/jocs.14483.

16. Patel, D. M., & Green, K. J. (2014). Desmosomes in the heart: A review of clinical and mechanistic analyses. *Cell Communication & Adhesion, 21*(3), 109–128. https://doi.org/10.3109/15419061.2014.938351.

17. Rehman, I., Nassereddin, A., & Rehman, A. (2023). Anatomy, thorax, pericardium. In *StatPearls* [Internet]. StatPearls Publishing. Retrieved from: https://www.statpearls.com/ArticleLibrary/viewarticle/30046 (accessed on 25 June 2024).

18. Roth, G. M., Bader, D. M., & Pfaltzgraff, E. R. (2014). Isolation and physiological analysis of mouse cardiomyocytes. *Journal of Visualized Experiments*, (91), e51109. https://doi.org/10.3791/51109.

19. Sallé, L., & Brette, F. (2007). T-tubules: A key structure of cardiac function and dysfunction. *Archives des Maladies du Coeur et des Vaisseaux, 100*(3), 225–230.

20. Schmitt, J. P., Kamisago, M., Asahi, M., Li, G. H., Ahmad, F., Mende, U., Kranias, E. G., MacLennan, D. H., Seidman, J. G., & Seidman, C. E. (2003). Dilated cardiomyopathy and heart failure caused by a mutation in phospholamban. *Science, 299*(5611), 1410–1413. https://doi.org/10.1126/science.1081578.

21. Sedmera, D., & McQuinn, T. (2008). Embryogenesis of the heart muscle. *Heart Failure Clinics, 4*(3), 235–245. https://doi.org/10.1016/j.hfc.2008.03.005.

22. Thompson, B. R., & Metzger, J. M. (2014). Cell biology of sarcomeric protein engineering: Disease modeling and therapeutic potential. *Anatomical Record, 297*(9), 1663–1669. https://doi.org/10.1002/ar.22999.

23. Towbin, J. A. (2014). Inherited cardiomyopathies. *Circulation Journal, 78*(10), 2347–2356. https://doi.org/10.1253/circj.CJ-14-0897.

24. Tran, D. B., Weber, C., & Lopez, R. A. (2022). Anatomy, thorax, heart muscles. In *StatPearls* [Internet]. StatPearls Publishing. Retrieved from: https://www.statpearls.com/ArticleLibrary/viewarticle/31898 (accessed on 25 June 2024).

25. Willott, R. H., Gomes, A. V., Chang, A. N., Parvatiyar, M. S., Pinto, J. R., & Potter, J. D. (2010). Mutations in Troponin that cause HCM, DCM AND RCM: What can we learn about thin filament function? *Journal of Molecular and Cellular Cardiology, 48*(5), 882–892. https://doi.org/10.1016/j.yjmcc.2009.10.031.

Chapter

ABDOMINAL MUSCLE

6

Contents

Introduction

Any of the three flat muscular sheets that make up the anterolateral walls of the abdominal cavity—the transverse, internal, and external oblique muscles—as well as the rectus abdominis muscle, which is added on either side of the midline, are collectively referred to as abdominal muscles. The lower ribs above, the iliac crest and pubis of the hip bone below, and the vertebral column behind are the locations of the first three muscle layers. Their fibers all unite in the direction of the midline, where they sheath the rectus abdominis before meeting the fibers of the opposing side at the linea alba. The crisscrossing of the fibers gives these relatively thin walls strength. The external oblique's fibers are oriented downward and forward, the internal oblique's upward and forward, and the transverse's horizontally forward. All of the aforementioned muscles are fibrous around the rectus abdominis, which runs from the pubis upward to the ribs. The inguinal canal, a passageway through the muscular layers, is formed in the groin area by a specific arrangement of these fibers that sits between the pubic bone and the anterior superior iliac spine. When the testes exit the abdominal cavity through its wall and enter the scrotum in males, this develops at birth. A fibrous cord from the uterus replaces this in females. Inguinal hernias can happen in this gap because it's a weak spot. In addition to providing the viscera with a tonic, elastic muscular support, the muscles of the abdominal walls also retract to pull the rib cage downward during expiration. They stiffen in response to strikes, creating a wall that shields the viscera from harm. These muscles participate in the expulsive actions of urinating, defecating, giving birth, vomiting, coughing, and singing when the glottis is closed and the thorax and pelvis are fixed. They begin to bend the trunk forward when the pelvis is immobilized. Subsequently, gravity sets in, the abdominal muscles loosen up, and the back muscles assume the load. On the other hand, preventing hyperextension involves the abdominal muscles. The lower limbs and pelvis can be raised by the abdominal muscles when the thorax is fixed. The vertebral column can be bent sideways by the muscles on one side, which also helps with rotation.

Orientation and Directional Terms:

Term	Definition	Illustration
Anterolateral	A ligament on the lateral aspect of the human knee, anterior to the fibular collateral ligament.	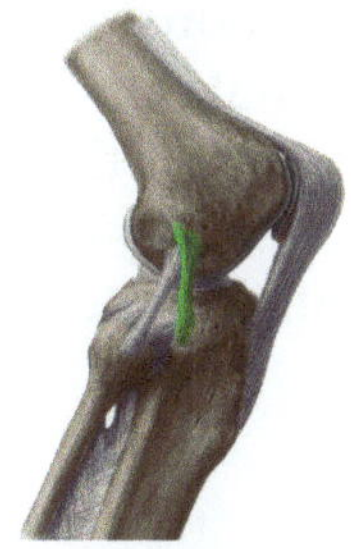
Femoral ring	The femoral ring is the opening at the proximal, abdominal end of the femoral canal, and represents the (superiorly directed/ oriented) base of the conically-shaped femoral canal.	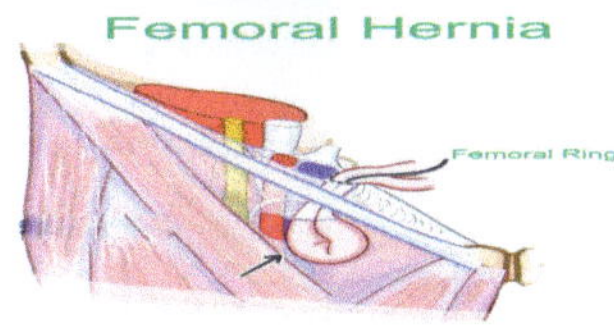
Motor protein	Motor proteins are a class of molecular motors that can move along the cytoskeleton of cells.	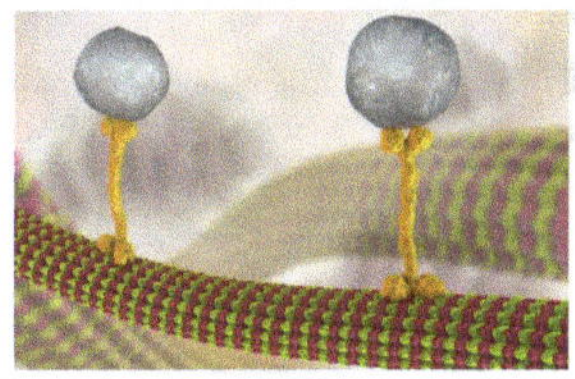
Phospho-rylation	Phosphorylation is the addition of a phosphoryl (PO3) group to a molecule. In biological systems, this reaction is vital for the cellular storage and transfer of free energy using energy carrier molecules.	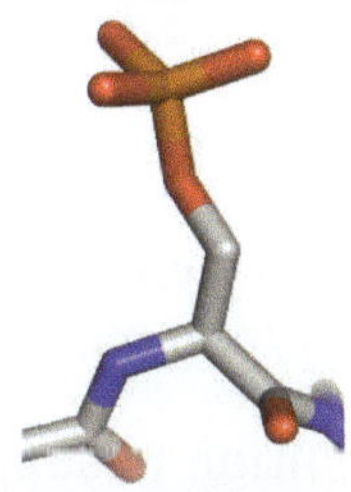
Umbilical hernia	A condition in which the intestine protrudes through the abdominal muscles at the belly button, owing to weakness in the cavity containing it.	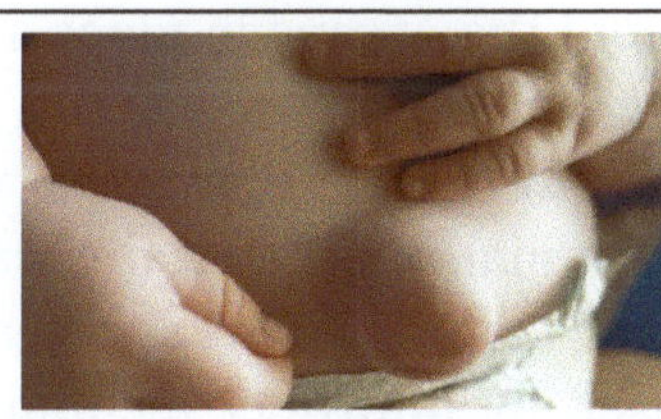

6.1. Anatomy of Abdomen and Pelvis

A section of the trunk that joins the thorax and pelvis is referred to as the abdomen. The viscera and abdominal cavity are enclosed by an abdominal wall made of muscle, fascia, and skin. In addition to housing and shielding the intra-abdominal organs, the abdominal wall can expand, create intra-abdominal pressure, and shift the vertebral column. Surgeons must have a thorough understanding of the anatomy of the abdominal wall to plan surgical access to the abdominal cavity and to comprehend the pathology that affects it. Patients' quality of life may be greatly impacted by congenital or acquired abdominal wall defects (Figure 6.1).

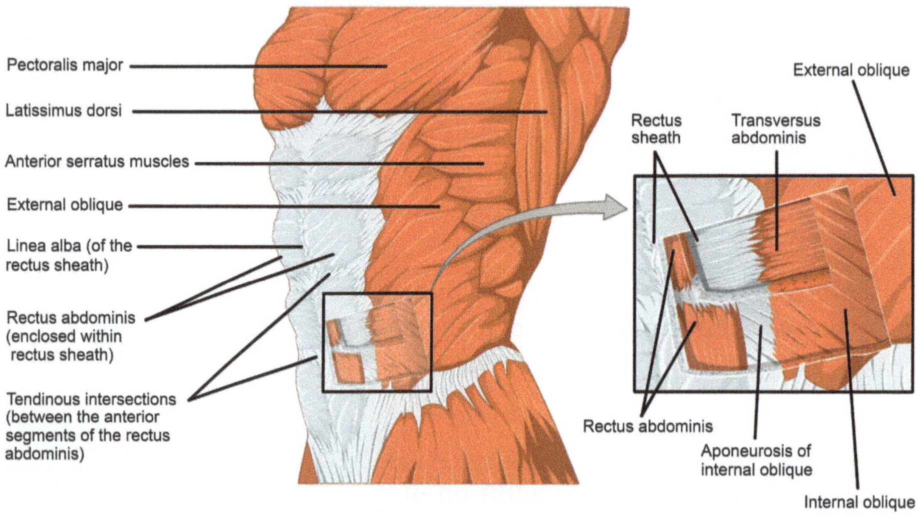

Figure 6.1. *Overview of the muscles of the abdominal wall.*

In addition to supporting the trunk and enabling movement, the abdominal muscles also serve to hold the organs in place and are distensible, or able to adapt to dynamic changes in the volume of the abdominal contents. The intrinsic back muscles and deep abdominal muscles together comprise the core muscles, which support and stabilize the body as well as safeguard the spine. Abdominal muscle strains can result from lifting heavy objects, laughing, sneezing, or coughing, overstretching, overuse, or a violent, poorly executed movement of the trunk. They can also be caused by improper technique when playing sports that require running, twisting, and jumping. The trunk is moved side to side by the coordinated action of the abdominal muscles. Additionally, they preserve the abdominal pressure that holds the organs in place. Also, the muscles in your abdomen aid in breathing. When these muscles contract, the contents of the abdomen are forced upward, placing pressure on the diaphragm. The same motion facilitates coughing and vomiting. A constant internal pressure is maintained by the abdominal muscles. This aids in the retention of the positions of the pancreas, liver, intestines, stomach, and other organs. Your abdominal muscles can compress, raising the pressure inside your abdomen. They aid in stools and urine passage and are utilized during childbirth in this way. Abdominal muscles.

Abdominal muscles are also needed to maintain posture and support your spine.

- **Rectus abdominis.** This pair of muscles lies in front of the abdomen. They arise from the fifth, sixth, and seventh ribs and attach to the pubic bone. These muscles have three horizontal tendons running across their front. These bumps give the "six-pack" appearance.
- **External oblique**. Also known as the obliquus externus abdominis, this muscle arises from the lower eight ribs and attaches to the hip bone. You have two of these muscles, one on each side. These are the outermost muscles of the abdominal wall and help you turn your trunk from side to side.
- **Internal obliques.** Also known as the obliquus internus abdominis, these are paired muscles lying on either side of the abdomen. They lie deeper than the external obliques but outside the transversus abdominis. They arise from the hip bone and attach to the lower six ribs. Along with your external oblique muscles, they enable you to twist and turn your trunk.
- **Transversus abdominis.** This is the deepest of the abdominal muscles. It arises from the lower six ribs and the hip bone and attaches to the pubic crest.
- **Pyramidalis.** This vertical muscle arises from the pubic bone and attaches to the linea alba, a structure between the two rectus abdominis muscles. The pyramidalis lies in front of the rectus abdominis and contributes to maintaining abdominal pressure (Huttinger et al., 2023; Tuma et al., 2023; Seeras et al., 2023; Zahouani & Mendez, 2023).

6.1.1. Structure and Function

The abdomen only has the lower ribs posteriorly and the vertebral column as skeletal support, whereas the thorax and pelvis have more. The superior and inferior pelvic bones are where the abdominal wall joins the skeletal structure. The trunk's flexibility and distensibility to accommodate dynamic changes in the volume of the abdominal contents are made possible by this relative bony deficiency. When performing surgical incisions, it is crucial to comprehend the various layers that comprise the abdominal wall.

From superficial to deep, these layers include:

- Skin
- Subcutaneous tissue, which can further subdivide into:
- Camper's fascia – a superficial fatty layer
- Scarper's fascia – a deep membranous layer
  - o Abdominal muscles, their investing fascia, and aponeuroses
  - o Transversalis fascia
  - o Parietal peritoneum

The abdominal wall carries out several essential tasks. It includes the scaffolding necessary for the growth and operation of the viscera in the abdomen. Each layer helps to shield the organs physically to some extent. Anterolateral and posterior components can be used to broadly categorize the abdominal muscles. The transversus abdominis, rectus abdominis, internal oblique, external oblique, and pyramidalis are the five paired muscles that make up the anterolateral muscles. The quadratus lumborum bilaterally and the psoas major are examples of posterior muscles. The trunk can move in various ways, including flexion, extension, lateral flexion, and rotation, thanks to the abdominal muscles. The production of intraabdominal and intrathoracic pressure, which is essential for sneezing, coughing, vomiting, and defecating, can be facilitated by simultaneous contraction of the abdominal muscles. When lifting large objects, this motion might also aid in stabilizing the trunk. The anterolateral muscles (apart from the transversus abdominis) function as accessory muscles of respiration when there is an increased physiological or pathological demand for airway ventilation. This is achieved by depressing the ribs, which results in active expiration.

Surface Anatomy: To accurately describe examination findings, the external surface of the abdominal wall can be divided into regions. The midclavicular point and the mid-inguinal point are the locations of vertical lines drawn along the midclavicular plane. Horizontal lines can be drawn through the intertubercular plane, which is parallel to the iliac tubercles, and the subcostal plane, which is the most inferior aspect of the anterior thoracic cage. The abdominal cavity is divided into nine regions by these two horizontal and two vertical lines. An alternative method is to draw a horizontal line across the transumbilical plane and a vertical median line that splits the abdomen into four quadrants. During laparoscopic surgery, when the peritoneal space is entered and inflated, the internal surface of the anterior abdominal wall is clearly visible. It is possible to see numerous folds and ligamentous landmarks. Situated along the free edge of the falciform ligament, the ligamentum teres is the vestige of the umbilical vein. After dividing the liver into the right and left anatomical lobes, it passes to the umbilicus by way of the inner surface of the anterior abdominal wall. Below the umbilicus, one can observe five folds or ligaments. The umbilicus to the bladder is connected by the median umbilical ligament, a remnant of the fetal urachus, which is located in the midline. The remnants of severed umbilical arteries are known as the medial umbilical ligaments, which are visible on either side of the median ligament. From the femoral ring to the arcuate line, the inferior epigastric vessels are transmitted by the lateral umbilical folds.

6.1.2. Embryology

The embryo changes morphology from a disc to a fetal shape at 3–4 weeks of gestation. This transition results in the endodermal and mesodermal disc layers folding in the opposite direction to form the gut tube and ventral body wall, and the ectodermal disc layer folding to form the neural tube. The mesoderm gives rise to the musculature and fascia of the abdominal wall. These four primary muscles come to mind when one thinks of abdominal muscles.

1. Transversus abdominis – the deepest muscle layer. Its main roles are to stabilize the trunk and maintain internal abdominal pressure.
2. Rectus abdominis – slung between the ribs and the pubis at the front of the pelvis. When contracting, this muscle has the characteristic bumps or bulges that are commonly called 'the six pack.' The main function of the rectus abdominis is to move the body between the ribcage and the pelvis.
3. External oblique muscles – these are on each side of the rectus abdominis. The external oblique muscles allow the trunk to twist but to the opposite side of whichever

external oblique is contracting. For example, the right external oblique contracts to turn the body to the left.

4. Internal oblique muscles – these flank the rectus abdominis and are located just inside the hip bones. They operate oppositely to the external oblique muscles. An example is twisting the trunk to the left requires the left side internal oblique and the right side external oblique to contract together.

6.1.3. Blood Supply and Lymphatics

The abdominal wall eventually draws blood from and empties into tributaries of the subclavian vessels superiorly. A branch of the subclavian artery's first segment is the internal thoracic artery. It descends posterior to the upper six costal cartilages in the thorax, between the transversus thoracis and internal intercostal muscles. It enters the abdomen through the foramina of Morgagni, also known as the sternocostal triangle, which is located at the anterior aspect of the diaphragm, directly behind the sternum. It becomes the superior epigastric artery as it enters the abdomen, where it gives off the musculophrenic artery. The musculophrenic supplies the anterolateral diaphragm and hypochondrium region by traveling inferolaterally along the subcostal margin. Running posterior to the rectus abdominis muscle in the rectus sheath, the superior epigastric supplies the rectus abdominis as well as the epigastric and umbilical regions. Except for the internal thoracic veins, which drain superiorly into the brachiocephalic veins, the venous drainage closely follows the arterial supply. Branches of the thoracic aorta, such as the subcostal and tenth and eleventh posterior intercostal arteries, supply blood to the lumbar and lateral abdominal wall. They travel circumferentially between the transversus abdominis and internal oblique muscles to reach the lateral abdomen. Before draining into the azygous vein on the right and the hemiazygous vein on the left, the tenth and eleventh posterior intercostal and subcostal veins travel alongside the arteries.

Subsequently, the external iliac artery supplies the anterior abdominal wall deeply, while femoral artery branches supply it superficially. It gives off the inferior epigastric and deep circumflex iliac arteries just before the external iliac descends into the femoral ring. To supply the deep suprapubic and umbilical regions, the inferior epigastric artery ascends the inner surface of the abdominal wall in the lateral umbilical folds on the deep surface of the rectus abdominis. It passes through the rectus sheath at the arcuate line and runs behind the rectus abdominis before anastomosing with the superior epigastric in the umbilical area. To supply the deep iliac fossa regions, the deep circumflex runs superolaterally along the inner surface of the wall, parallel to the inguinal ligament. The superficial circumflex iliac artery and the superficial epigastric artery emerge shortly after the femoral artery emerges from the femoral ring. The superficial iliac fossa region is supplied by the superficial epigastric, which ascends in the subcutaneous tissue and follows a recurrent path around the inguinal ligament. The principal veins that drain the anterior inferior abdominal wall travel along the same paths as their corresponding arteries. These veins may anastomose with paraumbilical vessels in the umbilical region, which travel from the umbilicus via the ligamentum teres to the portal vein. These anastomoses may become the location of a portosystemic shunt in cases of severe portal hypertension. In this scenario, they may enlarge and become visible on the abdominal surface as the "caput medusae" sign. Surgeons creating free flaps from the inferior abdominal wall for use in reconstructive surgery especially need to understand the anatomy of the superficial and deep epigastric vessels.

Branches of the abdominal aorta supply blood to the posterior abdominal wall. Among these are the inferior phrenic arteries, which supply the diaphragm and adrenal glands by running laterally and upward towards the diaphragmatic crus. The quadratus lumborum, internal oblique muscles, transversus abdominis, and four paired lumbar arteries emerge from the aorta at the level of L1–L4. They then proceed laterally through arches of tendinous origins of the psoas major. The lumbar vein drainage is more intricate. Ascended lumbar veins, which emerge from the common iliac veins and ascend on either side of the vertebral bodies, serve as a conduit for the connections between the four pairs of lumbar veins that travel alongside their artery counterparts. The azygous vein is formed when the left subcostal vein and the left ascending lumbar vein unite. The hemiazygos vein is formed when the right ascending lumbar vein unites with the right subcostal vein. The majority of lumbar veins communicate with the ascending lumbar veins as well as the IVC directly. The transumbilical plane divides the superficial lymphatic drainage of the skin and subcutaneous tissue of the anterolateral abdominal wall. Pectoral axillary nodes receive the drainage of superior lymph vessels. They empty into the superficial inguinal lymph nodes inferiorly. The deep blood vessels are followed by the anterolateral abdominal wall muscles' deep lymphatic drainage. Superior drainage travels to the parasternal lymph nodes via the superior epigastric vessels. The inferior drainage system travels to the external iliac lymph nodes along the inferior epigastric vessels. The intercostal and subcostal vessels lead the lateral wall drainage to the posterior mediastinum nodes. The lumbar vessels carry the lymphatic drainage of the posterior wall to the lateral aortic and retro-aortic nodes. The umbilicus can become the site of metastases from gastrointestinal tumors, particularly pancreatic cancer. This condition is known as a "Sister Mary Joseph's nodule" in clinical terms. Some theories explain how metastasis occurs, such as through the falciform ligament's lymphatic system (Huttinger et al., 2023; Tuma et al., 2023; Seeras et al., 2023; Zahouani & Mendez, 2023).

6.1.4. Muscle Actions

The abdominal muscles are connected by either a common site of connection or by fascia. The muscles have distinct orientations of muscle fibers and act in all three planes during movements. Control of the abdominal muscles involves sometimes intricate movements. Normally, a single muscle works in unison with other muscles rather than in isolation. There are almost endless variations in physical activity, all controlled by the brain. For example, during gait, the muscles of the abdomen cooperate to regulate the movement of the spine, pelvis, and rib cage. The upper and lower limbs counterrotate, and the arm and leg move in opposite directions from one another.

During normal gait, there is a time when:

- Rectus abdominis and external obliques on one side act eccentrically to decelerate the anterior pelvic tilt created by the extension of the hip on that side.
- The rectus abdominis and external obliques on the other side work eccentrically to control thoracic extension and rotation created by the extension of the shoulder.

Virtually all actions involve the abdominal muscles to some degree, from biking, running, and walking, to swimming, swinging a golf club, and playing chess. Even when the body is at rest, the abdominals (in concert with other core muscles) help keep it stable and balanced.

6.1.5. Nerves

Primarily, the T7–T12 intercostal nerves innervate the muscles of the anterolateral abdominal wall. Together with the remainder of the neurovascular bundle, they travel a circumferential path anteriorly between the transversus abdominis and internal oblique layers. The lumbar plexus supplies and runs adjacent to the posterior wall's psoas major and quadratus lumborum muscles as it emerges from the spinal cord. The lower fibers and conjoint tendon of the internal oblique and transversus abdominis muscles are likewise supplied by the lumbar plexus's iliohypogastric and ilioinguinal branches. Anterolateral abdominal wall regional anesthesia can be achieved with a "transversus abdominis plane" (TAP) block. A field block can result from local anesthetic infiltration into the potential space between the transversus abdominis and internal oblique, which anesthetizes several nerves running in this plane, including branches of nerve roots from T6-L1, such as the iliohypogastric and ilioinguinal nerves. An increasing body of research supports its use in various abdominal surgeries.

6.1.6. Muscles

6.1.6.1. Anterolateral Abdominal Wall Muscles

Anterior chest wall strength and movement receive contributions laterally by three layers of large flat paired muscles: the external oblique, internal oblique, and transversus abdominis. Anteromedially, these layers fuse to form a rectus sheath that encloses the rectus abdominis and pyramidalis muscles. In the midline, the combined aponeuroses of these muscles fuse to form the linea alba.

Ø **External Oblique:** The muscle closest to the skin on the anterolateral abdominal wall is the external oblique. Its fibers run inferomedially and originate from the fifth through twelfth ribs. Its fibers form an aponeurotic sheath as it gets closer to the midclavicular line. This sheath passes superficially across the rectus abdominis and ends at the linea alba in the midline. The vertebral column rotates and flexes laterally as a result of contraction of the internal oblique. The inguinal ligament, which connects the pubic tubercle to the ASIS, is formed by its inferior border.

Ø **Internal Oblique:** Close to the external oblique is this muscle. The vertebral column rotates and flexes laterally as a result of contraction of the external oblique. It originates from the iliac crest, lateral inguinal ligament, and lumbar fascia. Its fibers become aponeurotic and run superomedially, orthogonal to the external oblique. Its contributions to the rectus sheath vary depending on which of its lower and upper fibers are used. The rectus sheath is encased anteriorly and posteriorly by the division of upper fibers. All fibers travel anteriorly to the rectus abdominal muscle inferiorly. The rectus abdominis and transversalis fascia will not have an aponeurotic layer between them, resulting in a posterior deficiency of this section of the rectus sheath. The "arcuate line" refers to the inferior end of the posterior rectus sheath. Regardless of their connection to the rectus abdominis, every layer proceeds medially to connect with the linea alba in the midline.

- Ø **Transversus Abdominis:** The deepest anterolateral muscle is this one. It originates from the lumbar fascia, iliac crest, lateral inguinal ligament, and the fifth through tenth costal cartilages. Before becoming aponeurotic and entering the rectus sheath, its fibers run transversely. Its upper part contributes to the posterior rectus sheath by traveling posteriorly to the rectus abdominal muscles. Its aponeurosis runs anteriorly to the muscle below the arcuate line, adding to the anterior sheath. Abdominal contents are compressed when the transversus abdominis contracts. The conjoint tendon is formed by the transversus abdominis and the inferior edge of the internal oblique.
- Ø **Rectus Abdominis:** This long, narrow muscle runs parallel to the linea alba and vertically in the rectus sheath. It extends superiorly to attach to the fifth through seventh costal cartilages after emerging from the pubic symphysis and crest. It is a strong vertebral column flexor. Three tendinous intersections split each muscle belly into four distinct muscle segments. The anterior rectus sheath that covers the tendinous intersections has a tether to it. These could be noticeable and referred to as a "six-pack" in an athlete.
- Ø **Pyramidalis:** This muscle is a minor triangular muscle that sits anteriorly to the rectus abdominis in the inferior rectus sheath. Its origin is from the body of the pubis and tenses the linea alba when contracting. It is present bilaterally in 80% of people.

6.1.6.2. Posterior Abdominal Wall Muscles

a. *Quadratus Lumborum:* This muscle originates from the iliolumbar ligament and iliac crest and runs superomedially to insert into the twelfth rib and L1–4 transverse processes. Contraction can cause lateral flexion and extension of the vertebral column, and depression of the rib cage.

b. *Psoas Major:* This muscle originates from the transverse processes of T12 and L1–4 vertebrae and lateral surfaces of the intervening intervertebral discs. It runs inferiorly, joining the iliacus to insert into the lesser trochanter of the femur. The contraction causes flexion of the thigh.

6.1.7. Surgical Considerations

A surgeon must weigh the morbidity that the approach may cause against the ease of access needed to finish the procedure when planning the approach to the abdominal cavity. Different strategies will result in different outcomes regarding incisional hernias, wound healing, and cosmesis. The indication for operation and urgency will determine this balance. A sizable vertical midline incision will be made during an emergency exploratory laparotomy to provide rapid access and a wide view of the abdominal contents. Smaller, more precisely timed incisions will be made during elective procedures. Transverse cuts, e.g., the Pfannenstiel incision, which increases wound strength and reduces scarring and runs parallel to Langer's lines of skin tension, improves cosmesis. Since muscle transection will kill the muscle fibers, muscle splitting incisions made in line with the fibers are preferred over muscle cutting. As the risk of hernias increases with denervation and paralysis of the abdominal wall musculature, incisions must be carefully planned to avoid significant motor nerves. Traditional open surgical techniques are regularly being replaced by laparoscopic surgery. When compared to patients undergoing an equivalent open approach, patients undergoing laparoscopic surgery have a lower rate of postoperative wound infections and incisional hernias, as well as a shorter hospital stay.

6.1.8. Clinical Significance

Understanding the pathology and surgical repair potential of the abdominal wall necessitates an understanding of its working anatomy. The capacity of the abdominal wall to hold in stomach contents will be compromised by defects, which can show up clinically as an abnormal protrusion of tissue through an opening, known as a congenital or acquired hernia. Birth defects or weak areas in the developing embryo's abdominal wall can result in congenital hernias. They include the more common and benign umbilical hernia as well as the potentially fatal gastroschisis. Herniation of the abdominal contents through a patent umbilical ring following delivery is known as an umbilical hernia. Frequently, they resolve on their own without requiring surgery. When the contents of the abdomen rotate abnormally, they become outside the wall of the abdomen and are only covered by the peritoneum, resulting in an omphalocele. In the absence of proper care, it can be fatal and is frequently linked to other congenital malformations. Due to a failure in the fusion of the lateral body wall folds during embryonic development, the intestines lie outside the abdominal wall in gastroschisis without an overlying membrane. If this condition is not surgically corrected, it is fatal. Hernias of the abdominal wall that are acquired usually develop in weak spots and can lead to pain, constipation, and even strangulation. Usually, epigastric hernias appear in the midline, above the umbilicus, through the linea alba. Adult-acquired umbilical hernias typically necessitate surgical intervention and have a higher morbidity rate than their pediatric counterparts. Spigelian hernias typically develop above the arcuate line, at the semilunar line that separates the rectus sheath from the lateral border of the rectus abdominis. At the inferior border of the anterolateral muscles, inguinal hernias emerge through the superficial ring of the inguinal canal. Any incision made after surgery could result in an incisional hernia.

6.1.9. Strengthen Abdominal Muscles

Keeping your abdominal muscles strong is crucial to having a strong core. These muscles support your spine and pelvis when performing various movements. You should perform muscle-strengthening exercises at least two days a week and include exercises to strengthen your abdominal muscles:

- **Rectus exercise.** Lie on the floor with knees bent and feet slightly apart. Put your hands on your thighs and slide them toward your knees, raising your head and shoulders off the ground.
- **Obliques exercise.** Lie on the floor as before. Raise your head and shoulders and try to touch your knee with the opposite hand. Repeat on the other side.

  Repeat these as often as you can without pain, and try to increase the number of repetitions as you get used to the exercises.
- **Pilates.** This is a safe and effective

exercise technique for strengthening your core. Pilates is used for injury rehabilitation, too. You should have an expert fitness trainer to guide you in including abdominal exercises in your fitness plan. It is important to perform warming up and stretching exercises before and cooling down after any exercise program.

Apart from exercising regularly, some other measures help to keep your abdominal muscles healthy and safe:

- Be careful when lifting heavy objects.
- Tighten your abdominal muscles when sneezing or coughing.
- Eat a healthy diet with plenty of fruits and vegetables to prevent constipation.
- Maintain healthy body weight (Huttinger et al., 2023; Tuma et al., 2023; Seeras et al., 2023; Zahouani & Mendez, 2023).

6.2. Filament Evanescence of Myosin II and Smooth Muscle Function

The motor protein superfamily myosin transforms chemical energy from ATP hydrolysis into mechanical work. Muscle contraction and cell motility are made possible by the cyclic interaction of myosin heads with actin filaments. Every eukaryotic cell contains myosin. The superfamily was formerly thought to consist of >130 distinct members due to genetic variations and a total of 18 classes, each given a Roman numeral, as shown by an unrooted phylogenetic tree. The conserved myosin motorhead underwent phylogenetic analysis to support this classification. The myosin superfamily is made up of more than 70 classes, according to more recent research with better sequencing analysis, including that of the less conserved tail region. This review focuses on myosin II, which is present in smooth, cardiac, and skeletal muscle in addition to nonmuscle cells. This review focuses primarily on smooth muscle myosin II, but it also discusses some other myosin isoforms from other cell types and nonvertebrate organisms to give readers a complete understanding of the unique characteristics of smooth muscle myosin II. Myosin II, which was discovered by Kühne in 1864, has been the subject of the most research within the superfamily and is commonly known as the conventional myosin. It is the only class of myosin that can combine with actin to form functional filaments, which give muscle and nonmuscle cells their motility.

In smooth muscle, actin thin filaments and myosin thick filaments combine to form contractile units. The thick and thin filaments slide in relation to one another upon stimulation. Muscle contraction results from filament sliding shortening individual contractile units within the structural bounds of the contractile unit arrays. Myosin may predominantly exist as filaments in some types of smooth muscle, and smooth muscle function is not dependent on the assembly and disassembly of myosin filaments. Numerous lines of evidence in other types, like airway smooth muscle, lend credence to the idea that myosin exists in both relaxed and activated forms—monomeric and filamentous—and that cell function can be optimized by controlling the dynamic equilibrium between the pools of these two types of myosin. Organs with hollow walls are lined with smooth muscle. Some of them, like the bladder and stomach, experience frequent changes in volume, so the smooth muscle cells must be able to maintain optimal contractility over a wide range of lengths. Myosin filament evanescence has been proposed as one of the mechanisms underlying this mechanical plasticity. In order to allow muscle cells to adapt to a longer or shorter length while maintaining optimal overlap of the contractile filaments within each contractile unit, smooth muscle myosin filaments have the ability to "dissolve" into monomers or oligomers and to be added to or subtracted from existing contractile unit arrays during length changes. About 15% of the myosin in intact airway smooth muscle is nonmuscle myosin. Although nonmuscle myosin is not a component of the smooth muscle contractile unit, the recruitment of adhesion complexes to the cortical cytoskeleton of smooth muscle cells—which is essential for force transmission—seems to depend on its assembly from monomers into filaments. Similar to amoeba mobility, nonmuscle myosin also shows indications of filament evanescence; however, the regulatory mechanisms in amoeba are different from those in nonmuscle myosin in mammalian and vertebrate smooth muscle. We'll talk about this in more detail later.

Numerous variables, including pH, ionic strength, intracellular calcium concentrations, and the phosphorylation states of myosin light and heavy chains, control the reversible switching between the monomeric and filamentous forms of myosin in solution. It is well known that the dynamic process of filament formation and dissolution in intact muscle is significantly influenced by variations in cell length and other mechanical perturbations, as well as Rho-kinase (ROCK) activities within the cells. This review looks at the data supporting the existence and control of myosin evanescence, as well as the significance of this smooth muscle intrinsic feature and the possible consequences of dysregulation of myosin loss in illnesses.

6.2.1. Myosin II Structure and Filament Formation

Figure 6.2 demonstrates the structure of a mammalian smooth muscle myosin heavy chain (MHC), consisting of a globular head region, a helical rod region, and a nonhelical tail region. Each myosin head contains two light chains: the essential light chain (17 kD) and the regulatory light chain (RLC; 20 kD). Enzymatic digestion with trypsin or α-chymotrypsin can produce heavy meromyosin (HMM) and light meromyosin (LMM) fragments from myosin. Further digestion with papain or α-chymotrypsin breaks HMM into S1 and S2 subfragments, which are commonly used in biochemical assays. The S1 fragment contains ATP-binding and actin-binding sites crucial for ATP hydrolysis and actin-binding for muscle movement. The genetic codes of S1 in smooth and striated muscle myosin are mostly conserved, with some diversity in amino acid sequences. Studies on HMM fragments from smooth muscle have revealed mechanisms for phosphorylation-dependent myosin function regulation. The LMM fragment in skeletal and smooth muscle is responsible for myosin filament assembly in all muscle types. The rod portion of the myosin molecule has a highly repetitive amino acid sequence with alternating positively and negatively charged clusters, allowing for staggered assembly of adjacent rods and the formation of myosin heads on thick filaments. Skip residuals interrupt the charge repeats, affecting the rod's flexibility and coiled-coil structure, critical in myosin molecule assembly into thick filaments. A 29-residue segment near the C terminus of LMM plays a crucial role in myosin filament formation. Deletion of this assembly competence domain impairs thick filament self-assembly in full-length MHC.

The formation of myosin filaments may have an impact on mechanical plasticity, force production, and smooth muscle shortening. Therefore, controlling filament assembly has physiological ramifications. Myosin II's AA sequence plays a crucial role in determining the mechanism underlying the formation of the filaments. Cryoelectron microscopy demonstrates that every myosin molecule is made up of two entangled MHCs, as schematically depicted in Fig Sixth Point. There are four identified MHC isoforms in smooth muscle. Two isoforms in the motor domain close to the ATPase site differ in whether a 7-AA insert is present (in phasic smooth muscle) or absent (in tonic smooth muscle). The two isoforms, which differ slightly in the AA sequence between species, are known as SM-A (without insert) and SM-B (with insert).

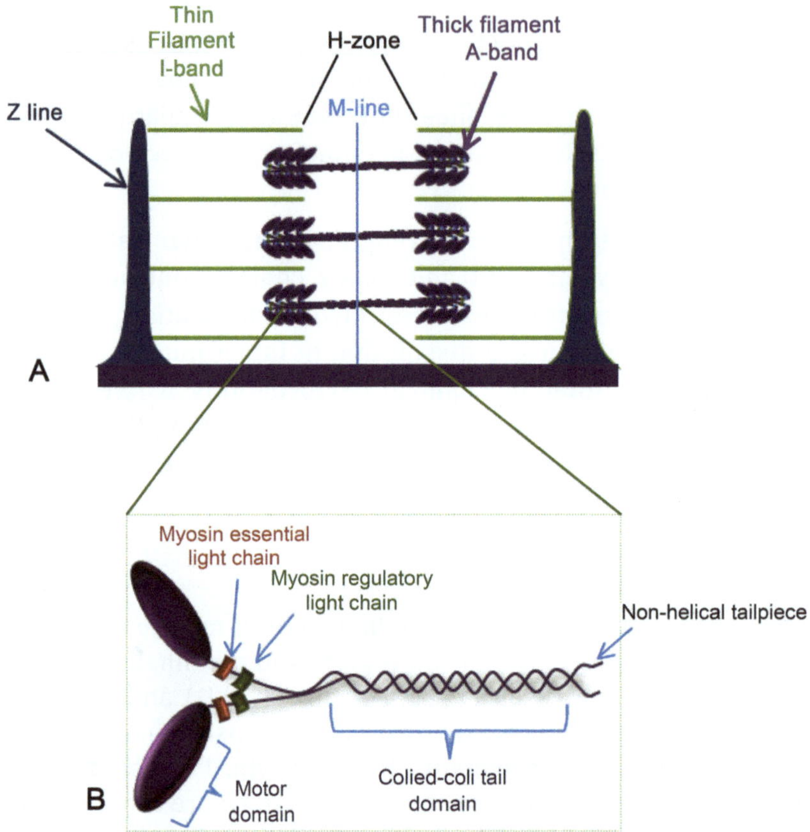

Figure 6.2. *Schematic diagram of a myosin II molecule. SM1 and SM2 heterodimers are drawn for illustration purposes only. Controversy exists about whether in living cells they exist as homodimers or homodimers and heterodimers by random chance.*

Source: Kachur TM, Pilgrim DB. Myosin Assembly, Maintenance and degradation in muscle: role of the chaperone UNC-45 in myosin thick filament dynamics. International Journal of Molecular Sciences. 2008; 9(9):1863–1875. https://doi.org/10.3390/ijms9091863.

In vitro motility tests have demonstrated that the insert (SM-B) can move actin twice as quickly as SM-A, but it has not been documented to be involved in myosin filament assembly. Two additional unique variants of smooth muscle MHC are present at the C terminus, resulting in isoforms of SM1 (204 kD) and SM2 (200 kD). Whether they exist as homodimers or as a random mixture of homodimers and heterodimers in living cells is a topic of controversy. SM1 in mammalian smooth muscle is 34 AAs longer than SM2 and has a total of 1,978 AAs. 1,979 AAs are present in the chicken (Figure 6.2) as a result of an additional residue in the tail area. 1,935 AAs make up the head and rod regions, with the remaining AAs found in the nonhelical tail. The location of alternative splicing, where the tail of SM1 has 43 AAs and the tail of SM2 has 9 AAs, is indicated by the 1,935th AA. Ikebe and colleagues used several monoclonal antibodies that targeted distinct amino acids (AAs) in the turkey gizzard smooth muscle myosin's C-terminal coiled-coil rod region. They found that the sequence essential for filament formation is found within a 28-AA segment (1,907–1,935) that is situated at the end of the LMM. As with cardiac myosin when the assembly competent domain is deleted, deletion of the segment increases the solubility of the truncated myosin rods. It is possible to totally prevent the formation of myosin filaments when an antibody (mm19) occupies this position. It has also been proposed that the nonhelical tail region right next to it regulates myosin II filament assembly in a significant way. When a 35-AA sequence in the nonhelical tail of vertebrate nonmuscle myosin is deleted, the critical concentration of rod polypeptides needed for filament assembly increases by a factor of 50. Myosin filaments lose some of their stability when the nonhelical tail is occupied. Differential effects of SM1 and SM2 isoforms' tailpieces on the assembly of myosin filaments in smooth muscle. Myosin filaments with the longer tailpiece of SM1 are found to be more stable (by four to five times) than filaments with the shorter tailpiece of SM2. Despite the fact that SM1 and SM2 can move actin, as demonstrated in unloaded muscle (Huttinger et al., 2023; Tuma et al., 2023; Seeras et al., 2023; Zahouani & Mendez, 2023).

6.2.2. Chemical Properties Influencing Myosin Filament Formation

Numerous variables affect the stability of myosin filaments in solution, but the concentration of monomeric myosin, ionic strength, pH, ATP concentration, and myosin phosphorylation state are the most crucial ones. Most organisms have an intracellular ionic strength of approximately 200–300 mM. Baseline intracellular pH has been reported to be 7.19 in porcine tracheal smooth muscle, 7.02–7.14 in sheep, ferret, and guinea pig cardiac muscle, and 7.38 in human skeletal muscle at rest. Purified unphosphorylated myosin's propensity to form filaments decreases with increasing ionic strength between 100 and 200 mM at pH 7.5 and in the presence of 4 mM MgCl2. Myosin is insoluble at ionic strengths less than 100 mM (i.e., myosin is only found in filamentous form). When the ionic strength exceeds 200 mM, the majority of myosin is present as monomers (i.e., soluble). Myosin filament formation can also be influenced by the presence of ATP. Myosin filaments break apart when unphosphorylated smooth muscle myosin is added to a solution containing MgATP. However, this ATP effect can be negated by bringing the pH below the physiological level. Lowering the pH from 7.0 to 6.5 or 6.2 eliminates the disassembling effect of MgATP on unphosphorylated smooth muscle myosin filaments at 150 mM ionic strength and 5 mM Mg2+. Lastly, the filaments may become more stable due to the phosphorylation of RLC brought about by the myosin light chain kinase/calmodulin-Ca+2 complex, preventing the filaments from disassembling even in the presence of ATP.

It has been proposed that the process of shifting dynamic equilibria between the polymeric myosin, the straight (6S) monomers, and the folded (10S) monomers forms the myosin filament (Figure 6.3), where 10S and 6S stand for the folded and straight monomers (10 and 6 Svedbergs, respectively) sedimentation rates in gel electrophoresis. Many forms of myosin can adopt an extended (6S) or folded (10S) conformation. These forms include smooth, cardiac, skeletal, and nonmuscle myosin. Without the assistance of a core or myosin-associated proteins, smooth muscle myosin self-assembles into flat sheets to form filaments in vitro. Myosin rods can interact with one another thanks to the extended 6S conformation, which enables filament formation. According to one theory, myosin filament formation requires the intermediate 6S conformation, and in order for filaments to form, the 10S must change into the 6S. This theory states that filament formation is favored by the RLC's phosphorylation, which changes the folded 10S into the extended 6S. The transition from the extended 6S to the folded 10S conformation is facilitated by RLC dephosphorylation. This theory highlights the pivotal function of RLC phosphorylation in the process of filament formation. A different theory places more emphasis on how ATP concentration and ionic strength affect the monomer conformation. RLC phosphorylation favors the 6S conformation, whereas MgATP favors the 10S conformation.

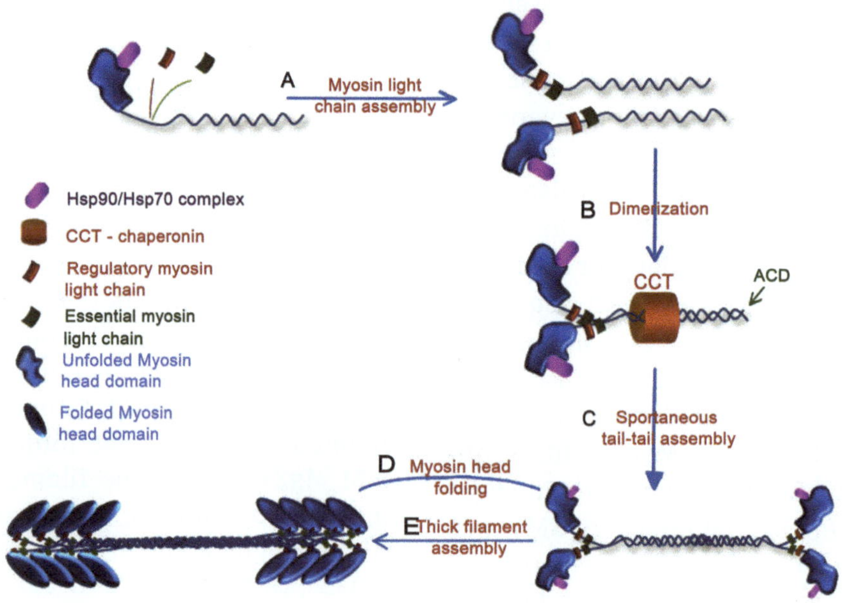

Figure 6.3. *Myosin maturation. (A) Nascent myosin molecules associate with the Hsp70/Hsp90 complex (purple). Myosin light chain assembly (green and red) and folding of the tail region occurs rapidly. (B) Dimerization of the myosin tails may require the chaperonin CCT (orange). (C) The assembly-competence domain (ACD) at the extreme C-terminus promotes tail-tail dimer formation. (D) Myosin head folding is the rate limiting step and can occur at any point in this cascade. (E) Assembly of myosin into thick filaments likely requires many different factors but does not require properly folded myosin heads. Note: the exact position of Hsp90 binding within the head domain is not known.*

Source: Kachur TM, Pilgrim DB. Myosin assembly, maintenance and degradation in muscle: role of the chaperone UNC-45 in myosin thick filament dynamics. International Journal of Molecular Sciences. 2008; 9(9):1863–1875. https://doi.org/10.3390/ijms9091863.

However, only in the range of 100–300 mM of salt concentration is the dependence of myosin monomer conformation on RLC phosphorylation seen. Regardless of whether the RLC is phosphorylated or not, all monomers unfold to become the extended 6S variety above 300 mM. Even when RLC is phosphorylated, below 100 mM, the monomers stay in the folded 10S conformation instead of going back to the extended 6S. In fact, it has been noted that 10S monomers can be phosphorylated and still remain folded, indicating that not all folded 10S must be changed to the extended 6S conformation in order to form filaments. This theory states that RLC phosphorylation plays a role in facilitating the assembly of myosin into antiparallel dimers of 6S myosin, which subsequently serve as the side-polar filament unit structures. The theory agrees with recent electron microscopy observations of different folded conformations in myosin in nonmuscle, skeletal, cardiac, and smooth muscle.

The current understanding of the process of myosin II filament formation in vitro, according to the two theories described above, is discussed. Unphosphorylated myosin from smooth, skeletal, cardiac, and nonmuscular muscle forms folded monomers (a folded three-segment structure with two hinge points) at ionic strength and pH around physiological levels. The formation of antiparallel folded dimers is possible with folded monomers. The resulting antiparallel folded tetramers are formed by antiparallel folded dimers (see top row of Figure 6.3). ATP blocks polymerization by promoting the folded 10S conformation because a particular tail region is needed for filament formation and is not visible in the folded conformation. In smooth muscle, ATP significantly lessens myosin polymerization compared to skeletal and cardiac muscle. This explains why the in vivo stability of smooth muscle myosin filaments is lower than that of striated muscle. The unfolding of any tertiary structures of monomers, dimers, or tetramers is favored by RLC phosphorylation, which counteracts the action of ATP. When RLC phosphorylation occurs, folded antiparallel tetramers unfurl, facilitating the binding and unfolding of additional folded tetramers. Later, as several unfolded tetramers combine, longer, mature filaments are formed. It's interesting to note that, in line with earlier research, smooth muscle myosin can also form filaments with a central bare zone in bipolar filaments during the initial moments of polymerization, while skeletal muscle myosin can form filaments without one.

Skeletal muscle myosin creates the well-known bipolar filaments after a few hours of polymerization, whereas smooth muscle myosin forms side-polar thick filaments. The previously mentioned opposing effects of ATP and RLC phosphorylation on filament formation still hold true, despite the fact that more recent research has identified distinct intermediate structures in the filament formation process. Atomic force microscopy has revealed that purified phosphorylated myosin filaments from bovine tracheal smooth muscle have a smaller diameter in solution than unphosphorylated filaments; this observation may be related to the phosphorylation-induced transformation of folded intermediate structures into straightened ones. Additionally, their resistance to physical agitation, like that caused by ultrasonication, is higher, which may indicate that the phosphorylated myosin filaments have a higher degree of structural integrity (Huttinger et al., 2023; Tuma et al., 2023; Seeras et al., 2023; Zahouani & Mendez, 2023).

6.2.3. Evidence for Two Intracellular Pools of Myosin

The polymerization and depolymerization of myosin in live cells can happen quickly. Research using immunoelectron microscopy has shown that when the chemotactic stimulant cAMP is exposed to live Dictyostelium discoideum amoeba, myosin filaments disappear completely within 2 minutes and then reappear within the next minute. This disappearance and reappearance of myosin filaments is due to a temporary cAMP-induced increase in phosphorylated MHC, which prevents the formation of myosin filaments. The rapid reappearance of myosin filaments suggests that there is a pool of myosin monomers already present in the cell, eliminating the need for new protein synthesis. The mechanism of myosin filament formation in Dictyostelium discoideum is different from that in vertebrate nonmuscle and smooth muscle cells. In *D. discoideum*, phosphorylation of certain residues in the tail region of MHC destabilizes filaments, while dephosphorylation promotes filament assembly. Although RLC phosphorylation has been shown to regulate motor function in D. discoideum, its role in myosin II filament formation is not well understood. In mammalian cells, RLC phosphorylation at multiple sites controls the assembly and disassembly of myosin filaments during processes like wound healing. Phosphorylation at a specific site prevents the interaction between RLC and myosin hexamers, leading to the disassembly of filaments. As the response to growth factor continues, another site of phosphorylation becomes dominant, driving the polymerization of myosin from a pool of soluble myosin.

A key process governing smooth muscle function is the dynamic interconversion between filamentous and monomeric populations in smooth muscle cells. Myosin molecules should primarily exist as monomers if in vitro results could be directly applied to living muscle cells, where MgATP is present at □5 mM and ionic strength is approximately 200 mM. Nonetheless, smooth muscle cells have been observed to contain filamentous myosin in both their relaxed and activated states. Based on the use of antibodies probing for monomers, it has been demonstrated in intact gizzard smooth muscle that there is no difference in the amount of monomeric myosin in the relaxed or contracted state and that there is no increase in monomer concentration when the muscle is relaxed after contraction. These findings have led to the following questions: does filamentous myosin exist in equilibrium with monomeric myosin within a smooth muscle cell, and could contractile states and other intracellular factors shift the equilibrium? These studies suggest that filamentous myosin predominates in cell structure and that the balance between filamentous and monomeric myosin is stable. Some studies, though, seem to indicate otherwise. It has been discovered that myosin polymerization happens during contractile activation and depolymerization occurs during relaxation in the anococcygeus muscle. It should be noted that there has been no discovery of myosin filament evanescence in guinea pig taenia coli. Thus, it would seem that the degree of change in the filament-monomer equilibrium linked to smooth muscle contraction and relaxation varies depending on the type of cell.

A sizable pool of monomeric myosin in dynamic equilibrium with filamentous myosin has been directly observed in cultured human airway smooth muscle. Two distinct pools of myosin can be identified in cultured human airway smooth muscle cells as filamentous myosin and 10S folded monomers. These pools are detected using two antibodies, one specifically against smooth muscle monomeric myosin and the other differentially against smooth muscle filamentous myosin, as well as a peptide that inhibits interaction between the head and tail of folded 10S monomer. Fifteen to twenty% of the total smooth muscle myosin can be switched from the monomeric pool to the filamentous pool and vice versa by adjusting the pH and buffer composition. In intact smooth muscle, different pools of monomeric and filamentous myosin have also been discovered. Researchers have found an inverse relationship between the resting muscle length and the baseline RLC phosphorylation level in preparations of smooth muscle in the airways. We discovered that muscle preparations fixed at longer resting lengths had significantly lower concentrations of monomers than muscle preparations fixed at shorter lengths, using immunostaining with the mm19 antibody specific for monomeric myosin. As smooth muscle cells that have adapted to a longer length have more contractile units, we hypothesize that myosin from the monomeric pool may be recruited into the contractile filament lattice, where filament formation is preferred. Depolymerization of myosin filaments may occur when smooth muscle cells adapt to a shorter length because fewer contractile units are required. We have discovered a baseline concentration of myosin monomers in resting muscle, and the monomer concentration in this pool is variable under physiological conditions, regardless of whether our interpretation is accurate.

Is the myosin filament length of smooth muscle uniform, as is the case with the bipolar thick filaments of striated muscle, for the pool of filamentous myosin? For rabbit vascular smooth muscle, the filament length was estimated to be approximately 2.2 μm by observing thick filaments in electron micrographs of serial cross sections with thicknesses of 400–500 nm. Subsequent investigations have revealed that the thick filament length, as determined by longitudinal sections of electron microscopy, is primarily less than 3 μm, although filaments as long as 8 μm have also been observed; in contracted chicken gizzard cells, the filament length has been measured in longitudinal sections to be approximately 1.6 μm. When measuring filament length in longitudinal sections, there is a chance that the length will be underestimated if the filament is not exactly parallel to the section's surface. Even though there is a chance that they underestimated the filament length, the discovery that some longitudinal section filaments are longer than 2.2 μm, which they took to be a constant length for the thick filaments they measured, suggests that there is disagreement over the length of myosin filaments in smooth muscle.

In a series of successive electron microscopic cross sections, scientists followed 16,587 thick filaments in both relaxed and activated states of rabbit carotid smooth muscle and ovine tracheal smooth muscle using serial sections that were about ten times thinner. Since a normal distribution of filament lengths has been seen in our measurements of myosin filaments made from purified tracheal smooth muscle myosin in solution, we had anticipated seeing one in our measurements as well. Surprisingly, we found that the in situ filament length frequency distribution had an exponential decay pattern, meaning that the distribution was biased toward short filaments (most of which were less than 500 nm long) and that the longer the filaments, the fewer of them were observed. This indicates that there are thick filaments of different lengths within the pool of filamentous myosin. There are deeper ramifications to the debate over whether smooth muscle myosin filaments are always the same length. A consistent length for the thick filaments in bipolar filaments, like those found in striated muscle, is essential to ensuring a consistent dimension for the contractile units. There is no need for a uniform length in side-polar filaments. The thick filament in a contractile unit that has thin filaments sandwiched between it can either be the same length as the contractile unit or it can be replaced by a number of shorter filaments arranged end to end inside the unit. Contractile unit configuration is thus determined by myosin filament structures, which can be either bipolar or side polar. Short filaments, such as myosin dimers and tetramers, which function as ratcheting motors, can also be more readily redistributed within the cytoskeleton when muscle cells change their shape in response to outside stimuli. Vanishing myosin filaments in smooth muscle both in rest and during contraction.

Smooth muscle's intracellular chemical environment is not conducive to the formation of myosin filaments, particularly when the muscle is relaxed, as was covered in earlier sections. Nevertheless, smooth muscle cells have myosin filaments regardless of whether the RLC is phosphorylated. The physical environment in smooth muscle cells promotes myosin polymerization, which could be one explanation for the puzzle. It is well known that close contact between myosin and actin facilitates the formation of myosin filaments within the actin filament lattice. In the relaxed state, actin and myosin can be cross-linked by the actin-filament-binding protein caldesmon, which stabilizes myosin filaments. In relaxed smooth muscle, telokin and 38k protein may also control the formation of myosin filaments. It has been proposed that 38k protein facilitates the assembly of dephosphorylated myosin into filaments, whereas telokin stabilizes dephosphorylated myosin. The concentration of myosin monomers also influences the formation of myosin filaments. Myosin polymerization will take place even in the absence of RLC phosphorylation if the concentration of monomeric myosin is high enough. In the actin filament lattice of smooth muscle, there may be a localized high concentration of myosin. Although the existence of myosin filaments in relaxed smooth muscle is widely accepted, and as was covered in the previous section, there is compelling evidence for the existence of both monomeric and filamentous myosin pools, it is reasonable to wonder if it is possible to increase the mass of filamentous myosin at the expense of monomeric myosin or vice versa. Dynamic equilibrium appears to exist in certain types of smooth muscle cells and not in others, as was covered in the previous section. The discussion that follows will mostly concentrate on airway smooth muscle, a type of cell that has a high degree of myosin evanescence.

The intracellular chemical environment of smooth muscle is not conducive to the formation of myosin filaments, particularly when the muscle is relaxed, as was covered in earlier sections.

6.2.4. Length Adaptation in Smooth Muscle

Smooth muscle can work over a very wide range of lengths, in contrast to striated muscle. In a full bladder, for instance, the length of a rabbit's bladder smooth muscle cell is more than seven times that of the cell when the bladder is empty. It is thought that a process known as length adaptation is responsible for smooth muscle's capacity to produce force over such a broad length range. The adaptive behavior with respect to length is maintained even in airway smooth muscle, which is not known to require a wide functional length range. The process by which smooth muscle recovers its contractility following a significant alteration in muscle length or other types of mechanical disturbance, such as force oscillation or length changes, is known as length adaptation. Length adaptation is known to cause a change in the length-force relationship of the muscle, though the underlying mechanism is not fully understood. In striated muscle, the sarcomeric structure governs the length-force relationship. Because the striated muscle's contractile apparatus has a static structure, the length-force relationship in this muscle type is also static. The observed changes in the length-force relationship in smooth muscle during length adaptation imply that the underlying structure of the contractile apparatus is amenable to easy modification. The structural malleability of smooth muscle's contractile apparatus is probably largely attributed to myosin evanescence.

Significant hints for understanding the mechanical function of striated muscle, including its force-generating capacity, can be found in alterations in the sarcomeric structure, such as the overlap between the thick and thin filaments. In striated muscle research, defining the sarcomeric structure change first has proven to be a fruitful strategy. This allows one to understand the corresponding functional change as the mechanical expression of the structural change. Smooth muscle's "smoothness" makes it difficult to see any evidence of an intracellular structural alteration that could account for the functional change. Therefore, in smooth muscle research, a reversal approach is frequently used, where changes in structure are predicted from available functional data. The linear increase in absolute shortening velocity and power output with adapted muscle length are two functional changes in smooth muscle associated with length adaptation, in addition to the previously mentioned shift in the length–force relationship. Isometric force stays constant before and after (but not during) length adaptation.

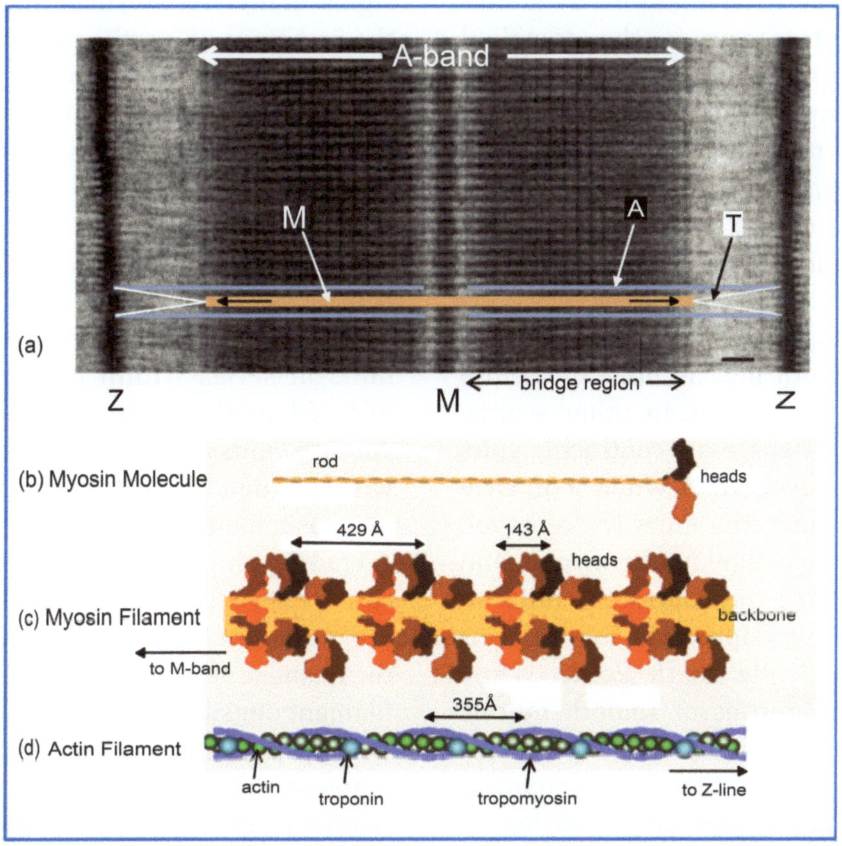

Figure 6.4. *(a) Electron micrograph of a vertebrate striated muscle sarcomere (here about 2.3 μm long) which runs between two Z-lines (Z) to which actin filaments (A) are attached. The A-band contains myosin (thick) filaments (M), cross-linked at the M-band, and which the actin filaments partly overlap. (b) Simplified diagram of a myosin II molecule; a long rod on the end of which are two myosin heads which bind and hydrolyze ATP and bind actin. Myosin molecules (b) aggregate to form myosin filaments (c); the rods are in the backbone and the heads are almost helically arranged on the filament surface. The head ends of the rods, myosin S2 (subfragment-2) can lift from the filament surface to enable myosin head attachment to actin. Actin (thin-) filaments (d) comprise a twisted helical array of globular (G-)actin monomers along which run two strands of tropomyosin on which is also the troponin complex.*

Source: Squire J. Special Issue: The actin-myosin interaction in muscle: background and overview. International Journal of Molecular Sciences. 2019; 20(22):5715. https://doi.org/10.3390/ijms20225715.

Take note that when speaking in terms of relativeness (i.e., following the normalization of velocity by muscle length), the power output and relative velocity would remain unchanged both prior to and following length adaptation. Furthermore, length adaptation does not change the force–velocity relationship in the muscle, indicating that the dynamics of actomyosin interaction in the so-called cross-bridge cycle remain unaltered. The most straightforward explanation for the structural alterations linked to length adaptation is that, although the fundamental makeup of individual contractile units does not change, the quantity of these units connected in series in an array spanning the length of the cell may vary. This explanation is supported by the observed differences in smooth muscle function before and after length adaptation. In other words, when a muscle lengthens, more contractile units are added to the array, and when a muscle contracts, some contractile units are removed from the array. This will allow the myosin and actin filaments inside the contractile units to remain optimally overlapped. In Figure., this is shown schematically. Sixth Point. While the mechanical properties of smooth muscle measured at various adapted lengths can be explained by this model, the mechanism responsible for the suggested alteration in the contractile apparatus's structure remains largely unidentified.

A description of the model of a contractile unit is provided in the text. For the purposes of illustration, the muscle cell contains two and three contractile units in series, adapted to 0.75 and 1.5 reference lengths ($L_{ref)}$, respectively. In comparison to smooth muscle adapted to a longer length (1.5 L_{ref}), which contains more filamentous myosin, smooth muscle adapted to a shorter length (0.75 $L_{ref)}$ has higher concentrations of monomers, dimers, and tetramers in both folded and straightened conformations outside of the contractile units. Since nonmuscle myosin intermediates are not involved in the adaptation process, they are not displayed. A contractile unit is indicated by "s" on the line. The finding that myosin filament mass decreased in response to length oscillation raises the possibility that mechanical strain is the first signal that causes myosin filament dissolution, the first stage of length adaptation. It's unclear if filament depolymerization results directly from shear strain or indirectly from a series of signals that the strain starts, like integrins and cAMP. In contrast to striated muscle, longitudinal sections of smooth muscle cannot be used by electron microscopy to identify individual contractile units. Therefore, it is not possible to verify by counting the number of contractile units in series within muscle cells that have been adapted to various lengths. Nonetheless, smooth muscle myosin filament density—which is determined by counting the number of myosin filaments per cell cross-sectional area, excluding the area occupied by organelles—can be precisely measured using electron micrographs of cell cross sections. Because both the filament number and length contribute to the filament density (i.e., the cross-sectional density of myosin filaments is a measure of myosin filament mass, and the probability of myosin filaments in a cell intersected by a random cross section is proportional to the number and average length of the filaments). Doubling the length of a smooth muscle cell results in a halving of the cell's cross-sectional area because the volume of the cell is conserved at different lengths of stretching. The filament density at any cell cross section in cells set at different lengths would be the same if we assume that the myosin filament mass is constant at different cell lengths and the filaments are uniformly distributed within the cell. In actuality, the filament density increases by approximately 67% when the muscle is stretched to twice its initial length. The same muscle that underwent the same length adaptation shows an identical increase in absolute shortening velocity and power output.

The model of adaptation suggests that similar to the linear relationships between absolute shortening velocity and power output and muscle length, there should be a linear relationship between myosin filament mass and muscle length. This presupposes that more myosin filaments must be synthesized, most likely from the monomeric myosin pool, if muscles adapted to a longer length require more contractile units (and vice versa for muscles adapted to a shorter length). An additional piece of evidence supporting the idea that muscles adapted to longer lengths have more contractile units (and therefore more myosin filaments), which leads to higher energy consumption, is the rate of ATP hydrolysis's linear relationship with muscle length. Subsequent research has directly demonstrated a linear decrease in the monomeric myosin concentration with adapted muscle length. This suggests that a reduction in the monomeric myosin pool is associated with the increased myosin polymerization observed at longer muscle lengths. It is reasonable to assume that myosin evanescence plays a major role in this process of length adaptation, even though it is unclear exactly how myosin monomers are recruited to actin filament lattices to form filaments and vice versa. In particular, myosin monomers and oligomers may be more readily redistributed to various intracellular locations to form filaments as a result of depolymerization.

6.2.5. Relevance to Asthma

We know that when airway smooth muscle is stretched to a sufficient extent, myosin filaments will temporarily depolymerize, causing the muscle's force production to temporarily decrease. This peculiar property of myosin filament lability in smooth muscle of the airways seems to be the cause of the phenomena of bronchodilation and bronchoprotection induced by DI, at least partially. Dilation induces bronchodilation in healthy subjects with bronchoconstriction. Additionally, it has been demonstrated that taking DIs right before a bronchochallenge can lessen the severity of a subsequently induced bronchoconstriction; this phenomenon is referred to as bronchoprotection. It's interesting to note that one of the main characteristics of asthma is that DI does not prevent bronchoconstriction in asthmatics. The mechanical characteristics of asthmatics' tracheal smooth muscle tissue were measured, and the results showed a different reaction. When airway smooth muscle from asthmatic patients is subjected to DI-mimicking oscillations, the reduction in force generation is less pronounced than in nonasthmatic controls. The clinical finding that asthmatics lack bronchoprotection is in line with this observation. Myosin filament stability is regulated by ROCK, according to an analysis of variables affecting myosin filament evanescence in living smooth muscle cells. Because ROCK inhibits myosin light chain phosphatase, it is known to promote RLC phosphorylation. RLC-phosphorylated myosin filaments, as previously noted, are more stable than unphosphorylated filaments, meaning that physical agitation does not quickly cause them to break down. Myosin filament stability is further increased by diphosphorylating RLC at the Ser19 and Thr18 sites. Myosin thick filament density in force-matched intact airway smooth muscle preparations is dramatically reduced upon inhibition of ROCK activity. The reason for this decrease in filament density could be that some filaments have entirely dissolved into monomers, while other filaments have only been reduced to shorter fragments that are undetectable under an electron microscope but still can generate force. The formation of myosin filaments and the control of filament length have been suggested to be mediated by ROCK as a result of these observations. The response of smooth muscle to mechanical oscillations, like those imposed by a DI, may be functionally affected by fragmented myosin filaments caused by ROCK inhibition. In asthmatics, pulmonary blood vessels and airway smooth muscle have been shown to have elevated ROCK protein expression, including both the ROCK1 and ROCK2 isoforms. It was also discovered that the smooth muscle of airways in asthmatics contained less of the protein p116Rip, which inhibits the RhoA-ROCK pathway. Both findings are consistent with a novel asthma phenotype characterized by increased ROCK signaling. This has numerous other effects on the stiffness and contractility of the smooth muscles in the airways (Huttinger et al., 2023; Tuma et al., 2023; Seeras et al., 2023; Zahouani & Mendez, 2023).

A Closer Look

Abdominal Exercises

Effective abdominal exercises are essential for building core strength, stability, and definition. Incorporating a variety of exercises that target different regions of the abdominal muscles can help achieve a balanced and sculpted midsection. Here's an overview of five effective exercises: crunches, planks, Russian twists, leg raises, and bicycle crunches, along with proper form and technique for each.

Crunches are classic abdominal exercises that primarily target the rectus abdominis, the front layer of abdominal muscles. To perform crunches, lie on your back with knees bent and feet flat on the floor, placing hands behind your head or crossed over your chest. Engage your core muscles and lift your shoulders off the floor, bringing your chest towards your knees while keeping your lower back pressed into the floor. Exhale as you crunch up and inhale as you lower back down. Avoid pulling on your neck or using momentum to lift yourself.

Planks are excellent for targeting not only the rectus abdominis but also the deeper stabilizing muscles of the core, including the transverse abdominis and obliques. Begin in a push-up position, with elbows directly beneath your shoulders and forearms resting on the ground. Keep your body in a straight line from head to heels, engaging your core muscles to prevent sagging or arching of the back. Hold this position for as long as you can while maintaining proper form and breathing rhythm.

Russian twists are effective for targeting the oblique muscles, which run along the sides of the torso. Sit on the floor with knees bent and feet lifted off the ground, leaning back slightly to engage the core. Hold a weight or medicine ball with both hands in front of your chest. Rotate your torso to the right, bringing the weight towards the floor beside your hip, then rotate to the left, bringing the weight across your body to the other side. Keep your core engaged and your back straight throughout the movement.

Leg raises primarily target the lower abdominal muscles, including the lower fibers of the rectus abdominis. Lie on your back with legs straight and hands placed under your glutes for support. Keeping your lower back pressed into the floor, lift your legs off the ground until they are perpendicular to the floor or as high as you can without arching your back. Slowly lower your legs back down towards the floor without letting them touch, then repeat the movement.

Bicycle crunches are a dynamic exercise that targets both the rectus abdominis and obliques. Lie on your back with knees bent and hands behind your head. Lift your shoulders off the floor and bring your right elbow towards your left knee while simultaneously straightening your right leg. Alternate sides, twisting your torso and bringing your left elbow towards your right knee while straightening your left leg. Focus on maintaining a smooth, controlled movement and engaging your core throughout. Incorporating these exercises into your workout routine, while ensuring proper form and technique, can help effectively target the abdominal muscles and contribute to a stronger, more defined core. Gradually increase the intensity, duration, and resistance as your strength and endurance improve, and remember to listen to your body and adjust the exercises as needed to prevent injury and maximize results.

Summary

- Abdominal muscles are the muscles of the anterolateral walls of the abdominal cavity, composed of three flat muscular sheets: external oblique, internal oblique, and transverse abdominis. In front on each side of the midline, they are supplemented by rectus abdominis.
- Around the rectus abdominis, which extends from the pubis upward to the ribs, the above muscles are all fibrous.
- The abdomen is a portion of the trunk connecting the thorax and pelvis. An abdominal wall formed of skin, fascia, and muscle encases the abdominal cavity and viscera. The abdominal wall not only contains and protects the intra-abdominal organs but can also distend, generate intrabdominal pressure, and move the vertebral column.
- The abdominal muscles form the abdominal walls, with the abdomen being the portion of the trunk connecting the thorax and pelvis. An abdominal wall is formed of skin, fascia, and muscle and encases the abdominal cavity and viscera.
- Superiorly, the abdominal wall ultimately receives blood from and drains to tributaries of the subclavian vessels. The internal thoracic artery is a branch of the first part of the subclavian artery. It descends between the internal intercostals and transversus thoracis muscles posterior to the upper six costal cartilages in the thorax.
- An understanding of the anatomy of superficial epigastric and deep epigastric vessels is particularly crucial for surgeons constructing free flaps from the inferior abdominal wall to use in reconstructive surgery.
- All the abdominal muscles have different muscle fiber orientations and act in all three planes during movements and are linked together by having a common site of connection or by fascia.
- Innervation of the muscles of the anterolateral abdominal wall derives primarily from the T7-T12 intercostal nerves. They run a circumferential route anteriorly with the rest of the neurovascular bundle between the layers of the internal oblique and transversus abdominis.
- Congenital hernias may occur due to weak spots in the neonatal abdominal wall or embryological malformations during development. They range from the common, more benign umbilical hernia to life-threatening gastroschisis.
- It's important to keep your abdominal muscles strong to maintain a solid core. These muscles help support your spine and pelvis during different movements.
- Myosin is a superfamily of motor proteins that convert chemical energy from ATP hydrolysis to mechanical work. The cyclic interaction of myosin heads with actin filaments enables muscle contraction and cell motility.
- The way myosin filaments are formed could affect smooth muscle shortening, force generation, and mechanical plasticity. Regulation of filament assembly therefore has physiological consequences.
- The stability of myosin filaments in solution is governed by many factors, the most important of which are monomeric myosin concentration, ionic strength, pH, ATP concentration, and the state of myosin phosphorylation.

References

1. Broyles, J. M., Schuenke, M. D., Patel, S. R., Vail, C. M., Broyles, H. V., & Dellon, A. L. (2018). Defining the anatomy of the tendinous intersections of the rectus abdominis muscle and their clinical implications in functional muscle neurotization. *Annals of Plastic Surgery, 80*(1), 50–53. https://doi.org/10.1097/SAP.0000000000001162.
2. Cherla, D. V., Moses, M. L., Viso, C. P., Holihan, J. L., Flores-Gonzalez, J. R., Kao, L. S., Ko, T. C., & Liang, M. K. (2018). Impact of abdominal wall hernias and repair on patient quality of life. *World Journal of Surgery, 42*(1), 19–25. https://doi.org/10.1007/s00268-017-4178-2.
3. Giambelluca, D., Caruana, G., Cannella, R., Picone, D., & Midiri, M. (2018). The "caput medusae" sign in portal hypertension. *Abdominal Radiology (NY), 43*(9), 2535–2536. https://doi.org/10.1007/s00261-018-1542-0.
4. Huttinger, R., Sugumar, K., & Baltazar-Ford, K. S. (2023). Spigelian hernia. In *StatPearls* [Internet]. StatPearls Publishing. https://www.ncbi.nlm.nih.gov/books/NBK519499/ (accessed on 25 June 2024).
5. Kössler-Ebs, J. B., Grummich, K., Jensen, K., Hüttner, F. J., Müller-Stich, B., Seiler, C. M., Knebel, P., Büchler, M. W., & Diener, M. K. (2016). Incisional hernia rates after laparoscopic or open abdominal surgery: A systematic review and meta-analysis. *World Journal of Surgery, 40*(10), 2319–2330. https://doi.org/10.1007/s00268-016-3520-6.
6. Lipa, J. E. (2007). Breast reconstruction with free flaps from the abdominal donor site: TRAM, DIEAP, and SIEA flaps. *Clinics in Plastic Surgery, 34*(1), 105–121. https://doi.org/10.1016/j.cps.2006.11.004.
7. Natsis, K., Piagkou, M., Repousi, E., Apostolidis, S., Kotsiomitis, E., Apostolou, K., & Skandalakis, P. (2016). Morphometric variability of pyramidalis muscle and its clinical significance. *Surgical and Radiologic Anatomy, 38*(3), 285–292. https://doi.org/10.1007/s00276-015-1548-0.
8. Sadler, T. W., & Feldkamp, M. L. (2008). The embryology of body wall closure: relevance to gastroschisis and other ventral body wall defects. *American Journal of Medical Genetics Part C: Seminars in Medical Genetics, 148C* (3), 180–185. https://doi.org/10.1002/ajmg.c.30176.
9. Seeras, K., Qasawa, R. N., Ju, R., & Prakash, S. (2023). Anatomy, abdomen and pelvis: anterolateral abdominal wall. In *StatPearls* [Internet]. StatPearls Publishing. https://www.ncbi.nlm.nih.gov/books/NBK482315/ (accessed on 25 June 2024).
10. Tsai, H. C., Yoshida, T., Chuang, T. Y., Yang, S. F., Chang, C. C., Yao, H. Y., Tai, Y. T., Lin, J. A., Chen, K. Y. (2017). Transversus abdominis plane block: An updated review of anatomy and techniques. *Biomed Research International, 2017*, 8284363. https://doi.org/10.1155/2017/8284363.
11. Tuma, F., Lopez, R. A., & Varacallo, M. (2023). Anatomy, abdomen and pelvis: inguinal region (inguinal canal). In *StatPearls* [Internet]. StatPearls Publishing. https://www.ncbi.nlm.nih.gov/books/NBK482318/ (accessed on 25 June 2024).
12. Yendluri, V., Centeno, B., & Springett, G. M. (2007). Pancreatic cancer presenting as a Sister Mary Joseph's nodule: case report and update of the literature. *Pancreas, 34*(1), 161–164. https://doi.org/10.1097/MPA.0b013e31802eedac.

13. Zahouani, T., & Mendez, M. D. (2023). Omphalocele. In *StatPearls* [Internet]. StatPearls Publishing. https://www.ncbi.nlm.nih.gov/books/NBK470308/ (accessed on 25 June 2024).

14. Zens, T., Nichol, P. F., Cartmill, R., & Kohler, J. E. (2017). Management of asymptomatic pediatric umbilical hernias: A systematic review. *Journal of Pediatric Surgery, 52*(11), 1723–1731. https://doi.org/10.1016/j.jpedsurg.2017.07.003.

Chapter

MUSCLE TISSUE

7

Contents

Introduction

One of the four main categories of animal tissue is muscle, which is a soft tissue. Skeletal muscles contract because of the muscle tissue that surrounds them. The process of myogenesis, which occurs during embryonic development, is how muscle is formed. Actin and myosin, two unique contractile proteins found in muscle tissue, work together to produce movement. Two regulatory proteins, troponin and tropomyosin, are present along with numerous other muscle proteins. The type and location of muscle tissue in the body vary. Skeletal or striated muscle, smooth muscle (non-striated muscle), and cardiac muscle are the three types found in vertebrates. The body moves because of the elongated, multinucleate muscle cells known as muscle fibers that make up skeletal muscle tissue. The perimysium and tendons are additional tissues found in skeletal muscle. Without conscious thought, smooth and cardiac muscle contract involuntarily. These muscle types can become activated through peripheral plexus innervation, endocrine (hormonal) activation, and interactions with the central nervous system. Skeletal or striated muscle can only contract voluntarily when the central nervous system is involved. Reflexes are a type of unconsciously contracted skeletal muscle, but they also originate from central nervous system activation, even though cortical structures are not engaged until after the contraction has taken place. Depending on the type of muscle and its precise location, different muscle types respond differently to hormones and neurotransmitters like nitric oxide, acetylcholine, noradrenaline, and adrenaline. Muscle tissue can also be subcategorized based on factors like myoglobin, mitochondria, myosin ATPase, and other components.

Orientation and Directional Terms:

Term	**Definition**	**Illustration**
Embryonic development	Embryonic development starts with the fertilization of an egg cell by a sperm cell. Once fertilized, the ovum becomes a single diploid cell known as a zygote.	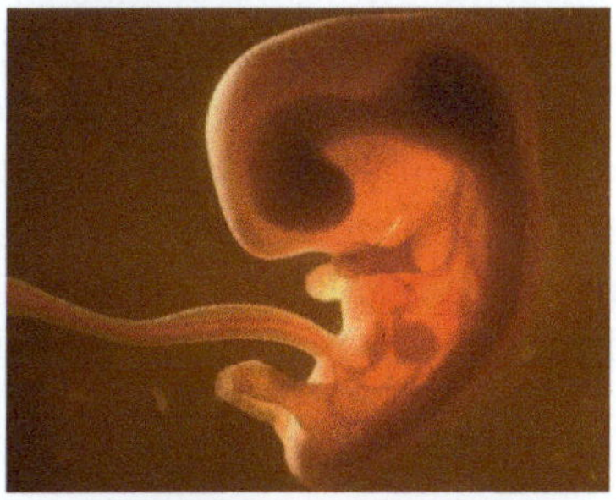
Epimysium	It is a layer of dense irregular connective tissue which ensheaths the entire muscle and protects muscles from friction against other muscles and bones. It also allows a muscle to contract and move powerfully while maintaining its structural integrity.	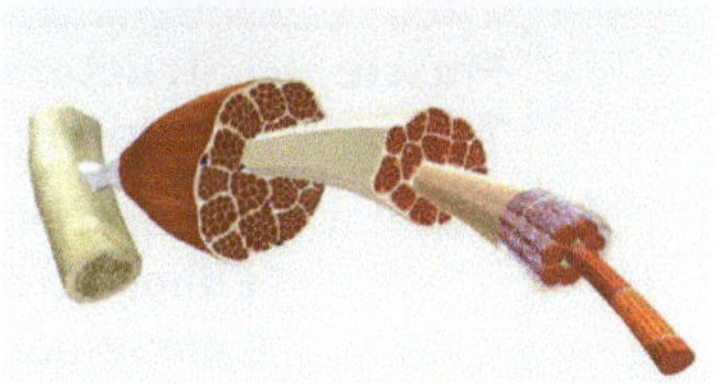
Gap junction	Gap junctions are clusters of intercellular channels that allow direct diffusion of ions and small molecules between adjacent cells.	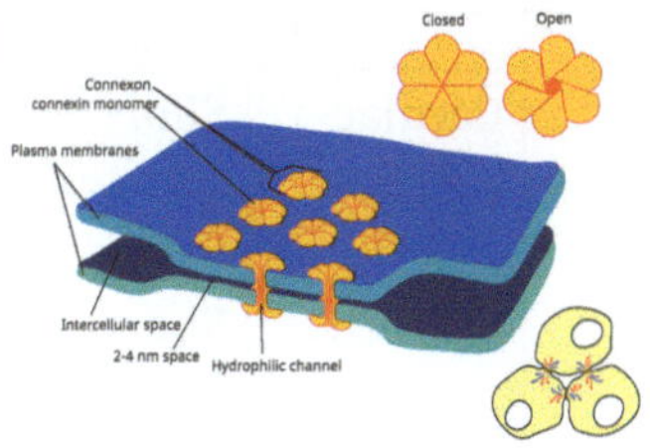
Myofilament	Myofilaments are the three protein filaments of myofibrils in muscle cells. The main proteins involved are myosin, actin, and titin. Myosin and actin are the contractile proteins and titin is an elastic protein.	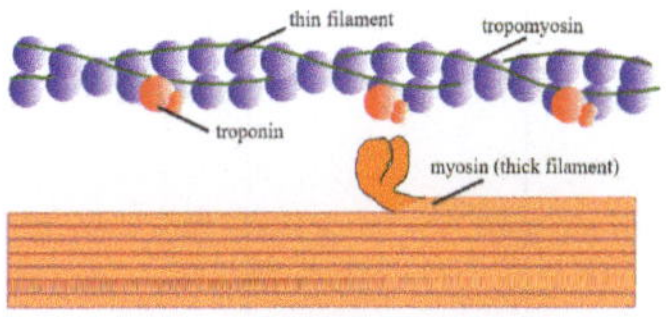
Sarcopenia	Sarcopenia is a type of muscle loss that occurs with aging and/or immobility. It is characterized by the degenerative loss of skeletal muscle mass, quality, and strength.	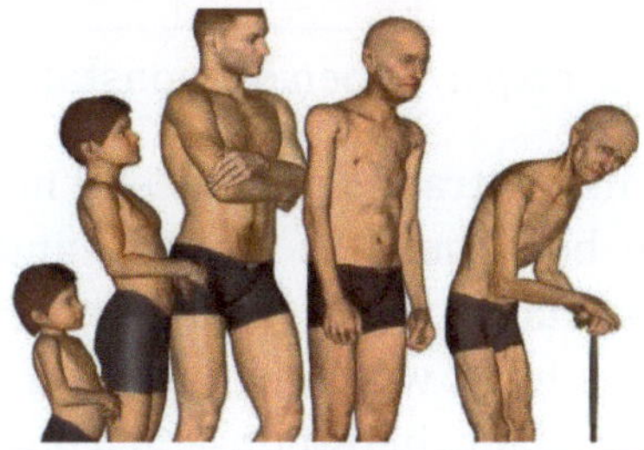

7.1. Basics of Muscle Tissue

The characteristics of muscle tissue permit movement. Because they are excitable, muscle cells react to external stimuli. Because they can shorten and produce a pulling force, they are contractile. Muscle contraction drives the motion of the bones when it is attached between two movable objects, like two bones. Certain muscle movements are voluntary, denoting that they are controlled consciously. For instance, someone chooses to open a book and peruse the anatomy chapter. Some movements, like the contraction of your pupil in bright light, are involuntary, meaning you are not conscious of them. Skeletal, cardiac, and smooth muscle tissue are the three categories into which it is divided based on structure and function (Table 7.1).

Table 7.1. *Comparison of the Structure and Properties of Muscle Tissue Types*

Muscle Type	**Structural elements**	**Function**	**Location**
Skeletal	Long cylindrical fiber, striated, many peripherally located nuclei	Voluntary movement, produces heat, protects organs	Attached to bones and around entry & exit sites of the body (e.g., mouth, anus)
Cardiac	Short, branched, striated, single central nucleus	Contracts to pump blood	Heart
Smooth	Short, spindle-shaped, no evident striation, a single nucleus in each fiber	Involuntary movement, moves food, involuntary control of respiration, moves secretions, regulates the flow of blood in arteries by contraction	Walls of major organs and passageways

Source: https://open.oregonstate.education/aandp/chapter/4-4-muscle-tissue/.

The contraction of skeletal muscle, which is affixed to the bones, enables voluntary movements of the body such as walking and expressing emotions on the face and in the posture. Skeletal muscle makes up forty percent of your body mass. As a result of their contraction, skeletal muscles produce heat, which helps maintain thermal homeostasis. Skeletal muscle contractions that occur uncontrollably in response to a body temperature that is below normal cause shivering. The myoblasts that come from the mesoderm give rise to the muscle cell or myocyte. Throughout life, the number of myocytes stays mostly constant. Bundles of skeletal muscle tissue are encircled by connective tissue. Muscle cells appear striated and have numerous nuclei squeezed along the membranes when viewed under a light microscope. The actin and myosin contractile proteins, as well as the structural proteins that link the contractile proteins to connective tissues, alternate on a regular basis, resulting in striation. Each long muscle fiber is formed by the fusion of numerous myoblasts, which causes the cells to become multinucleated. The heart's contractile walls are made of cardiac muscle. Under a microscope, cardiomyocytes—the cells that make up the heart muscle—also have striated appearances. Cardiomyocytes are single cells with a single nucleus located in the center, in contrast to skeletal muscle fibers.

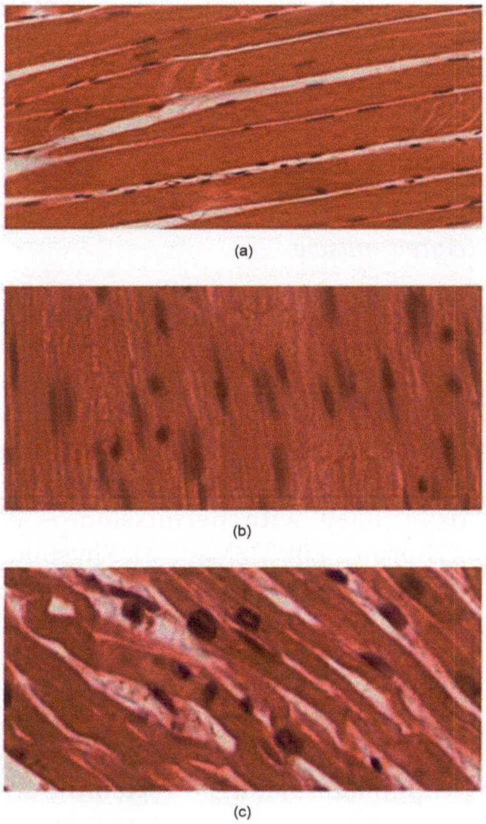

Figure 7.1. *Muscle Tissue: (a) Skeletal muscle cells have prominent striation and nuclei on their periphery. (b) Smooth muscle cells have a single nucleus and no visible striations. (c) Cardiac muscle cells appear striated and have a single nucleus.*

Source: https://open.oregonstate.education/app/uploads/sites/157/2019/07/414_Skeletal_Smooth_Cardiac-350x589.jpg

Cardiomyocytes are distinguished by their ability to contract on their own intrinsic rhythm in the absence of outside stimulation. Intercalated discs are specialized cell junctions that allow cardiomyocytes to adhere to one another. Gap junctions and anchoring junctions are both present in intercalated discs. Heart muscle fibers with attached cells branch out and function as a syncytium, enabling the cells to coordinate their movements. The heart muscle is controlled involuntarily and pumps blood throughout the body. Internal organ movements that are not voluntary are caused by contractions of smooth muscle tissue. It creates the blood vessels, airways, and contractile elements of the reproductive, urinary, and digestive systems. With a single nucleus and a spindle shape, every cell lacks visible striations (Figure 7.1).

7.1.1. Structure of Muscular Tissue

The epimysium, a tough connective tissue that resembles cartilage, envelops the bundles of muscular tissues. The epimysium envelops the bundle of nerve cells that run in long fibers known as fascicles. The perimysium is a layer of protection that envelops the fascicles. It permits blood and nerves to reach each individual fiber. The endomysium, another layer of defense, envelops the fibers. The contraction of various muscle parts is aided by these layers and muscles. As they contract, the various bundles slide past one another. The tendons that are connected to the periosteum, the connective tissue that envelops the bones, are connected to the epimysium. When the muscles contract, this facilitates the skeleton's movement. The epimysium exerts a force on the organs and regulates everything from food processing to circulation through its connections with other connective tissues.

7.1.2. General Features of Muscle and Movement

Multi-cellular animals rely on muscles to propel their movements and sustain their posture. Their unique appearance is recognizable as fish flesh or meat. In many animals, muscle is the most abundant tissue; in fish, for instance, it comprises 50–60% of the body mass, whereas in antelopes, it accounts for 40–50%. Voluntary muscles are those that can be controlled consciously. Other muscles are referred to as involuntary muscles because the organism cannot consciously control them. For instance, in vertebrates, peristalsis is the mechanism by which muscles in the walls of the intestines move food along, and constriction and relaxation of the muscles in the walls of small blood vessels regulate the flow of blood to various parts of the body. These muscles also contract rhythmically in the heart, pumping blood throughout the body. Because of the increased or decreased blood flow to the skin, blushing and paling are visible consequences of muscle changes in the blood vessels. Animals move using more than just their muscles. Instead, many unicellular organisms known as protozoa (also called protists) move by actively beating their cell surface processes, known as flagella or cilia, to propel them through water. Certain unicellular organisms possess the ability to move like amoeboids, wherein the contents of the cell flow outward into projections known as pseudopodia from the cell body.

A few ciliated protozoans move with the help of rods known as myonemes, which can shorten quickly. Multicellular animals also depend on nonmuscular means of locomotion. Cilia beat to facilitate swimming in many microscopic organisms. Certain flatworms and tiny mollusks use their cilia to enable them to crawl along their undersides. Cilia are used by certain invertebrates that obtain their food by filtering particles from water and creating the necessary water currents. White blood cells in higher animals use amoeboid movements, and respiratory tract lining cells' cilia clear foreign particles from the sensitive membranes.

Each long, thin cell, or fiber, that makes up a muscle is a bundle of smaller fibrils (Figure 7.2). Each fibril contains thin filaments of actin and other proteins as well as relatively thick filaments of the protein myosin. The filaments in a muscle fiber slide past one another as it lengthens or shortens, as seen in Figure 7.2.

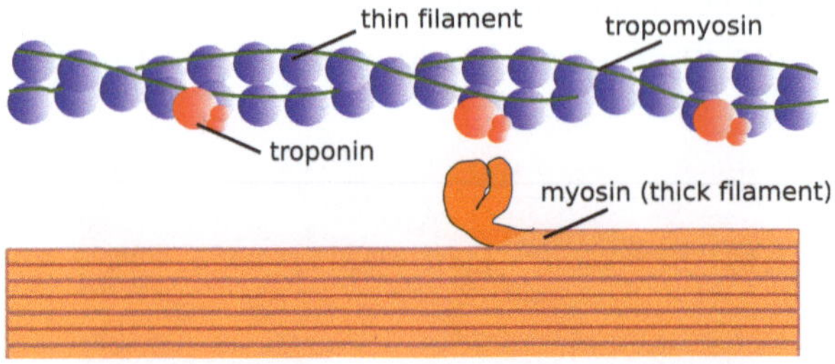

Figure 7.2. *The arrangement of the myofilaments in a striated muscle.*

Source: By Mikael Häggström. When using this image in external works, it may be cited as: Häggström, Mikael (2014). "Medical gallery of Mikael Häggström 2014." WikiJournal of Medicine 1 (2). DOI: 10.15347/wjm/2014.008. ISSN 2002-4436. Public Domain. or By Mikael Häggström, used with permission. - Walter F., PhD. Boron (2003) Medical Physiology: A Cellular And Molecular Approach, Elsevier/ Saunders, pp. 1,300 ISBN: 1-4160-2328-3. Page 29, Public Domain, https://commons.wikimedia.org/w/index.php?curid=3426065.

The thick filaments are 1.6 micrometers (0.0016 millimeters) long in vertebrate striated muscle but up to six micrometers long in some arthropods.

The filaments' length is essentially constant. The cross bridges in active muscles cause tension (i.e., projections that attach to the thin filaments and apply force to them from the thick filaments). Cross bridges repeatedly detach and reattach in new positions as the filaments slide past each other and the active muscle lengthens or shortens. Their maneuver resembles pulling in a rope with both hands. Most other cells are only a fraction of a millimeter long, but some muscle fibers can reach lengths of several centimeters. Several nuclei are spaced out along the length of these long fibers because one nucleus cannot sufficiently service them.

Chemical energy from food metabolism is needed by muscle to perform its functions. A portion of the chemical energy used by muscles to contract and carry out mechanical work is transformed into work, while the remainder is lost as heat. Both the chemical energy used and the mechanical energy absorbed by the action—such as slowly lowering a weight—are transformed into heat when muscles lengthen while exerting tension. In warm-blooded animals, muscle plays a crucial role in producing heat. Muscle contractions that cause the body to warm up are called shivering. Comparably, before taking off, some insects vibrate their wings to warm their muscles to the optimal temperature.

7.1.3. Diversity of Muscle

Animal species and even individual parts of the same animal have different muscle fiber compositions. Muscles vary in structure and activity, in addition to being classified as voluntary or involuntary. The myofilament arrangement varies among muscles. The three main types of muscles are smooth muscle, where the filaments are arranged randomly, obliquely striated muscle, where the filaments are staggered to create oblique bands, and striated muscle, where the filaments are organized in transverse bands as shown in Figure 7.2. Except for the cardiac muscle, which is involuntary but striated, all voluntary muscles in vertebrates are striated, while all involuntary muscles are smooth. Only a few groups of invertebrates, including mollusks, annelids, and nematodes, have obliquely striated muscles. The thick filaments of these muscles contain both myosin and the protein paramyosin. The stimuli needed to activate each muscle vary. Voluntary muscles in vertebrates rely on electrical signals called action potentials in their nerves to start each contraction. Action potentials in the nerves of certain involuntary muscles merely alter the muscle's inherent contraction rhythm. These muscles contract spontaneously. All insects' leg muscles and many of their wing muscles need action potentials to begin each contraction; however, some insects' wing muscles are made of fibrillar muscle, which only sometimes needs action potentials to sustain its fast, rhythmic contractions. These wings are affixed to their bodies in a way that causes them to vibrate at a resonant frequency, much like a guitar string does when it is plucked at its resonance frequency. Fibrillar muscles contract when they are active to keep the resonant system vibrating. The capacity of each muscle to withstand stress varies. The long, thick filaments in muscles that are subjected to high stresses carry more cross bridges. As a result, compared to other muscles, there are more cross bridges. This implies that greater stresses can be applied and that more force can be transferred from each thick filament to the nearby thin filaments. When fibers are being forced to stretch, more stress can be applied than when they are staying constant in length. Conversely, when fibers are shortening, less stress can be applied.

The ways in which muscles regulate their forces are different. The majority of the fibers in mammals' voluntary muscles are only able to be turned on or off, and varying numbers of fibers can be activated to produce varying degrees of force. On the other hand, the force that every muscle fiber produces varies in many other muscles. In these muscles, force is modulated by altering the overall intensity of muscle activation rather than by varying the number of fibers activated. The ranges of lengths over which muscles can function vary. Though some striated muscles are exceptional, smooth muscles typically function over larger ranges of length than striated ones. A single muscle in the chameleon's tongue has the ability to contract to a sixth of its maximum length. Additionally, there are differences in the rates at which muscles shorten and develop force. A muscle shortens at a rate of one length per second if it shortens by a tenth of its length in a tenth of a second. Maximum rates of shortening differ between muscle fibers within an animal and between species. For instance, at 37°C, the maximum shortening speeds of two mouse limb muscles are 24 and 13 lengths per second. Finally, the metabolism of muscles varies. They can either produce the adenosine triphosphate (ATP) they need as their immediate energy source through anaerobic processes, which do not require oxygen, or through oxidative reactions, in which food is oxidized to carbon dioxide and water. For brief spurts of intense activity, like sprinting, vertebrates and crabs use the anaerobic process of glycolysis, which converts the carbohydrate glycogen to lactic acid. After the activity spike, there is a recovery phase during which some of the lactic acid is oxidized by oxygen, which releases the energy required to convert the remaining lactic acid back to glycogen. This method of utilizing anaerobic metabolism has the benefit of allowing the burst's intensity of activity to be unrestricted by the blood's ability to supply oxygen to the muscles.

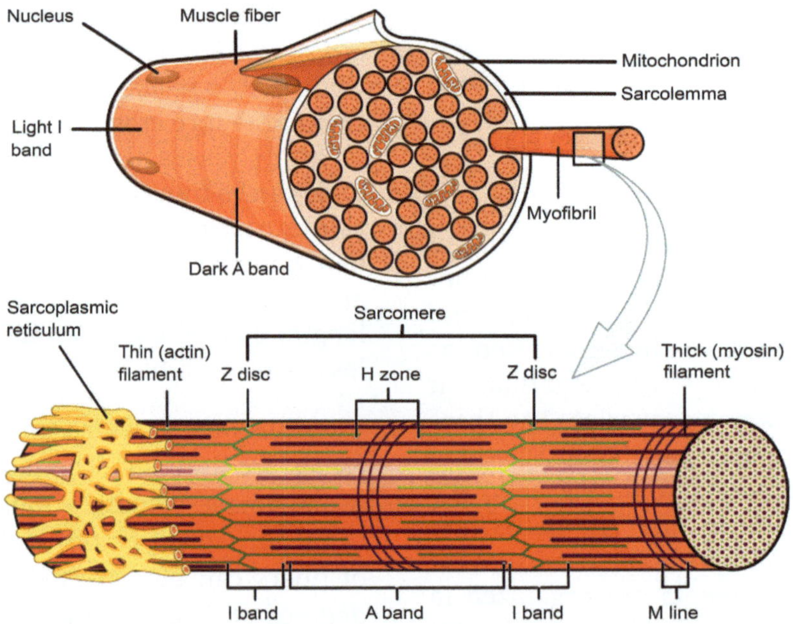

Figure 7.3. *The Arrangement of the Myofilaments in Obliquely Striated Muscle.*

Source: By OpenStax – https://cnx.org/contents/FPtK1zmh@8.25:fEI3C8Ot@10/Preface, CC BY 4.0, https://commons.wikimedia.org/w/index.php?curid=49885687.

Many muscle fibers in vertebrates only carry out glycolysis or oxidative metabolism, however some carry out both functions. Owing to the pigment myoglobin's presence, oxidative fibers are typically red in color. The majority of fish exhibit a clear distinction between a narrow band of red muscle running along the side of the body and the main mass of white swimming muscle. The red (oxidative) muscle powers slow swimming, while the white (glycolytic) muscle powers quick swimming bursts. Red and white muscles can also be easily distinguished in domestic chickens, where the dark meat of the legs is made up of red fibers and the pale meat of the breast is primarily made up of white fibers. The primary muscles of the wings, which chickens only use for sporadic, brief flights, are the breast muscles. Some avian athletes, such as hummingbirds, primarily have red breast muscles (Figure 7.3).

7.1.4. Muscles that Work Skeletons

An illustration of a basic system where muscles operate a rigid skeleton is a clamshell. The shell's two rigid sections are hinged together (Figure 7.4). They can be left open or closed to safeguard the animal inside. Just inside the hinge is the inner hinge ligament, a block of rubbery protein. The inner hinge ligament is compressed when the adductor muscle contracts, closing the shell. The ligament recoils elastically upon relaxation, causing the shell to open again. The fact that only one muscle is used to operate this system makes it unique. The majority of other skeletal systems require antagonistic pairs of muscles, meaning that each muscle is paired with another muscle that has the opposite function. The human ankle serves as an illustration of this antagonism. The soleus muscle extends the ankle, while the tibialis anterior muscle flexes the ankle, lifting the toes. This pair of muscles is antagonistic. In this instance, the gastrocnemius is an additional muscle that works in tandem with the soleus to facilitate ankle extension. However, the gastrocnemius crosses the ankle as well as the knee, affecting both joints.

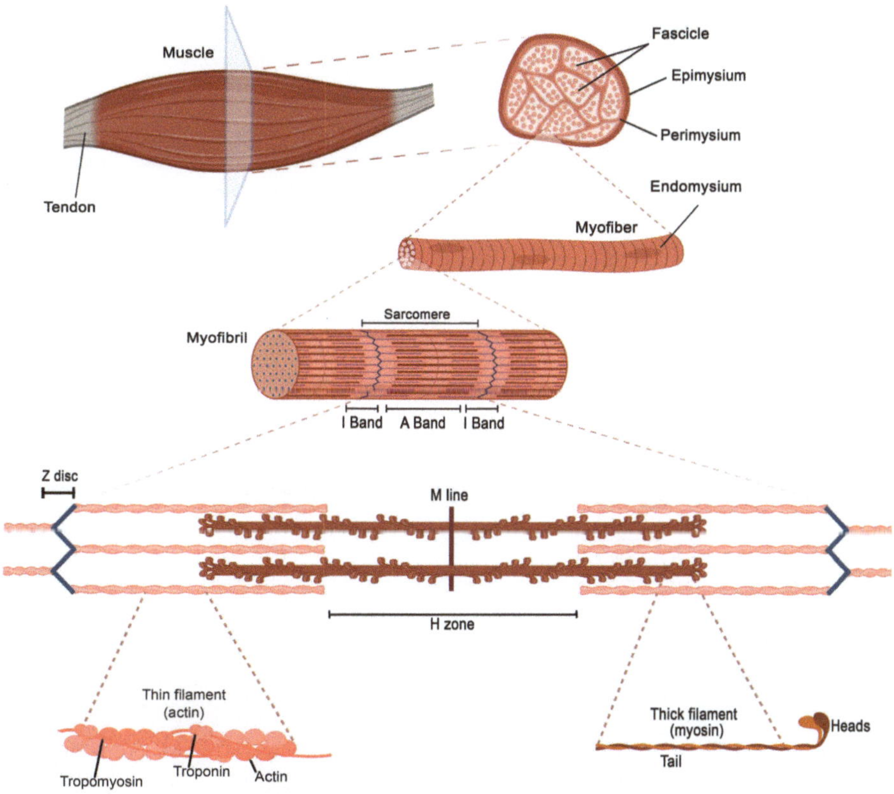

Figure 7.4. *Rigid skeletons worked by muscles.*

Source: Zuccaro E, Marchioretti C, Pirazzini M, Pennuto M. Introduction to the special issue "skeletal muscle atrophy: mechanisms at a cellular level." Cells. 2023; 12(3):502. https://doi.org/10.3390/cells12030502.

Ankles are not just hinge joints. They can display inversion (the sole of the foot facing the other leg) or eversion (the opposite movement) in addition to flexion and extension. The peroneus muscles, which are antagonistic and evert the ankle, and the tibialis posterior, which inverts it, regulate these movements. A hinge, like the clam joint or the human knee, can only move in one direction, which is called flexion/extension, or one degree of freedom of movement. The human ankle has two degrees of freedom due to its ability to move in two different ways: flexion/extension and inversion/eversion. The human hip is a ball-and-socket joint that offers three degrees of freedom. For every degree of freedom, the majority of animal joints contain at least two muscles (an antagonistic pair).

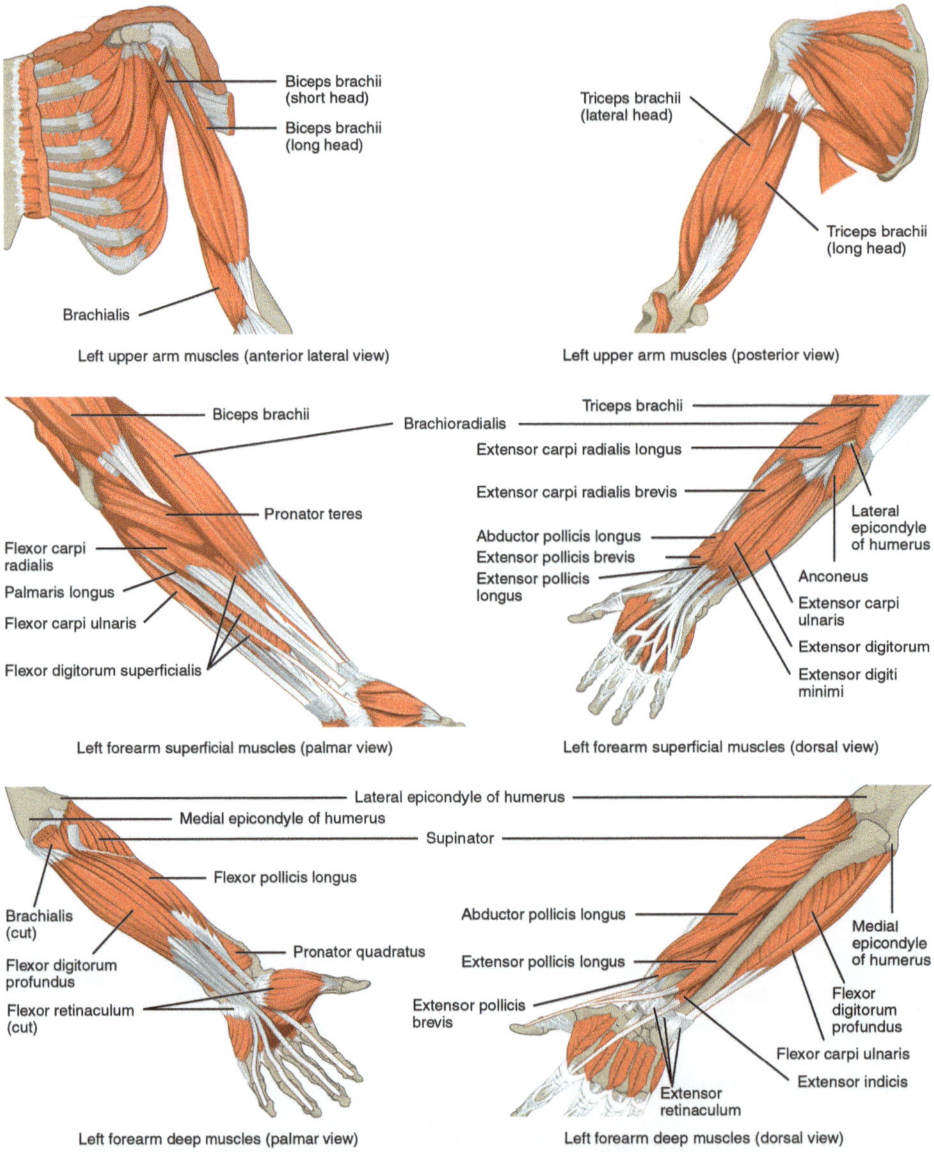

Figure 7.5. *Muscles of the human forearm (anterior view, superficial layer).*

Source: https://commons.wikimedia.org/wiki/File:1120_Muscles_that_Move_the_Forearm.jpg

Muscle fibers are rarely as long as the corresponding muscle, but many muscles, including the biceps in the arm, are made up of comparatively long fibers that are almost exactly parallel to one another. Just at their extreme ends are these parallel muscles connected to tendons or apodemes (chitinous rods that act as sites for muscle attachment in arthropods). This configuration works well for rapid, large movements because muscle fibers can contract to approximately one-third of their resting length. When relatively short fibers attach diagonally to a tendon that extends deep into the muscle, the shoulder deltoid muscle in humans is said to be pennate. The majority of the hamstring muscles, which are located at the back of the thigh, are parallel, but the ankle muscles depicted in Figure 7.4B are pennate. Arthropod leg muscles are mostly pennate, but the adductor muscles of clam shells are parallel. When comparing a pennate muscle to a parallel muscle of the same mass, the pennate muscle may have many more shorter fibers. Because of this, the parallel-fibered muscle can shorten considerably but only exert a relatively small force, whereas the pennate muscle can exert a greater force but cannot shorten greatly. Pennate muscle can have an effect similar to that of a longer lever arm in a particular structure. Because there isn't enough room for large muscles or long lever arms in the slim legs of arthropods, many of the muscles are pennate. The elastic properties of tendons and apodemes. Mammalian tendons act as springs in their legs, storing and returning energy lost during foot strike and body deceleration as an elastic strain energy in the tendons and an elastic recoil upon landing. It is these tendons that reduce the energy cost of running. For instance, an apodeme in locusts' hind legs is a crucial elastic component of the catapult mechanism that propels them forward (Figure 7.5).

7.1.5. Types of Muscle Tissue and Fibers

Muscle cells are specialized for contraction. Muscles allow for motions such as walking, and they also facilitate bodily processes such as respiration and digestion. The body contains three types of muscle tissue: skeletal muscle, cardiac muscle, and smooth muscle (Figure 7.6)

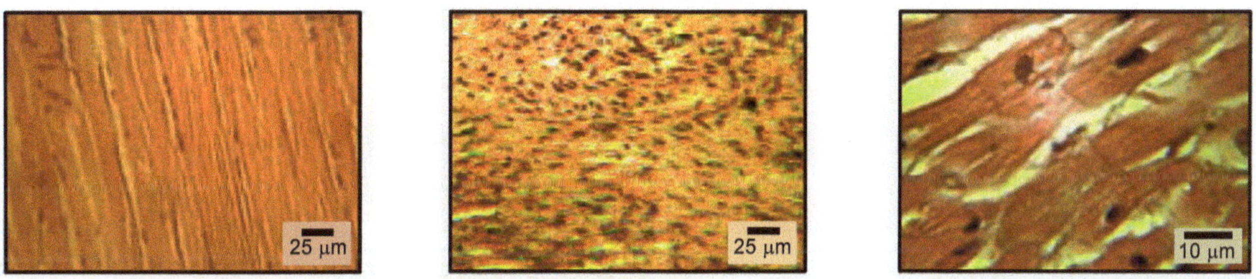

Skeletal muscle | Smooth muscle | Cardiac muscle

Figure 7.6. *The body contains three types of muscle tissue: skeletal muscle, smooth muscle, and cardiac muscle, visualized here using light microscopy. Smooth muscle cells are short, tapered at each end, and have only one plump nucleus in each. Cardiac muscle cells are branched and striated, but short. The cytoplasm may branch, and they have one nucleus in the center of the cell.*

Source: https://s3-us-west-2.amazonaws.com/courses-images/wp-content/uploads/sites/1223/2017/02/08002620/Figure_38_04_01-1024x248.jpg.

Skeletal muscle tissue gives rise to skeletal muscles, which are attached to the skin or bones and regulate all conscious movements, including walking. Skeletal muscle is also referred to as voluntary muscle because it is thought-controlled. Under a microscope, skeletal muscle tissue appears striped or striated. Skeletal muscles are long and cylindrical in shape. The regular arrangement of contractile proteins (myosin and actin) is what causes the striations. A globular contractile protein called actin works with myosin to contract muscles. Multiple nuclei can be found in a single cell in skeletal muscle. Smooth muscle tissue surrounds blood vessels and the respiratory tract in addition to the walls of hollow organs like the stomach, bladder, and intestines. Smooth muscle is referred to as involuntary muscle since it lacks striations, has a single nucleus per cell, is tapered at both ends, and is not subject to voluntary control. Only the heart contains cardiac muscle tissue, and cardiac contractions are responsible for both blood pressure maintenance and blood pumping throughout the body. Similar to skeletal muscle, cardiac muscle has striations, but unlike skeletal muscle, cardiac muscle is referred to as involuntary muscle since it is not under conscious control. It is branched, has one nucleus per cell, and can be identified by the intercalated disks that surround it.

7.1.5.1. Skeletal Muscle Fiber Structure

A skeletal muscle cell is a single skeletal muscle fiber. With diameters of up to 100 μm and lengths of up to 30 cm, these cells are enormous. The sarcolemma is the name of the plasma membrane found in skeletal muscle fibers. The action potential conduction site, which initiates muscle contraction, is the sarcolemma. Myofibrils are long, cylindrical structures that run parallel to the muscle fiber within each muscle fiber. Since myofibrils only have a diameter of about 1.2 μm, hundreds to thousands of them can be found inside a single muscle fiber. Myofibrils run the entire length of the muscle fiber. Their ends are attached to the sarcolemma, causing the entire muscle cell to contract as the myofibrils shorten (Figure 7.7).

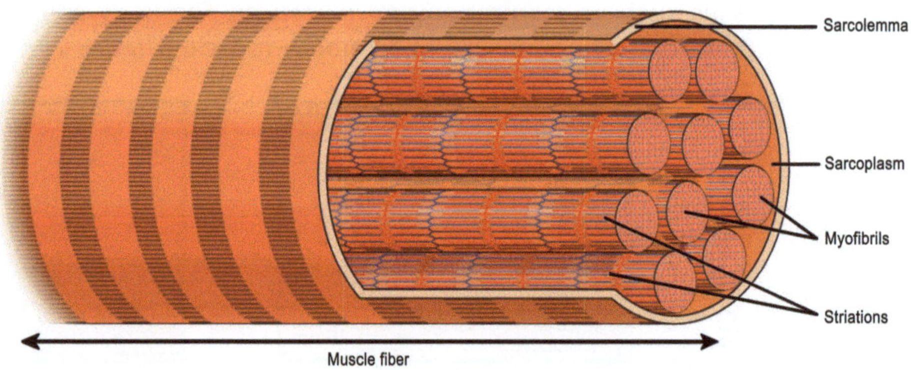

Figure 7.7. *A skeletal muscle cell is surrounded by a plasma membrane called the sarcolemma with a cytoplasm called the sarcoplasm. A muscle fiber is composed of many fibrils, packaged into orderly units.*

Source: https://s3-us-west-2.amazonaws.com/courses-images/wp-content/uploads/sites/1223/2017/02/08002651/Figure_38_04_02–1024x401.jpg,

The actin and myosin protein bands that repeat along the length of myofibrils give skeletal muscle tissue its striated appearance. Myofibril alignment results in the appearance of striations or bands throughout the cell. Dark A bands and light I bands repeat along myofibrils (Figure 7.8).

A dense line known as a Z disc or Z line runs vertically through the center of each I band. The Z discs delineate the boundaries of skeletal muscle's functional units known as sarcomeres. One complete A band and two halves of an I band, one on either side of the A band, are found in a single sarcomere, which is the area between two successive Z discs. Sarcomeres, which run the length of a myofibril, are what cause the myofibrils and muscle cells to shorten as a result of their individual contraction (Figure 7.8).

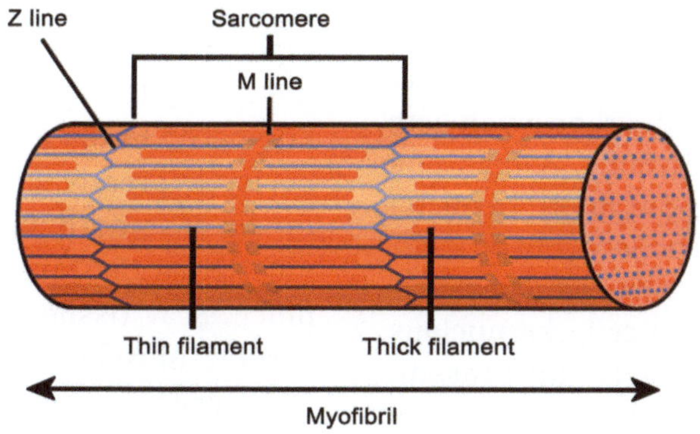

Figure 7.8. *A sarcomere is the region from one Z line to the next Z line. Many sarcomeres are present in a myofibril, resulting in the striation pattern characteristic of skeletal muscle.*

Source: https://s3-us-west-2.amazonaws.com/courses-images/wp-content/uploads/sites/1223/2017/02/08002716/Figure_38_04_03.jpg.

Myofilaments are the smaller structural units that make up myofibrils. The two primary filament types are thick filaments and thin filaments, each of which has a unique composition and distribution. Thick filaments are limited to a myofibril's A band. The entire length of the I band and a portion of the A band are covered in thin filaments, which are attached to the protein alpha-actinin found in the Z disc. Because there is little space between the thick and thin filaments, the area where they overlap appears dense. There is a central region of the A band that only has thick filaments; thin filaments do not extend all the way into the A bands. The H zone is the central area of the A band that appears somewhat lighter than the rest of the band. Thick filaments are held together by accessory proteins at the M line, a vertical line that runs through the center of the H zone. Myofilaments are held in place by the Z disc and the M line, which preserves the myofibril's structural organization and layering. Desmin, or intermediate, filaments attach to the Z disc and connect myofibrils to one another. The components of thick and thin filaments are proteins. The protein myosin makes up thick filaments. Whereas the heads of myosin molecules align on either side of the thick filament where the thin filaments overlap, the tails of individual myosin molecules join together to form the central region of a thick filament close to the M line. The actin protein is the main building block of thin filaments. Tropomyosin and troponin are the other two constituents of the thin filament. Myosin attachment sites are found on actin. When the muscles are at rest, strands of tropomyosin block the binding sites and stop actin-myosin interactions. There are three globular subunits that make up troponin. Three subunits bind: one to actin, one to tropomyosin, and one to Ca^{2+} ions.

7.2. Development and Regeneration of Muscle Tissue

The majority of the body's muscle tissue develops from embryonic mesoderm. Next to the neural tube, paraxial mesodermal cells form somite cells, which are blocks of cells. While skeletal muscles in the head and limbs develop from general mesoderm, all other skeletal muscles, with the exception of those in the head and limbs, develop from mesodermal somites. Myoblasts are produced by somites. A myoblast is a kind of stem cell that forms muscles. It can migrate to various parts of the body and then fuse with other myoblasts to form myotubes, or syncytiums. A myotube has a continuous cytoplasm but multiple nuclei due to its formation from various myoblast cells. Skeletal muscle cells are multinucleate because, in the mature skeletal muscle cell, the nucleus of each contributing myoblast is still present. Nevertheless, because the myoblasts that make up cardiac and smooth muscle cells do not fuse, these cells are not multinucleate. Early in development, gap junctions form in the cardiac and single-unit smooth muscle. Acetylcholine receptors are first found on the majority of the myoblast surface in skeletal muscles, but growth factors are released upon spinal nerve innervation, which promotes the development of motor end-plates and NMJs. Electrical signals that are sent through the muscle when neurons become active affect the distribution of fast and slow fibers in the muscle.

Satellite cells aid in the repair of skeletal muscle cells, even though the quantity of muscle cells is fixed during development. As a form of stem cell, satellite cells are comparable to myoblasts; however, because they are integrated into muscle cells, satellite cells help with the synthesis of proteins needed for growth and repair. These cells are found outside the sarcolemma and are stimulated by growth factors released by the muscle fibers in response to specific types of stress to proliferate and fuse with muscle cells. Although they mainly aid in the repair of damage to living cells, satellite cells have a very limited ability to regenerate muscle fibers. Fibrosis is the process by which muscle fibers are replaced by scar tissue when a cell sustains damage beyond what satellite cells can restore. Muscle that has suffered significant damage loses strength and is unable to produce the same amount of power or endurance as it did prior to the damage because scar tissue is unable to contract. Some small blood vessels contain a type of stem cell called a pericyte, which has the ability to regenerate smooth muscle tissue. Compared to skeletal and cardiac muscle tissue, pericytes greatly facilitate the regeneration and repair of smooth muscle cells. Just like skeletal muscle, cardiac muscle does not regenerate very much. Scar tissue takes the place of the dead cardiac muscle tissue and is non-contractile. The accumulation of scar tissue impairs the heart's contractile power, which prevents the heart from pumping. However, blood-derived stem cells that sporadically penetrate cardiac tissue may cause some modest regeneration.

7.2.1. Muscular Tissue Location

The entire body, from head to toe, is made up of muscle tissue. Tendons are found in the arms, legs, abdomen, chest, back, and face. They serve as the link between skeletal muscles and bones. These muscles control voluntary motions such as running, walking, and making facial expressions. The walls of internal organs such as the stomach, intestines, bladder, and blood vessels are lined with smooth muscles, which are also referred to as involuntary muscles. They facilitate the passage of food through the digestive system, control the flow of urine, and alter blood vessel diameter to lower or raise blood pressure. The heart alone contains cardiac muscle, which is in charge of pumping blood throughout the body. It functions automatically to keep the blood flowing and make sure that all tissues receive nutrition and oxygen.

7.2.2. Function and Developmental Role of Various Muscular Tissue

Muscle tissue is a type of soft tissue that forms the majority of tissues found in the muscles of the human body. Alongside muscle tissue, muscles also contain connective tissues like tendons, which connect skeletal muscles to bones, and sheaths of connective tissue that surround muscle tissues. Only muscle tissue itself has cells capable of contracting. There are three main types of muscular tissue.

7.2.2.1. Skeletal Muscle Tissue

About 40% of the body's mass is made up of skeletal muscle, which is necessary for posture, movement, facial expressions, and voluntary actions. For these purposes, it adheres to bones and contracts. By producing heat during contraction, skeletal muscle also contributes significantly to thermal regulation. This is especially true when shivering, an involuntary reaction to a low body temperature, occurs. Myoblasts from the mesoderm layer give rise to skeletal muscle cells, or myocytes, which are arranged into bundles encircled by connective tissue. The arrangement of the contractile proteins myosin and actin, as well as the structural proteins that connect them to connective tissues, gives the appearance of striated skeletal muscle cells when viewed under a light microscope. As a result of myoblast fusion during the formation of muscle fibers, they are multinucleated.

7.2.2.2. Functions of Skeletal Muscle Tissue

The skeletal system, also known as the musculoskeletal system, has several functions:

1. *Support:* It provides structural support for the body and serves as an attachment point for muscles and tendons.
2. *Movement:* It facilitates movement by providing a framework for muscles to act upon.
3. *Protection:* It protects internal organs from damage.
4. *Mineral storage:* It stores minerals and fat, releasing them when needed.
5. *Blood cell production:* It produces blood cells, primarily in the red marrow of bones.
6. *Endocrine regulation:* It produces osteocalcin, a hormone that regulates cellular responses to insulin stimuli.

7.2.2.3. Smooth Muscle Tissue

The muscle tissue that lines internal organs and structures like blood vessels is called smooth muscle. It contracts to facilitate the function of these vessels and organs. Unlike skeletal muscles, which we can control, smooth muscles contract involuntarily. Hormones, the autonomic nervous system, and other elements are involved in this. Actin and myosin filaments are present in smooth muscle cells, also known as myocytes, but unlike skeletal muscles, they are not arranged in sarcomeres. Instead, they alternate and are spaced apart.

Smooth muscle has several key functions in the body:

1. **Uterine Wall:** It helps the uterus stretch during pregnancy and contract during childbirth.
2. **Contractions and Stretching:** Unlike skeletal muscle, smooth muscle can sustain long contractions and stretch while maintaining its ability to contract.
3. **Control of Air Passages:** It regulates the diameter of air passages, aiding in efficient respiration.
4. **Blood Flow and Pressure:** It regulates blood flow and pressure by constricting or dilating blood vessels.

5. **Gastrointestinal Motility**: It facilitates digestion by moving food through the digestive tract.
6. **Urinary System Function:** It helps control the flow of urine in the urinary system.
7. **Lymphatic System Function:** It propels lymph fluid through the lymphatic system.
8. **Control of Pupil Size:** It regulates the size of the pupil in the eyes.
9. **Hair Erection:** It raises hairs in hair follicles in the skin.

7.2.2.4. Cardiac Muscle Tissue

The contractile walls of the heart are composed of cardiomyocytes, which are cells that make up cardiac muscle. These cells have a single nucleus and are striated. Unlike skeletal muscle, cardiomyocytes can contract on their own initiative without outside assistance. They are joined by gap junctions and intercalated discs that act as anchors. Because of this configuration, the cells can coordinate their contractions to produce long, branching fibers. The heart muscle works without conscious thought to pump blood throughout the body.

Functions of cardiac muscle include:

1. Pumping Blood: It delivers oxygen and nutrients to cells and removes waste.
2. Involuntary Movements: Contractions are automatic and cannot be controlled consciously.
3. Rhythmic Contractions: Cardiac muscle contracts and relaxes rhythmically to pump blood.
4. Contractility: It is responsible for the heart's ability to contract and pump blood.
5. Cell Response: Cardiac muscle cells respond to nervous impulses.
6. Locomotion: Involved in movement or locomotion.
7. Excitation-Contraction Coupling: Links the muscle cell's action potential to contraction.
8. Pacemaker Potential: Produced by changes in membrane permeability and currents.

7.3. Current Strategies for the Regeneration of Skeletal Muscle Tissue

The most prevalent tissue in the human body, making up between 40 and 45% of the body's total mass, is skeletal muscle. This type of striated muscle tissue is mainly in charge of producing a sequence of distinct uniaxial forces that permit locomotion. It is controlled voluntarily by the somatic nervous system. Thankfully, skeletal muscle tissue can heal itself from injuries quite well. However, severe injuries involving loss of volumetric muscle (VML) lead to irreversible functional impairments. Interventional treatment is necessary for VML because it cannot be healed naturally. Because it severely limits musculoskeletal functionality, it can have a major impact on the quality of life. The most common causes of skeletal muscle damage are traumatic injuries, tumor resections, and degenerative genetic diseases that result in muscle fiber atrophy, such as juvenile Charcot-Marie-Tooth disease, amyotrophic lateral sclerosis (ALS), and Duchenne muscular dystrophy (DMD). Skeletal muscle is made up of connective tissue, blood vessels, nerves, and hierarchically arranged muscle fibers, or myofibers. Depending on the location and function of the muscle, myoblasts fuse to form elongated, cylindrical, multi-nucleated fibers called myotubes, which range in diameter from 10 to 100 μm. These fibers are then called myofibers. The functional unit of skeletal muscle is represented by them. Sarcomeres, the repeating contractile units of skeletal muscle, are found on multiple myofibrils within each muscle fiber, which is a skeletal muscle cell. Thin filament actin and thick filament myosin are two contractile proteins found in sarcomeres. The sarcoplasm, a type of cytoplasm, and the plasma membrane encircle the muscle fiber. The nuclei of mature myofibers align with the periphery beneath the sarcolemma. Parallel myofibers in skeletal muscle tissue are bundled into fascicles that are encased in perimysium. Every muscle fiber in the contraction is supplied by a somatic motor neuron. These large, highly protein-rich cells can produce large amounts of proteins and enzymes required for their proper function because they have multiple nuclei.

Muscle regeneration is primarily regulated by extracellular matrix (ECM) proteins and secreted factors, and it depends on a diverse population of resident muscle stem cells, also known as satellite cells (SCs), interstitial cells, and blood vessels. Tissue engineering uses a mix of cells, scaffolds, and growth factors to restore or regenerate damaged or lost skeletal muscle tissue. Scaffolds made of three-dimensional (3D) biomaterials can be used to guide and control tissue regeneration locally. These scaffolds provide cells with an artificial extracellular matrix (ECM) that resembles tissue. Additionally, bioactive substances like proteins and growth factors can be added to scaffolds to encourage the synthesis of the cell's own extracellular matrix (ECM) and support cell adhesion and proliferation. A range of well-known and cutting-edge biomaterials have been used to create scaffolds that offer the necessary mechanical, structural, physicochemical, and biological qualities. As a result, a variety of multifunctional biomaterials have been developed that can carry out a number of crucial tasks, including drug delivery, stem cell fate regulation, and cell guidance.

7.3.1. Strategies for Skeletal Muscle Regeneration

One benefit of the skeletal muscle engineered constructs, which can facilitate muscle regeneration, is their capacity to integrate functional striated muscle structures into the injured region of the host. Skeletal muscle has been produced and regenerated in recent years through the use of in vitro, in vivo, and in situ muscle engineering techniques (Figure 7.9). Every strategy has benefits and drawbacks of its own. In vitro cell differentiation into myotubes is a common step in the in vitro skeletal muscle engineering technique. Prior to implantation, preconditioning in a bioreactor optimizes the tissue structure. The goal of this approach is to create functional, mature, contractile constructs for transplantation. Furthermore, cocultures of cells or multipotent cells are frequently employed to promote and aid in the development of blood vessels and neuromuscular junctions (NMJs). But the primary obstacles to in vitro skeletal muscle tissue engineering are the size needed, the intricacy of the structure, the lack of myotube alignment, the inability to generate enough contractile force, and the high cell density needed to induce differentiation into aligned myotubes. Therefore, obtaining large constructs for VML repair remains a challenge. Furthermore, in order to guarantee the supply of nutrients and oxygen to highly metabolically active cells in large constructs, successful vascularization is a crucial parameter. Furthermore, the cells used in in vitro skeletal muscle engineering must not induce rejection reactions, and the biomaterials chosen must be biocompatible.

To create a local niche at the transplantation site, the in vivo strategy depends on the transplantation of cells, either with or without a scaffold. The goal of this approach is to promote in vivo myoneural junction, muscle, and vasculature regeneration.

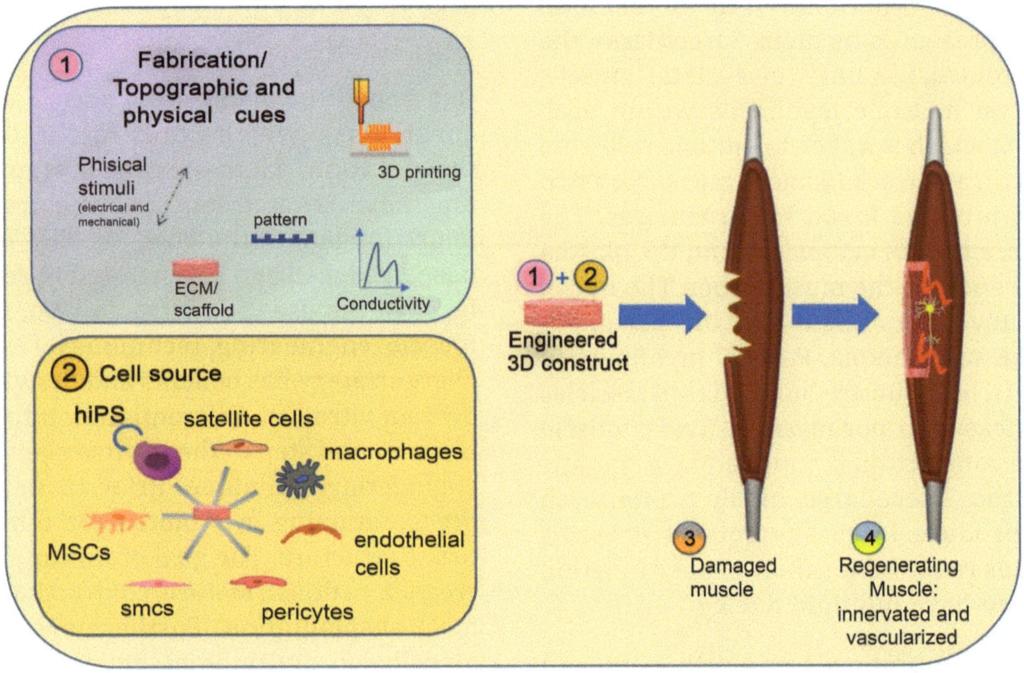

Figure 7.9. *Muscle tissue engineering. (1) Tissue engineering technologies (fabrication/topographic and physical cues) are needed to generate a 3D muscle-like construct together with (2) different cell types: satellite cells, macrophages, endothelial cells, pericytes, smcs, MSCs. The 3D engineered tissue is applied to a damaged muscle (3) in order to induce muscle regeneration (4) including a functional innervated and vascularized muscle.*

Source: Reid G, Magarotto F, Marsano A, Pozzobon M. Next stage approach to tissue engineering skeletal muscle. Bioengineering. 2020; 7(4):118. https://doi.org/10.3390/bioengineering7040118.

By avoiding the need for extensive processing of cell-loaded constructs, in vivo engineering can guarantee the functional characteristics of the cells and encourage the development of new tissue in vivo. The primary benefits of this system are lower costs and complexity. Acellular biomaterials serve as models for in situ engineering techniques that promote skeletal muscle endogenous regeneration. These biomaterials can be engineered to produce particular topographies, release bioactive and chemotactic molecules, draw in cells from the site of injury, and activate and stimulate their infiltration to promote the regeneration of the NMJ, muscle, and vasculature. Technological developments in tissue engineering and biomaterial science, which encompass scaffold fabrication methods, are critical to the development of the in situ engineering approach. The primary benefit of this approach is that it may make it possible to produce a clinician-friendly off-the-shelf product. To comprehend the relationships between the biomaterial and the healing responses, this strategy also calls for sophisticated biomaterials and in-depth research (Qazi et al., 2015; Liu et al., 2018).

7.3.2. Cell Types for the Regeneration of Skeletal Muscle

The most popular method for enhancing skeletal muscle regeneration is cell therapy. Using the right cell source is crucial to achieving a successful course of treatment. Various cell candidates have been reported for skeletal muscle regeneration (Figure 7.10) and their transplantation for the treatment of muscle injury has been investigated. These cell candidates include SCs, myoblasts, muscle-derived stem cells (MDSCs), pericytes, and mesoangioblasts, bone marrow-derived mesenchymal stromal cells (BM-MSCs), or adipose tissue-derived stem cells (ADSCs), and induced pluripotent stem cells (iPSCs).

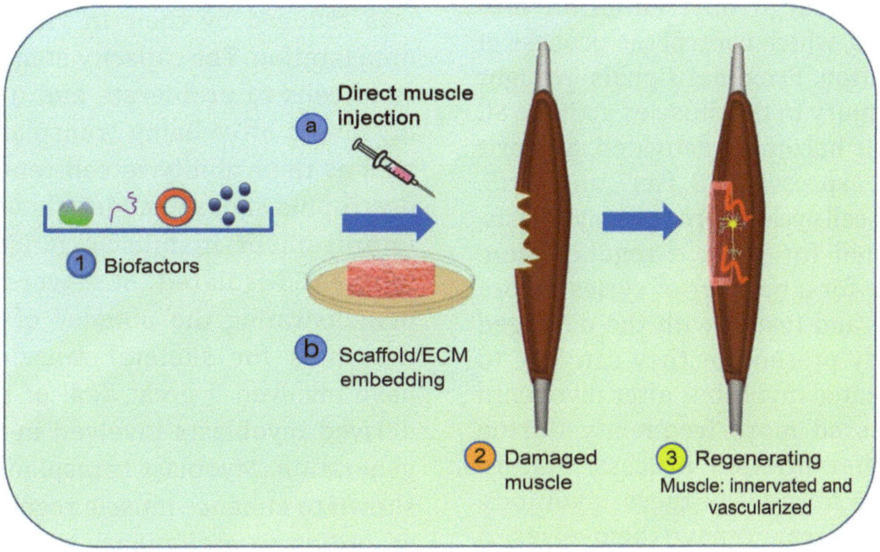

Figure 7.10. *Biochemical stimuli to enhance muscle regeneration. (1) Growth factors, cytokines, small molecules, miRNA are biofactors known to improve the regeneration process (3) of a damaged muscle (2). The biofactors can be delivered to a damaged muscle by (a) direct injection or (b) previous embedding in a scaffold. The factors can be also vehicled by plasmid or virus to enhance the release and possibly achieve innervated and vascularized muscle.*

Source: Reid G, Magarotto F, Marsano A, Pozzobon M. Next Stage approach to tissue engineering skeletal muscle. Bioengineering. 2020; 7(4):118. https://doi.org/10.3390/bioengineering7040118.

Obtaining enough cell numbers for the application is essential for an effective cell-based treatment. In addition, the applied cells should not cause rejection reactions, which would eliminate the need for long-term immunosuppressive medications. They should also maintain viability, preserve myogenic potential during in vitro culture, improve muscle function permanently following transplantation, interact and integrate both structurally and functionally with the host tissue, and replenish and renew stem cell niches located within the tissue.

7.3.2.1. Satellite Cells (SCs) and Myoblasts

Skeletal muscle growth and regeneration are attributed to SCs, the muscle stem cells. They are situated close to blood capillaries and between the basal lamina and sarcolemma of myofibers. Near neuromuscular and myotendinous junctions, SC density is higher. They also express myogenic factor 5 (Myf5) and the transcription factors Pax7 and Pax3. The most crucial indicator for preserving SC function is Pax7, which is expressed primarily by proliferating and quiescent SCs. About 30% of the sublaminal nuclei on myofibers in early postnatal muscles are made up of

SCs, whereas in healthy adults, this percentage drops to only 2–7%. In the juvenile growth phase of muscle development, SCs can multiply and supply nuclei for the developing myofibers. Adult SCs are typically quiescent during mitosis. After being triggered, they move to the site of damage and undergo differentiation into skeletal myoblasts, which control the process of muscle regeneration. Proximal signals brought on by illness or injury to the muscles activate SC myogenesis. After becoming activated, SCs exit the basal lamina, express MyoD, Pax7, and Myf5, and go through a cell cycle to produce myoblasts, which are needed for muscle regeneration. Myoblasts divide for a number of cycles before exiting the cycle and fusing with the damaged myofibers already present, or they can fuse to form multi-nucleated myotubes after myogenin (Myf4) is expressed more frequently during the terminal differentiation process. Mature myofibers can be formed by these myotubes. Because stem cells can renew themselves, a tiny percentage of them stay in a quiescent state to add new stem cells to the population. Therefore, following repeated cycles of injury and regeneration, the number of satellite cells stays constant throughout life.

The surrounding niche, which is made up of fibroblasts, endothelial cells, immune cells, and inflammatory cells, is highly receptive to SCs. It has been demonstrated that these cells mediate SC differentiation and proliferation. Specifically, it has been documented that fibroblasts play a major role in modulating the SC niche and that, following injury, a lack of fibroblasts may cause smaller regenerated fibers to form. Murphy et al.'s study demonstrated that SC expansion during repair is regulated by fibroblasts, and that fibroblast-SC interaction can enhance muscle regeneration. Considering the critical role SCs play in muscle regeneration, many studies have looked into transplanting SCs into injured muscles. In this study, after being transplanted into the same host environment, stem cells derived from various hindlimb muscles produced distinct behavioral traits. Following their transplantation into mice lacking dystrophin, these cells promoted the repair of fibers and increased the number of stem cells. Notably, the ability of SCs to regenerate was reduced by their in vitro growth before implantation. The capacity of individual isolated stem cells to proliferate and differentiate into myofibers after being transplanted in vivo, as well as their ability to self-renew after that. A dystrophic mouse model showed measurable improvement in muscle function after only 900 FACS-isolated SCs were transplanted, demonstrating the potency of SCs. Cell-based therapies for skeletal muscle regeneration have involved a great deal of research on SC-derived myoblasts involved in skeletal muscle generation. Myoblast transplantation has been shown to enhance muscle regeneration in mice, according to preliminary trials. In dystrophin-deficient mdx mice, Partridge and colleagues showed that intramuscular injection of normal myoblasts produced myofibers that expressed dystrophin through fusion with host muscle fibers. Several additional investigations involving myoblast transplantation into mdx mice verified enhanced muscle regeneration.

Furthermore, research was done on the application of tissue-engineered scaffolds for stem cell delivery. For example, stem cells were embedded in in situ photo-cross-linkable hydrogels based on hyaluronan by Rossi and colleagues. When hydrogels containing recently isolated stem cells were transplanted into a mouse model, the quantity of new myofibers and functional recovery were higher than when hydrogels containing muscle progenitor cells or hydrogels alone were used. Collagen I, fibrin, or PEG-fibrinogen gels were recently used by Prüller and colleagues to encapsulate various sources of human and murine myogenic cells. Human immortalized C25Cl48 myoblasts, primary in vitro expanded stem cell-derived myoblasts from EDL muscle, mouse skeletal myoblast cell line C2C12, and recently isolated murine soleus myofibers were employed. Large multinucleated myotubes were primarily formed by C2C12 myoblasts in collagen I and fibrin hydrogel. Nevertheless, stem cells created aligned, multinucleated, contractile myotubes in collagen I and fibrin hydrogels. While the muscle niche in vivo facilitates muscle regeneration following the transplantation of recently isolated muscle stem cells, the regenerative capacity of these cells is quickly reduced when they are cultured in vitro on rigid tissue culture plates. The heterogeneity of the SC population and the challenges associated with isolation persist, despite the possibility that transplanting SCs could be an effective therapeutic approach. Variations can be seen in the gene expression, proliferation rate, myogenic differentiation capacity, and self-renewal ability of stem cells (SCs) from both different and identical muscles. For example, compared to limb muscle, the masseter muscle has been reported to have a lower capacity for regeneration. Furthermore, the myogenic potential of newly isolated stem cells is significantly reduced in vivo by their expansion in vitro, making it challenging to obtain an adequate number of cells to promote regeneration. For instance, it has been demonstrated that isolated SCs' proliferative and myogenic potential is greatly diminished even after a 3-day culture period.

Various approaches have been taken to date to deal with these shortcomings. For example, Mooney and colleagues were able to sufficiently regenerate muscle tissue by seeding enriched populations of myoblasts into alginate hydrogels. Growth factor delivery and scaffold composition and architecture also had a major impact on the long-term survival of myoblasts. Several myoblast-incorporated tissue-engineered scaffolds have been created thus far to treat VML brought on by trauma, tumor removal, or degenerative illnesses. This group then created three distinct constructs to examine the impact of the cell composition of the porcine bladder matrix scaffold on functional recovery. The constructs were made of cells that resembled myoblasts, myotubes, or a combination of myoblasts and myotubes. One construct was produced by the short-term, non-bioreactor preconditioned cellular proliferation of rat muscle-derived cells, which produced primarily myoblasts. To produce myotubes primarily, the second type of construct was created by long-term cell differentiation and preconditioning in a bioreactor. The second type of construct was treated similarly to generate the third type of construct, but during bioreactor preconditioning, rat muscle-derived cells were applied twice to primarily create myotubes and myoblasts, simulating exercise. The first and second type constructs showed comparable functional recovery following implantation into the mouse VML injury model, whereas the third type of constructs encouraged an accelerated and prolonged functional recovery with twice the magnitude of functional recovery as the other constructs. In addition, they observed a 2- to 3-fold increase in functional recovery when the second type of constructs were implanted into a Lewis rat tibialis anterior muscle VML defect model, as opposed to acellular matrix scaffolds made of porcine bladder without cells (Qazi et al., 2015; Liu et al., 2018).

7.3.2.2. Mesenchymal Stromal Cells (MSCs)

Multipotent stem cells called mesenchymal stromal cells (MSCs) can differentiate into mesodermal cells like chondrocytes, adipocytes, and osteoblasts. The role of MSCs in skeletal muscle regeneration has been shown in several investigations. However, the effectiveness of the myogenic differentiation of human MSCs has been called into question. MSCs are essential for angiogenesis and peripheral nerve regeneration, both critical for the repair of skeletal muscle. They can also contribute to the formation of ectodermal and endodermal tissues in addition to skeletal muscle. MSCs are easily isolated from a variety of tissues, including Wharton's jelly, bone marrow, adipose tissue, and the placenta. Crucially, MSCs exhibit immune evasion traits. MHC I and MHC II are usually not expressed by culture-expanded MSCs. However, MHC class I and class II can be expressed much more when MSCs are exposed to IFN-γ or differentiate into mature cell types. The use of MSCs for local and systemic administration in the repair of skeletal muscle is gaining a lot of attention.

Because of their potential for myogenic repair, bone marrow-derived MSCs (BM-MSCs) are a valuable type of adult stem cells that are non-hematopoietic and multipotent. By co-culturing with myoblasts, applying myogenic media, or responding to biophysical stimuli, they can differentiate into myoblasts. Prior research indicates that BM-MSCs support myogenesis after local (e.g., injection into the muscle) and systemic delivery (e.g., intravenous or intra-arterial injection) is used. As an illustration, consider the number of mature muscle fibers and the cross-sectional area of muscle fibers 28 days after injury in comparison to the non-treated group. By suppressing inflammatory cytokines and upregulating the anti-inflammatory cytokine IL-10, the intramuscular injection of BM-MSCs into the muscle injury site lowered local immune responses and accelerated muscle fiber regeneration. Furthermore, we observed enhanced angiogenesis, and fibrosis was inhibited by BM-MSCs through downregulating transforming growth factor-beta 1 (TGF-β1) and lowering collagen synthesis at the site of soft tissue injury. Significantly, the number of transplanted BM-MSCs and the rate of muscle recovery after intramuscular BM-MSC injection in rats with severe skeletal muscle injury were found to have a logarithmic dose-response relationship. Upon transplanting BM-MSCs into the peritoneal cavity of DMD model mice that had severe muscle degeneration, Maeda and colleagues showed enhanced muscle recovery. The importance of CXCL12 for muscle regeneration was also determined by them. The expression of MyoD, myogenin, α-sarcomeric actin, and MMP-2 in myoblasts as well as the activation of SCs were demonstrated by Sassoli and colleagues involving platelet-rich plasma (PRP). Comparing PRP alone to PRP plus BM-MSC, it was discovered that the latter was less effective.

They also revealed that myoblast response was guided by BM-MSCs through paracrine activation of AKT signaling. The enhanced green fluorescent protein (eGFP) transgenic SD rats were used by Natsu and colleagues to isolate BM-MSCs, which they then implanted into the injured muscle region of the SD rats by embedding the cells in a fibrin scaffold. The myofiber maturation and functional recovery one month post-transplant were both enhanced by transplanted BM-MSCs. Transplanted bone marrow-derived myofibroblasts (BM-MSCs) underwent differentiation into muscle progenitor cells but did not fuse or differentiate into myofibers. This suggests that inflammatory cells may have an indirect role in skeletal muscle regeneration. Better skeletal muscle regeneration and vascularization were observed when BM-MSCs and ECM scaffold were combined, as opposed to when decellularized ECM was used alone.

This led to enhanced recovery of both structure and function. BM-MSCs and MSCs derived from skeletal muscle co-cultured in another study led to the fusion of both co-cultured cell types within 24 hours, and after 5 days of cultivation, myotube-like cells were found (Qazi et al., 2015; Liu et al., 2018).

Similar to bone marrow-derived mesenchymal stem cells (BM-MSCs), adipose-derived stem cells (ADSCs) are a multipotent MSC source that is readily expandable, adult, and abundant. A straightforward liposuction technique can be used to extract them from adipose tissue with high yield, and a myogenic medium containing factors that induce myogenesis can be used to differentiate them into myoblasts. Other methods include co-culturing with myoblasts, genetic modification of ADSCs, or biophysical stimuli. Notably, when Pax7, Myf5, and MyoD are expressed, they show myogenesis potential comparable to SCs. A small percentage of recently harvested ADSCs spontaneously differentiate into myogenic cells, as shown by Di Rocco and colleagues, indicating their inherent myogenic potential. Only when the ADSCs were cultured close to myoblasts did they fuse into myotubes. They found that in mdx mice with ischemic skeletal muscle, the injection of recently isolated ADSCs led to fusion with muscle fibers to achieve muscle recovery and significantly restored dystrophin expression. Similarly, in mouse models of muscular dystrophy, injection of ADSCs into the site of injury was demonstrated to control inflammation, improve angiogenesis, enhance muscle repair, and restore dystrophin expression. In a different study, Kesireddy compared the ability of ADSCs and muscle-derived progenitor cells (MDCs) seeded onto decellularized porcine urinary bladder matrix scaffolds to regenerate skeletal muscle using a mouse VML injury model. Histological examination revealed that the two constructs seeded with ADSCs or MDCs had comparable capacities for regeneration, exhibiting neotissue formation indicators like cell fusion, fiber formation, and scaffold remodeling. However, compared to the donor MDCs, ADSCs had a relatively small contribution to the creation of new hybrid myofibers, according to immunohistochemical analyses of the donor cells labeled with lentivirus Cherry. However, ADSCs seemed to play a role in vascularization, which could make up for the less effective myofiber formation.

The in vitro differentiation capacity and isolation efficiency of MSCs from skeletal muscle tissue (MC-MSCs), bone marrow (BM-MSCs), and adipose tissue (ADSCs) were examined by Meligy and colleagues. After being isolated, 5-azacytidine was added to MSCs to stimulate myogenic differentiation. According to immunocytochemical analyses, BM-MSCs had the lowest proliferation rate and ADSCs the highest. Furthermore, myogenin expression was found to be a useful tool for evaluating MSC differentiation potential. The myogenin expression level of MC-MSCs was the highest at 93%, followed by that of BM-MSCs (83.3%) and AD-MSCs (77%). MC-MSCs had the lowest percentage of cells expressing CD44 and CD90, while AD-MSCs had the highest percentage. AD-MSCs are the most readily available cells and exhibit the highest growth as well as the highest percentage of stem cell marker expression, although MC-MSCs demonstrated the highest myogenic differentiation potential.

7.3.2.3. Muscle Derived Stem Cells (MDSCs)

Adult skeletal muscle contains a unique population of stem cells called MDSCs. The preplating technique was used to isolate these cells based on their adherence to collagen-coated flasks. Specifically, stem cell and satellite cell markers are expressed by late-adhering cells and early-adhering cells, respectively. As a result, they are negative for the hematopoietic stem cell markers CD45, CD43, and c-kit, but positive for myogenic markers like desmin, myogenin, and MyoD, and stem cell markers like Flk-1 and Sca-1. Crucially, they retain their myogenic potential and can expand up to 30 passages, self-renew, and differentiate into myotubes. Additionally, they exhibit high rates of survival in hypoxic environments, a high potential for proliferation and differentiation, and resistance to oxidative stress. In contrast to SCs, MDSCs are a precursor of SCs that can differentiate into different mesodermal lineages in addition to the myogenic lineage. When an injury affects the muscle-tendon interface, or myotendinous junction, as well as the muscle-associated tendon, MDSCs may be especially helpful. After being injected locally or systemically, MDSCs stimulated muscle regeneration and produced hybrid fibers that expressed dystrophin in the dystrophic mouse model. According to a study by Qu-Petersen and colleagues, transplanting MDSCs produced 10 times more dystrophin+ myofibers than transplanting SCs. When MDSCs were injected intra-arterially into immunosuppressed dystrophic dogs, the outcome was improved clinical benefits, including enhanced myofiber regeneration, long-term dystrophin expression, SC replenishment, and increased walking ability. Matthias and colleagues recently used an in situ fibrin gel cast to transplant MDSCs into a model of muscle loss injury. The ability of transplanted MDSCs in fibrin gel to engraft, form new myofibers, increase muscle mass, decrease fibrotic tissue, encourage the formation of new vessels, and restore muscle SCs was discovered.

In a clinical trial, tacrolimus was used to suppress the patient's immune system while a high-density injection of in vitro-cultured normal muscle precursor cells was administered to the DMD patient. Eighteen months after transplantation, donor-derived dystrophin expression was still observed. Additionally, a normalized profile of pro-inflammatory cytokines and reduced creatine kinase levels were noted. The trophic, paracrine, and immunomodulatory activity of BM-MSCs suggests that they may enhance the regenerative potential of skeletal muscle-derived stem/progenitor cells. Therefore, by fusing with skeletal muscle fibers that are degenerating in vivo, both cell types may contribute to the recovery of skeletal muscle.

7.3.2.4. Pericytes

Pericytes are stem cells that are found in the walls of capillaries and microvascular structures. These cells interact with capillary endothelial cells to modify microcirculation; they are located beneath the microvascular basal lamina. Pericytes can differentiate into adipogenic, chondrogenic, and myogenic cells. They have been isolated from a variety of tissues, including skeletal muscle, adipose tissue, and the pancreas. Pericytes typically express myogenic markers only after differentiation and neither Pax7 nor MyoD. Two primary subpopulations of pericytes have been identified: type 1 (nestin–NG^{2+}) and type 2 (nestin+NG2+). Type 2 pericytes are known to promote the development of new muscle, whereas type 1 pericytes are implicated in the accumulation of fat. Pericytes have been shown by Dellavalle and colleagues to play a role in tissue regeneration, the development of skeletal muscle fibers, and the SC pool during postnatal growth. The creation of a large number of differentiated muscle fibers expressing human dystrophin following injection into immunodeficient SCID–mdx dystrophic mice demonstrated the myogenic potential of pericytes. They also demonstrated that it is possible to grow pericytes that have been isolated from both normal and dystrophic human skeletal muscle to produce enough cells to treat a young patient. For DMD therapy, these cells can be differentiated into skeletal muscles and transduced with viral vectors to express dystrophin. Adult pericytes shared characteristics with juvenile pericytes in terms of morphology and capacity to form colonies. They could no longer form myotubes and capillary-like structures, which limited their myogenic potential as they aged. The myogenic and angiogenic activity of adult pericytes was remarkably enhanced both in vitro and in vivo by their culture on a PEG-based hydrogel. Thus, it was hypothesized that PEG-based 3D hydrogels would stimulate the renewal of myogenic potential by imitating the rigidity and mechanical cues of the muscle extracellular matrix. (Qazi et al., 2015; Liu et al., 2018)

7.3.2.5. Induced Pluripotent Stem Cells (iPSCs)

Yamanaka factors are reprogramming factors that can be introduced into somatic cells to generate iPSCs in vitro. They are capable of self-renewing indefinitely in culture and can differentiate into nearly every type of cell. Because iPSCs can differentiate into myogenic cells, they present an appealing option for myogenic regeneration. Significantly, ethical issues and rejection responses are among the main drawbacks of using human embryonic stem cells (ESCs) that are addressed by the use of patient-specific iPSCs. You can create iPSCs, e.g., either from the skin biopsy-extracted fibroblasts from the patient or from non-invasively obtained renal epithelial cells from urine. These iPSCs can expand a patient's autologous cells in vitro in large quantities, allowing them to be differentiated into autologous myocytes later on. Their proliferative capacity is limitless. Pax7 or MyoD overexpression can be used to induce iPSCs to differentiate into myogenic cells. As an alternative, transgene-free differentiation can be carried out using small molecules. But using this approach to create a pure, expandable myogenic population is challenging. Using genome-integrating vectors specifically for reprogramming has the potential to cause genetic abnormalities and instability as well as encourage the growth of tumors. Thus, the creation of iPSCs and myogenic differentiation devoid of genetic alterations are the main areas of study for researchers. To create functional skeletal muscles in vitro and to fuse these cells with pre-existing myofibers following in vivo transplantation, many studies have been conducted on the myogenic differentiation of iPSCs. Darabi et al. produced induced pluripotent stem cells (iPSCs) from human fibroblasts and activated Pax7 to facilitate the cells' differentiation into myogenic progenitors capable of in vitro proliferation. Dystrophin-positive myofibers were formed and contractility was increased when these myogenic progenitors were transplanted into dystrophic mice. Conditional expression of Pax7 in human ESCs and iPSCs produced large numbers of myogenic progenitors, and improved muscle fiber formation was observed after engraftment in immunodeficient dystrophic mice.

Tetracycline-inducible myogenic differentiation 1 (MYOD1) piggyBac (PB) vector-based myogenic differentiation protocol for iPSCs that is repeatable. Their method produced a population of uniform skeletal muscle cells with a high differentiation efficiency (70–90%). Muscle fibers and satellite-like cells were successfully generated by realizing important embryonic signaling events, such as the alteration of both Wnt and bone morphogenetic protein (BMP) pathway signaling, thanks to a serum-free myogenic differentiation protocol that Chal and colleagues recently developed. To obtain myogenic progenitors from human ESCs and iPSCs, Hosoyama and colleagues used free-floating spherical culture (EZ spheres) in a defined culture medium. Myogenic progenitors from human induced pluripotent stem cells (iPSCs) were observed after 6 weeks of culture in a medium containing high concentrations of fibroblast growth factor-2 (FGF-2) and epidermal growth factor (EGF). After an additional 2 weeks of terminal differentiation, multinucleated myotubes expressing Pax7, MyoD, MHC, and myogenin were discovered. In the same way, the EZ sphere-derived myogenic progenitors' time course for muscle differentiation and sarcomere formation. According to what they said, iPSCs needed to differentiate into myogenic progenitors for at least six weeks to produce mature skeletal myotubes with well-organized sarcomeres. Borchin et al. have effectively triggered the Wnt signaling pathway for myogenic cell production by using a small-molecule GSK3β inhibitor (CHIR99021). The resulting PAX3+/PAX7+ skeletal muscle precursors that could differentiate into mature myocytes were purified thanks to the use of fluorescence-activated cell sorting (FACS). After that, van der Wal and colleagues changed Borchin's differentiation protocol, using CHIR99021 at a higher concentration (3.5 μM) for a longer time (5–6 days), which produced a higher yield of Pax7+ cells. Using C-Met+/Hnk1− cells, FACS was used to purify Pax7+ cells. The resultant cells underwent differentiation into multinucleated myotubes exhibiting a high index of fusion. Additionally, they showed their effective role in myofiber formation following intramuscular engraftment into mice pre-injured muscles *in vivo.*

Human iPSCs that were dystrophic were first cultured in a myogenic medium before being transfected with an adenoviral vector to express MyoD. By following this two-step protocol, multinucleated myotubes were formed in vitro. By fusing with preexisting muscle fibers, the transplantation into the muscle of Rag/mdx mice resulted in the regeneration of muscle. Recently, a transgene-free protocol using skeletal muscle-derived extracellular vesicles (EVs) cargo and GSK-3 inhibitor was developed for the myogenic differentiation of iPSCs derived from muscular pericytes or fibroblasts.

Myogenic marker expression was found to be elevated in vitro after 30 days, indicating expanded muscle differentiation. Differentiated iPSCs were then injected into mice muscles, whereupon they integrated with the host myofibers that were regenerating. Furthermore, the used EVs functioned well as biological "shuttles" that delivered bioactive molecules to cause iPSC differentiation.

7.3.3. Biomechanical Strategies for the Generation of Skeletal Muscle Tissue

Clinical application of skeletal muscle tissue engineering is possible, and it permits precise myogenesis modeling and drug treatment assessment. However, the poor generation of contractile forces, myotube alignment, low packing density, and poor cell survival in large constructs seriously limit the clinical applicability of tissue-engineered skeletal muscle. In vitro myogenesis that mimics native tissue requires close emulation of the natural cell niche in vivo. Post-mitotic, terminally differentiated cells make up adult myofibers. Therefore, adaptive mechanisms that cause an accumulation of contractile fiber proteins through either increased protein synthesis or decreased protein degradation are in charge of controlling the remodeling of skeletal muscle. Numerous in vivo adaptations, such as the control of protein synthesis and degradation, DNA and RNA content, and protein accumulation, were brought about by muscle training and stretching. Mechanically stimulating skeletal muscle primarily modifies the muscle fiber's molecular engine and causes remodeling, or changes in muscle mass and volume, e.g., phenotypic variations in myosin isoform expression. These alterations enable the muscle to modify its contractile characteristics to meet the necessary requirements. Given that mechanical stimulation has a major impact on the behavior of skeletal muscle cells, researchers have studied it extensively. To replicate the environment of the muscle matrix, human craniofacial muscle-derived cells were cultured in a sponge composed of a three-dimensional collagen network. These constructs were then subjected to strain regimes of either cyclical ramp strain or rapid ramp stretch. Increased expression of the mechanoresponsive gene matrix metalloproteinase-2 (MMP-2) in cultures exposed to continuous as opposed to cyclic strain indicated the remodeling of the extracellular matrix (Qazi et al., 2015; Liu et al., 2018).

Using a mechanical cell stimulator, muscle cells in collagen matrix were subjected to repeated cycles of stretching and relaxing (MCS). Eight days later, construct elasticity had increased two to three times, myofiber area had increased by 40%, and mean myofiber diameter had increased by 12%. Sakiyama and associates demonstrated that the application of a mechanical stimulus can influence the properties of muscle fibers in addition to myoblast growth and differentiation. After mechanically stretching C2C12 myoblasts, the levels of myosin heavy chain (MHC) isoform mRNA expression were assessed at various intervals. The findings demonstrated that following stretching, MHC-2b expression first rose and then fell. Without stretching, MHC-2d expression grew over time, but with stretching, it became hardly noticeable. Furthermore, the stretching group exhibited a significantly higher level of MHC-2a expression. These findings suggest that mechanical stimulation modifies MHC isoform levels, which in turn affects muscle function. In a different investigation, the C2C12 myoblasts' cyclic mechanical stretch raised the levels of the protein β1D-integrin, which controls myogenesis and mechanotransduction, and triggered the cytoskeletal signaling proteins RhoA and focal adhesion kinase (FAK). Mouse BM-MSCs were seeded on silicone sheets coated with fibronectin and exposed to cyclic 10% uniaxial strain in this investigation. The skeletal myogenic marker genes (myogenin, Myf5, and myogenic regulatory factor 4 (MRF4)) were upregulated when the cells were cultured in a myogenic medium, but not the smooth muscle marker genes (myocardin and α-smooth muscle actin). In addition, within five days, the cells developed into multinucleated myotubes in the direction of applied tension.

7.3.4. Scaffold Topographies for Improved Generation of Muscle Tissue

The ability of cells to respond to topographic properties at the micro/nanometer scale has increased the significance of micro/nanostructures in recent years. In light of this, several bioengineering techniques are used to analyze the creation of muscle tissue with topographical cues. Consequently, a variety of fabrication methods were used, including solvent casting, electrospinning, hot embossing, photolithography, soft lithography, solvent stretching, or active stretching of scaffolds. The geometric structures of the scaffolds in muscle tissue vary; these include pits, pillars, wrinkles, and combinations of fibrous scaffolds with micro- and nanostructures. Electrospun fibers mimic the nanoscale characteristics of a native extracellular matrix (ECM), allowing them to replicate and regenerate tissue environments in three dimensions. To regulate the commitment of muscle cells to a specific lineage, they can also be manufactured in an anisotropic or isotropic manner. Furthermore, micro- and nanoscale fibers can be created from a range of synthetic and biopolymers. It is possible to evaluate the characteristics of electrospun nanofibers in relation to topographical effects, including their random and aligned structures, variable thicknesses, and nanoscale micropores. To enhance the length of myotubes, skeletal muscle scaffolds with uniaxially patterned structures have been created using the electrospinning technique. For instance, when C2C12 cells were cultured on aligned PLLA nanofibrous scaffolds, the uniaxially patterned electrospun PLLA fibers could increase the length of myotubes by approximately three times compared with random fiber mats. As part of a multifaceted approach to improve elastic fiber formation, aligned nanofiber scaffolds can also be utilized in the development of tissue-engineered vascular grafts (TEVGs). In order to improve the quality of TEVGs, substrate topography and biochemical additives can work in concert to promote the formation of elastin fibers by cultured cells (umbilical artery smooth muscle cells) on the aligned fibers. In addition to directing cell orientation and the synthesis of newly synthesized extracellular matrix fibers, electrospun fibrinogen nanofibers with aligned topography also increased the synthesis of elastin and phenotypic contractile proteins (Figure 7.11).

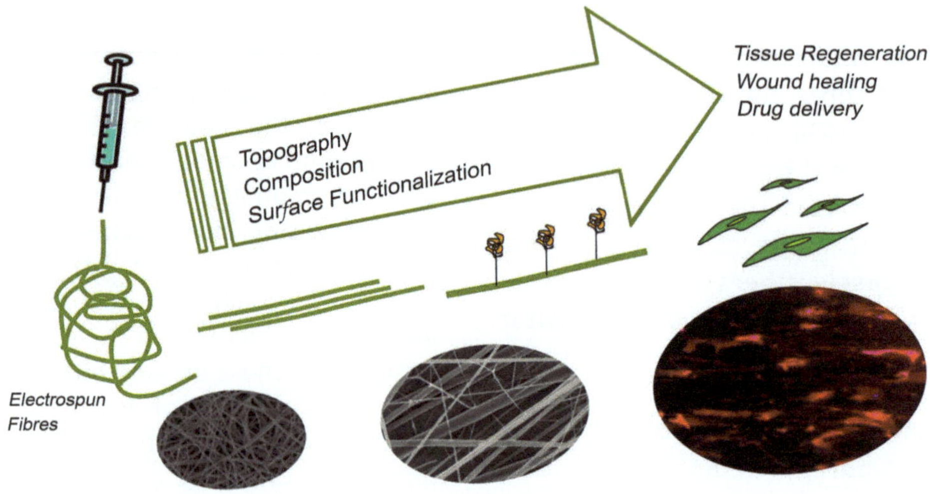

Figure 7.11. *Substrate electrospun fibers with different topographies direct the cell morphology and phenotype.*

Source: Ferraris S, Spriano S, Scalia AC, Cochis A, Rimondini L, Cruz-Maya I, Guarino V, Varesano A, Vineis C. Topographical and biomechanical guidance of electrospun fibers for biomedical applications. Polymers. 2020; 12(12):2896. https://doi.org/10.3390/polym12122896 –.

It is possible to mimic the features and operations of blood vessels through research on tubular scaffolds. To restore and regenerate blood vessels, three distinct tissue layers—the adventitia, media, and intima—with varying structures and purposes are needed at the same time. ECs can benefit from the topographical guidance provided by the axial nanofibers in the inner layer, while smooth muscle cells can benefit from the mechanical strength and topographical guidance provided by the circumferentially aligned nanofibers in the outer layer. To replicate the form and functionality of natural blood vessels, a study was conducted. Fibers that were slanted and circumferentially aligned formed the middle inner and outer layers, while random fibers made up the outermost layer. Furthermore, 100% random fiber layers were used to create tubular scaffolds. The scaffold hydrophilicity was increased by the PEG incorporation. According to the results, the scaffolds with aligned fibers not only had better mechanical qualities, but they also promoted HUVEC viability and cellular proliferation. To guide 3D cell alignment and replicate the anisotropic structure of the heart, scaffold design is crucial for cardiac tissue regeneration. The challenge of simulating the three-dimensional anisotropy of cardiac muscle remains despite numerous studies aimed at controlling cell alignment and elongation. PCL patches for cardiac muscle were created by hybridizing random and aligned nanofibers simultaneously using an electrolyte solution as a collector in the electrolyte-assisted electrospinning (ELES) process. Random nanofibers can offer suture- and handling-friendly mechanical support, whereas aligned nanofibers enhance cardiomyocyte alignment and the creation of a three-dimensional anisotropic structure. To engineer 3D cardiac anisotropy and regulate cell orientation, additional research produced 3D hybrid scaffolds with core and shell structures. GelMA hydrogel was used to encase the nanofiber PCL/SF/CNT yarn network, resulting in the creation of 3D hybrid conductive scaffolds. In GelMA hydrogel with GFP-expressing ECs, cardiomyocytes were embedded after being seeded on a yarn network. In addition to improving cardiomyocyte alignment and elongation, these scaffolds facilitated cardiomyocyte maturation and function.

For skeletal muscle tissue engineering, scaffolds with core-shell structures have also been studied. For instance, coaxial electrospun poly(acrylic acid)/poly(vinyl alcohol) (PAA/PVA) hydrogel and PCL solution containing multiwalled carbon nanotubes have been used as the shell and core layers, respectively. While the hydrogel shell can activate, the multiwalled carbon nanotubes in the PCL core layer function as an internal electrode and boost conductivity. In comparison to the scaffolds without hydrogel, the scaffolds with a hydrogel shell showed a higher number of multinucleated cells with interacting actin filaments. Another effective method for creating 3D topographies at the micrometer and submicrometer scales is micropatterning technology. This approach can be used to engineer aligned myoblasts and myotubes using cell-culture substrates. The myotube alignment was caused by the seeding of murine C2C12 myoblasts inside the microchannels. In contrast, hydrogels without patterns showed no evidence of alignment. Additionally, the electrical stimulation produced myotubes with a larger diameter and further enhanced myotube alignment. This work showed that micropatterns can be used to change the behavior and destiny of cells, including elongation, differentiation, and cell-cell contact and signaling. As an alternative, different surface topographies can also be produced by applying photolithography and/or soft lithography as micropatterning techniques. In one study, compared to cells grown on non-patterned substrates, the cultivation of human iPSC-derived myogenic progenitors on PDMS-based micropatterned substrates produced larger fiber diameters, more myogenin-positive nuclei, and increased nuclear fusion. Another method for creating microstructured scaffolds in skeletal muscle tissue engineering is freeze-drying. These scaffolds were used to cultivate rat L6 skeletal myoblasts, which produced multilayered muscle bundle tissue. Depending on the size of the microgrooves and cell density, the myoblasts aligned and formed myotubes in this tissue. Nevertheless, the expression of myogenic genes remained unaffected by alterations to the groove sizes. Cell organization, differentiation, and alignment may be impacted by the grooves' size, ridge structure, and material composition. Micro-sized hydrogels can be used as micropatterned substrates in muscle tissue engineering and are highly effective at guiding cells into a biomimetic tissue architecture in vitro. For example, two kinds of micropatterned methacrylated gelatin hydrogel substrates were made with different ridge patterns (50 and 100 μm) and the same grooves (100 μm). The findings demonstrated that compared to wider ridge micropatterns, smaller ridge micropatterns produce more myotubes that are aligned in the groove direction.

The endeavor to create biocompatible and biodegradable scaffolds for skeletal muscle tissue engineering through 3D printing has greatly intensified in the last few years. Three-dimensional bioprinting allows scaffolds to be created layer by layer, controlling cellular alignment and reconstructing the desired tissue structure in an anatomically realistic manner. Recently, a uniaxially oriented patterned structure was created using 3D bioprinting by combining fibrillated PVA with decellularized ECM methacrylate (dECM-MA) from swine skeletal muscles as a bioink. In this way, topographical cues and tissue-specific biochemical cues from the dECM-MA were combined. Myoblasts from the C_2C1_2 cell line were integrated, and this alignment led to a high degree of myotube formation. Furthermore, myogenic gene expression (MyoD1, MYH2, and MyoG) was upregulated in dECM-based scaffolds as compared to GelMA scaffolds with the same topographical cues. The 3D bioprinted muscle constructs demonstrated de novo muscle formation in a VML rat model, showed densely packed and aligned myotubes throughout the construct, and maintained high cell viability without producing a hypoxic environment. Additionally, prevascularized muscle constructs were produced through coaxial nozzle printing using vascular and muscle dECM bioinks. This led to improved de novo muscle fiber formation, vascularization, innervation, and an 85% functional recovery in VML injury. It has also been demonstrated that appropriate nozzle size and extrusion pressure selection are beneficial for cell orientation in 3D printing technology. By increasing the extrusion pressure and decreasing the extrusion nozzle diameter, Distler and colleagues demonstrated the rise in shear force using an extrusion bioprinting technique. Additionally, they observed an increase in the frequency of F-actin orientation in the direction of the 3D-printed oxidized alginate-gelatin hydrogel (Figure 7.13C,D). Furthermore, when the pressure was reduced and the extrusion nozzle's diameter stayed the same, the orientation of the C_2C1_2 cells also decreased.

To obtain the uniaxially aligned PCL bundles, the fibrillated PVA was leached from a mixture of PVA and PCL. The findings showed that MHC expression indicated myogenic differentiation and that C_2C1_2 cells were properly oriented along the microfibril direction (Qazi et al., 2015; Liu et al., 2018). Table 7.2 summarizes a few in vivo tissue engineering approaches.

Table 7.2. *In Vivo Tissue Engineering Approaches*

In Vivo			
Scaffold	**Model**	**Main Findings**	**References**
Neuro-Muscular Compartment			
SMUs and ENC	VML in sheep	3 months post implant, sheep treated with SMU recovered muscle mass and tetanic force production.	Novakova et al. (2020) [21]
Collagen-GAG scaffold	VML in mouse	Increased hypertrophy in treated mouse 2 and 6 weeks post implant. increased running speed on a treadmill after 6 weeks compared to sham mice.	Panayi et al. (2019) [22]
Dex-AT and CECS hydrogel.	VML in rat, injectable hydrogel with C2C12 and HUVEC-GFP.	1 and 4 weeks post treatment, cells were proportionally released over time. Higher myofiber density was present in animals treated with hydrogel and cells when compared with animals treated with hydrogel alone.	Guo et al. (2019) [23]

Porcine muscle ECM sponge and bioink. Descending aorta ECM bioink for bioprinting.	VML in rat and ECM with hSKMs and HUVEC.	3 scaffolds were compared: (1) muscle ECM sponge with hSKMs (2) ECM hydrogel used as bioink with hSKMs (3) gelatin granules mold for muscle and aorta ECM seeded with hSKMs and HUVEC. 4-weeks after implant, scaffold number 3 produced better cell viability, myotube formation, angiogenesis and muscle strength recovery in respect to the other scaffolds.	Choi et al. (2019) [24]
Muscle tissue plug	Rat VML.	3 different alignment (0°,45°,90°) of muscle defect plug were implanted. The best tissue regeneration was achieved with aligned muscle plug (0°): increased expression of myogenic genes 2 weeks after implant; a peak of tetanic torque force and reduced collagen deposition after 12 weeks.	Kim et al. (2020) [25]
Subcutaneous implant of PCL fibers	Rat VML, sciatic nerve and abdominal artery defects.	In vivo implant of depleted PCL ECM allows: (1) muscle tissue regeneration with reduction of collagen deposition; (2) good axon diameter, thickness of myelin sheets; (3) vascular regeneration with good morphology of vascular microchannels	Zhu et al. (2019) [26]
Fibrinogen, gelatin, hyaluronic acid and glycerol bioink in PCL pillar	VML in rat and bioink with hMPCs	8-weeks post implant, muscle strength, vascularization and number of NMJs were higher in comparison with rats treated with bioink without cells (printed and non-printed).	Kim et al. (2018) [27]
PCL bioprinting	VML in rat and scaffold with hMPCs co-cultured with hNSCs.	Analysis were performed at 4 and 8 weeks. Pre-innervated scaffold ameliorated functional muscle regeneration, NMJs formation and reduce fibrotic tissue deposition compared to rat treated with scaffold seeded with hMPCs alone.	Kim et al. (2020) [20]
Vascular Compartment			

BAM in fibrin hydrogel	Subcutaneous injection on the fascia of the *latissimus dorsi* muscle of hydrogel and BAM with and without HUVEC-GFP	(1) BAM alone, (2) BAM co-cultured with HUVEC-GFP and (3) BAM with HUVEC in fibrin hydrogel (two-stage approach). 14 days post treatment, myotube length and area, vessel length and branching were evaluated. The number 3 construct gave better results.	Gholobova et al. (2020) [28]
PLLA and PLGA scaffold	Abdominal wall defect in mouse and PLLA/PLGA with satellite and lung microvascular cells.	Scaffolds with satellite cells alone and scaffolds with both cell types were implanted in immunocompetent and immunocompromised mice. 18 days post implantation, the pre-vascularized scaffold inserted in immunocompromised mice showed better neovascularization and myogenesis in respect to the immunocompetent.	Perry et al. (2019) [29]
Fibrinogen hydrogel	VML in rat and hydrogel with BMDMs.	After 15 days, implantation of gel with muscle cells+BMDMs shows increased vascularization, muscle area and muscle strength compared with implantation of gel containing only muscle cells.	Juhas et al. (2018) [30]
Tetronic-tyramine hydrogel RGD	C2C12-VEGF cell sheets	Ischemic model with myoblasts sheets: promoted the formation of capillaries and arterioles in ischemic muscles, attenuated the muscle necrosis and fibrosis progressed by ischemia, and prevented ischemic limb loss.	Lee et al. (2014) [15]

Abbreviations: BAM: Bio Artificial Muscle with human skeletal muscle cells; BMDMs: Bone Marrow Derived Macrophages; CECS: N-carboxyethyl chitosan; Dex-AT: Dextran-graft-aniline tetramer-graft-4; ENC: Engineered Neural Conduit; GAG: Glycosaminoglycans; hMPCs: human Muscle Precursor Cells; hNSCs: human Neural Stem Cells; hSKMs: human Skeletal Muscle Cells; NMJs: Neuromuscular Junction; PLGA: Poly Lactic-co-Glycolic Acid; PLLA: Poly L-Lactic Acid; SMUs: Small Muscle Units.

Source: Reid G, Magarotto F, Marsano A, Pozzobon M. Next stage approach to tissue engineering skeletal Muscle. Bioengineering. 2020; 7(4):118. https://doi.org/10.3390/bioengineering7040118.

A Closer Look

Muscle Aging and Sarcopenia

As individuals age, muscle tissue undergoes significant changes, leading to declines in muscle mass, strength, and function—a phenomenon commonly referred to as sarcopenia. Sarcopenia is characterized by the gradual loss of skeletal muscle mass and quality, accompanied by reductions in muscle strength, power, and endurance. Several factors contribute to age-related muscle loss, including changes in hormonal profiles, decreased physical activity, altered protein metabolism, and impaired neuromuscular function. Additionally, chronic inflammation, oxidative stress, and changes in mitochondrial function also play a role in the development of sarcopenia.

One of the primary manifestations of sarcopenia is the loss of muscle mass, a process known as muscle atrophy. With advancing age, there is a gradual decline in the number and size of muscle fibers, as well as alterations in muscle architecture and composition. This loss of muscle mass contributes to declines in muscle strength and function, leading to decreased mobility, increased risk of falls, and impaired activities of daily living. Furthermore, sarcopenia is associated with a higher risk of frailty, disability, and mortality in older adults.

Several risk factors predispose individuals to sarcopenia, including age, gender, genetics, and lifestyle factors. Advancing age is the most significant risk factor for sarcopenia, with muscle mass declining at a rate of approximately 1–2% per year after the age of 50. Additionally, hormonal changes, such as reductions in testosterone, growth hormone, and insulin-like growth factor 1 (IGF-1), contribute to age-related muscle loss. Other risk factors include sedentary behavior, poor nutrition, chronic diseases (e.g., diabetes, cardiovascular disease), and medications that affect muscle metabolism.

Preventing or mitigating age-related muscle loss and frailty requires a multi-faceted approach targeting various aspects of muscle health. Regular physical activity, particularly resistance training and aerobic exercise, is essential for preserving muscle mass, strength, and function. Resistance training, in particular, stimulates muscle protein synthesis and promotes muscle hypertrophy, helping to counteract age-related declines in muscle mass and strength. Moreover, engaging in activities that challenge balance, coordination, and flexibility can help reduce the risk of falls and improve functional mobility in older adults.

Optimizing nutrition is another key component of sarcopenia prevention and management. Adequate protein intake, along with essential amino acids, is crucial for supporting muscle protein synthesis and maintaining muscle mass. Consuming a balanced diet rich in high-quality protein sources, such as lean meats, poultry, fish, dairy products, legumes, and nuts, can help meet the increased protein requirements of older adults. Additionally, ensuring sufficient intake of vitamins and minerals, particularly vitamin D and calcium, is important for bone health and muscle function.

Summary

- Muscle is a soft tissue, one of the four basic types of animal tissue. Muscle tissue gives skeletal muscles the ability to contract. Muscle is formed during embryonic development, in a process known as myogenesis.
- Muscle tissue varies with function and location in the body. In vertebrates, the three types are skeletal or striated muscle; smooth muscle (non-striated); and cardiac muscle.
- Muscle tissue is characterized by properties that allow movement. Muscle cells are excitable; they respond to a stimulus. They are contractile, meaning they can shorten and generate a pulling force.
- Skeletal muscle is attached to bones and its contraction makes possible locomotion, facial expressions, posture, and other voluntary movements of the body. Forty percent of your body mass is made up of skeletal muscle.
- The fascicles are surrounded by a protective layer known as perimysium. It allows the flow of nerves and blood to the individual fibers.
- Muscle powers the movements of multicellular animals and maintains posture. Its gross appearance is familiar as meat or as the flesh of fish. Muscle is the most plentiful tissue in many animals; for example, it makes up 50 to 60% of the body mass in many fishes and 40 to 50% in antelopes.
- Muscle fibers differ from species to species of animal and between parts of the same animal. Apart from the distinction between voluntary and involuntary muscles, muscles differ in structure and activity.
- Muscle cells are specialized for contraction. Muscles allow for motions such as walking, and they also facilitate bodily processes such as respiration and digestion.
- Most muscle tissue of the body arises from the embryonic mesoderm. Paraxial mesodermal cells adjacent to the neural tube form blocks of cells called somites.
- Muscle tissue is found throughout the body, spanning from head to toe. Tendons connect skeletal muscles to bones and can be found in the arms, legs, abdomen, chest, back, and face. These muscles regulate voluntary movements like walking, running, and facial expressions.

References

1. Basurto, I. M., Mora, M. T., Gardner, G. M., Christ, G. J., & Caliari, S. R. (2021). Aligned and conductive 3D collagen scaffolds for skeletal muscle tissue engineering. *Biomaterials Science*. https://doi.org/10.1039/D1BM00147G.
2. Carnes, M. E., & Pins, G. D. (2020). Skeletal muscle tissue engineering: Biomaterials-based strategies for the treatment of volumetric muscle loss. *Bioengineering, 7*(3), 85. https://doi.org/10.3390/bioengineering7030085.
3. Cezar, C. A., & Mooney, D. J. (2015). Biomaterial-based delivery for skeletal muscle repair. *Advanced Drug Delivery Reviews, 84*, 188–197. https://doi.org/10.1016/j.addr.2014.09.008.

4. Forcina, L., Cosentino, M., & Musaro, A. (2020). Mechanisms regulating muscle regeneration: Insights into the interrelated and time-dependent phases of tissue healing. *Cells, 9*(5), 1297. https://doi.org/10.3390/cells9051297.

5. Jarvinen, T. A., Jarvinen, M., & Kalimo, H. (2013). Regeneration of injured skeletal muscle after the injury. *Muscles, Ligaments and Tendons Journal, 3*, 337–345. https://doi.org/10.32098/mltj.04.2013.16.

6. Liu, J., Saul, D., Boker, K. O., Ernst, J., Lehman, W., & Schilling, A. F. (2018). Current methods for skeletal muscle tissue repair and regeneration. *Biomed Research International, 2018*, 1984879. https://doi.org/10.1155/2018/1984879.

7. Qazi, T. H., Mooney, D. J., Pumberger, M., Geissler, S., & Duda, G. N. (2015). Biomaterials based strategies for skeletal muscle tissue engineering: Existing technologies and future trends. *Biomaterials, 53*, 502–521. https://doi.org/10.1016/j.biomaterials.2015.02.110.

8. Smoak, M. M., & Mikos, A. G. (2020). Advances in biomaterials for skeletal muscle engineering and obstacles still to overcome. *Materials Today Bio, 7*, 100069. https://doi.org/10.1016/j.mtbio.2020.100069.

9. Xing, F., Li, L., Zhou, C., Long, C., Wu, L., Lei, H., Kong, Q., Fan, Y., Xiang, Z., & Zhang, X. (2019). Regulation and directing stem cell fate by tissue engineering functional microenvironments: Scaffold physical and chemical cues. *Stem Cells International, 2019*, 2180925. https://doi.org/10.1155/2019/2180925.

Chapter 8

MUSCLE ADAPTATIONS

Contents

Introduction

The complex physiological alterations that take place in skeletal muscle as a result of repetitive physical activity or exercise training are known as muscle adaptations. The intricate interactions between metabolic processes, gene expression patterns, and cellular signaling pathways orchestrate these adaptations, which ultimately result in improvements in muscle structure, function, and performance. Optimizing exercise programming, improving athletic performance, and advancing general health and well-being all depend on an understanding of muscle adaptations. Hypertrophy, or the expansion of individual muscle fibers leading to an increase in muscle size, is one of the main responses of the muscles to exercise. In reaction to mechanical strain, metabolic stress, and muscle damage brought on by exercise, hypertrophy develops. Lifting weights or doing exercises with your body weight is known as resistance training, and it is a powerful stimulus for muscle hypertrophy. Muscle fibers undergo microtrauma and stress during resistance training, which sets off a series of molecular reactions that promote protein synthesis and muscle growth. In this process, muscle stem cells called satellite cells—which are in charge of both muscle growth and repair—are activated. These cells multiply, differentiate, and fuse with pre-existing muscle fibers, which causes the muscles to enlarge and undergo hypertrophy. Exercise training causes structural changes in muscle tissue in addition to hypertrophy, which improves the muscle's ability to produce force, withstand fatigue, and facilitate movement. These adaptations include modifications to the structure and composition of structural proteins like myosin and actin, as well as increases in the quantity and size of myofibrils, the contractile units that make up muscle fibers. Exercise also encourages the growth of mitochondria, which are cellular organelles that produce energy through aerobic metabolism. By increasing the muscle's capacity to produce ATP (adenosine triphosphate), the main energy unit of cells, this increase in mitochondrial density improves endurance and delays the onset of fatigue during prolonged exercise.

Additionally, muscle tissue undergoes biochemical changes brought on by exercise training that enhance its functionality and metabolic efficiency. The expression of enzymes involved in lipid metabolism, oxidative phosphorylation, and glycolysis is increased by regular exercise, which makes it easier to use fats and carbohydrates as energy substrates during physical activity. Exercise training also improves muscle tissue's ability to buffer lactate and other metabolic byproducts, which helps to postpone the onset of muscle fatigue and increase exercise tolerance. Moreover, adaptations brought about by exercise go beyond the cellular and biochemical levels and include systemic modifications that enhance the general performance and functionality of muscles. These include improvements in oxygen delivery, which improves the delivery of nutrients and the elimination of waste from muscle tissue, and increases in muscle blood flow and capillarization, or the development of new capillaries. Exercise also stimulates the release of growth factors that are important for muscle growth, repair, and neuroplasticity, such as brain-derived neurotrophic factor (BDNF) and insulin-like growth factor 1 (IGF-1).

Orientation and Directional Terms

Term	Definition	Illustration
Basal lamina	Basal laminae are thin, flexible sheets of ECM which are made by and underlie epithelial cells.	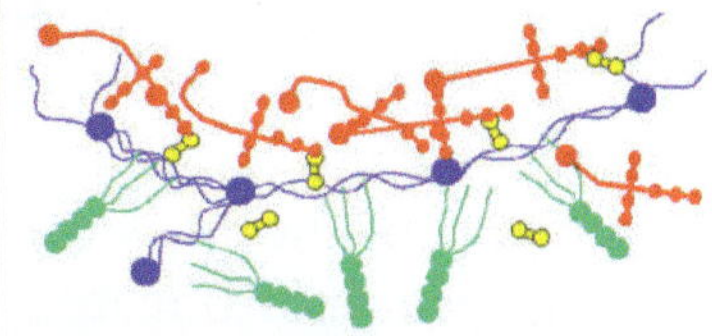
Gynecomastia	An increase in the amount of breast gland tissue in boys or men. An imbalance of the hormones estrogen and testosterone causes it.	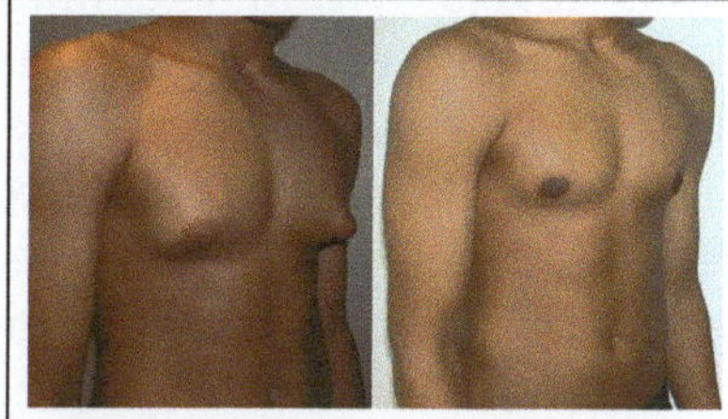
Muscle lineage	A bundle of skeletal muscle fibers running parallel to each other, enveloped by a collagenous sheath called the perimysium.	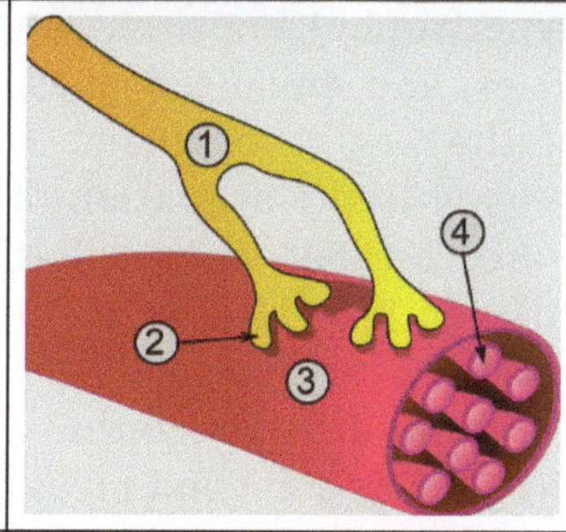
Myogenesis	Myogenesis is the formation of skeletal muscular tissue, particularly during embryonic development.	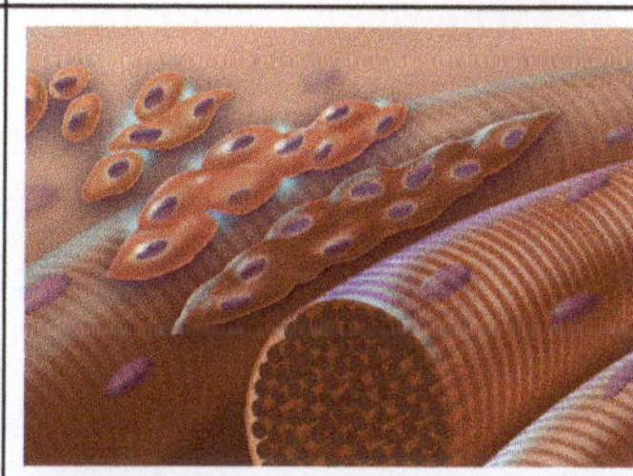
Precursor cells	Precursor cells are stem cells that have developed to the stage where they are committed to forming a particular kind of new blood cell.	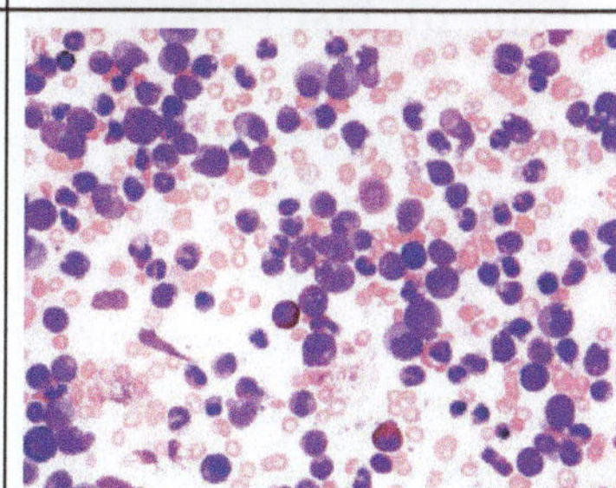

8.1. Muscle Adaptations to Exercise

Muscle adaptations to exercise encompass a complex array of physiological changes orchestrated by the body in response to the demands imposed by physical activity. These adaptations are multifaceted and occur at various levels within the muscular system, ranging from molecular alterations within muscle cells to changes in whole muscle structure and function. At the cellular level, exercise induces a cascade of signaling pathways that regulate gene expression and protein synthesis, leading to adaptations such as increased muscle fiber size (hypertrophy), improved muscle contractile properties, and enhanced energy metabolism. One of the key mechanisms driving muscle hypertrophy is the activation of satellite cells, which are resident stem cells that proliferate and differentiate into new muscle fibers in response to mechanical stress. Moreover, exercise promotes the synthesis of contractile proteins such as actin and myosin, contributing to greater force production and muscle strength.

Beyond cellular adaptations, exercise elicits changes in muscle architecture and composition. Regular resistance training, for instance, leads to alterations in muscle fiber type distribution, with a shift towards a greater proportion of fast-twitch fibers, which are capable of generating higher force outputs. Concurrently, there is an increase in the number and size of myofibrils within muscle fibers, enhancing their capacity for force generation and contraction. These structural adaptations are further complemented by improvements in neuromuscular coordination and efficiency, as the nervous system learns to recruit motor units more effectively and synchronize muscle contractions to optimize performance during exercise.

In addition to hypertrophic and structural adaptations, exercise stimulates the enhancement of muscle metabolic pathways to meet the increased energy demands associated with physical activity. Aerobic exercise, such as endurance training, promotes mitochondrial biogenesis, leading to greater mitochondrial density within muscle cells and improved oxidative capacity. This enables more efficient utilization of fuels such as glucose and fatty acids, resulting in prolonged endurance and delayed onset of fatigue during prolonged exercise. Furthermore, exercise training induces adaptations in muscle glycogen storage and utilization, facilitating rapid energy production during high-intensity efforts.

Importantly, the magnitude and specificity of muscle adaptations to exercise are influenced by various factors including the type, intensity, duration, and frequency of training, as well as individual genetic predispositions and nutritional status. Progressive overload, achieved by gradually increasing the intensity or volume of training, is a fundamental principle driving muscle adaptation, as it continuously challenges the muscles to adapt to greater demands over time. Furthermore, the concept of specificity dictates that the adaptations elicited by exercise are specific to the type of activity performed, highlighting the importance of tailoring training programs to match the desired outcomes.

8.1.1. Muscle Hypertrophy

Mass gain in muscles is referred to as muscular hypertrophy. Typically, this shows up as a gain in muscle mass and power. Muscle hypertrophy usually results from strength training, like lifting weights. Sarcoplasmic and myofibrillar hypertrophy are the two forms of muscle hypertrophy. Some people might modify their training regimens to focus on various forms of muscle growth. Some people, for instance, will train with the goal of maximizing either muscle strength or size. An increase in muscle mass is referred to as muscular hypertrophy or muscle growth. Muscle hypertrophy can be classified into two categories: myofibrillar, or an increase in myofibrils, and sarcoplasmic, or an increase in the storage of muscle glycogen. Movement is made possible by the skeletal muscles, which are attached to the bones by tendons. Skeletal muscles are composed of bundles of muscle fibers called myocytes. Myofibrils, which are found in every myocyte, enable muscle contraction. The term "myofibrillar hypertrophy" describes an increase in myofibril count. Muscle density and strength increase as a result. Sarcoplasmic fluid can be found in muscles as well. The fluid that envelops the muscle fibers is a source of energy. It is composed of water, creatine phosphate, glycogen, and adenosine triphosphate. More fluid flows to the muscles during exercise to supply energy. The term "sarcoplasmic hypertrophy" describes this fluid's increased volume. It doesn't increase strength, but it can give the appearance of larger muscles.

8.1.1.1. What Causes Muscular Hypertrophy?

People can gain muscle through both sarcoplasmic and myofibrillar hypertrophy with strength training. Training against resistance that progressively rises over time is required for this. This puts strain on the muscles, causing the body to repair the damaged muscle fibers. When you challenge your muscles in this way on a regular basis, they adapt by becoming stronger and bigger. By concentrating on strength training, engaging in a variety of activities, and getting enough sleep, people can train to promote muscle growth. On the other hand, some illnesses can prevent muscle hypertrophy. For instance, a form of muscular dystrophy called myofibrillar myopathy usually results in muscle weakness in mid-adulthood. The hands and feet are typically where the symptoms first appear before spreading to the center of the body.

8.1.1.2. Factors Affecting Hypertrophy

Muscle hypertrophy can be influenced by dietary factors, training variables, and biological factors (like sex and DNA). Genetic variations among individuals explain a significant amount of the variation in current muscle mass. A classical twin study design, akin to those in behavioral genetics, estimated that approximately 45% of the variance in the proportion of muscle fibers and 53% of the variance in lean body mass are heritable. In males, hypertrophy happens more quickly during puberty. In the late teens, natural hypertrophy typically ends at full growth. Since testosterone is one of the body's primary growth hormones, men typically have approximately 60% more muscle mass than women and, on average, find it much easier to achieve hypertrophy. Increasing testosterone levels, as in anabolic steroids, will improve outcomes. It is also regarded as a performance-enhancing substance, and using it can result in competitors' suspensions or exclusions from contests. In most nations, testosterone is also classified as a medicinally regulated substance, meaning that it is unlawful to possess without a prescription. Gynecomastia, cardiac arrest, and testicular atrophy can all result from using anabolic steroids.

In the long run, anabolism and consequently muscle hypertrophy benefit from a positive energy balance, which occurs when more calories are consumed than burned. Athletes training for muscle hypertrophy exhibit elevated protein synthesis, which can be attributed to an increased protein requirement. On the other hand, there is disagreement among scientists as to whether strength-trained athletes need more protein. Training factors including frequency, intensity, and total volume have a direct impact on the development of muscle hypertrophy in the context of strength training. Muscular hypertrophy can be achieved by progressively increasing each of these training factors.

8.1.1.3. How to build muscle and increase muscle size

Lifting weights requires both mechanical damage and metabolic exhaustion in order to build muscle. Lifting a heavy weight requires the muscles' contractile proteins to produce force in order to overcome the weight's resistance. As a result, the muscles may sustain structural damage. Muscle protein damage caused by mechanical means triggers the body's repair mechanism. Muscle size increases as a result of the damaged muscle protein fibers. When your muscles run out of ATP, the energy molecule that powers your contractions, mechanical fatigue sets in. They can no longer lift the weight correctly or are unable to sustain muscle contractions. Gaining muscle can also result from this. It takes both metabolic exhaustion and mechanical injury to achieve muscular hypertrophy. To achieve the desired effects, you don't always have to push your muscles to the point of "failure," which is when you can't complete a repetition. A 2010 study discovered that significant metabolic stress on the muscles along with a moderate level of muscle tension are necessary for maximum gains. Exercises involving shortening (concentric) movements at fast-to-moderate speeds for one to three seconds and elongating (eccentric) movements at slower speeds (two to four seconds) have been shown to be very effective by researchers. A bicep curl exercise where you raise the weight to your shoulder is an example of a concentric movement. Eccentric would be the return to the starting position.

8.1.2. Endurance Training

An overall increase in exercise capacity and performance is supported by adaptations that endurance training causes in the musculoskeletal and cardiovascular systems (Brooks, 2011). Increased mitochondrial biogenesis and capillary density, two local adaptations found in skeletal muscle, help the body use and transport oxygen to produce energy, delaying the onset of muscle fatigue during prolonged aerobic performance. The primary organelle for producing energy is the mitochondria, which uses substrates from the tricarboxylic acid cycle (TCA) to generate adenosine triphosphate (ATP) via the electron transport system (ETS). Recent research has started looking into how different exercise intensity paradigms affect mitochondrial content and function in relation to adaptations in mitochondrial biogenesis brought on by exercise. Experiments utilizing long slow-distance (LSD) training, sprint interval training (SIT; approximately 30 sec maximal bouts), and high-intensity interval training (HIIT; 1–4 min all-out bouts) have been used to examine the impact of exercise volume and intensity on mitochondrial adaptations. Conventional LSD training requires a person to maintain a submaximal workload for an extended amount of time or to successfully complete a set distance or time with a power output that is higher than average. HIIT and SIT, on the other hand, call for the person to execute repeated bouts at nearly maximal intensity for a brief amount of time while reducing their training volume. Numerous investigations have demonstrated parallels in the adaptations for mitochondrial markers (e.g., skeletal muscle oxidative capacity, and peroxisome proliferator-activated receptor γ coactivator 1α [PGC-1α]) in both training models; as a result, HIIT/SIT has been suggested as a time-efficient method for improving aerobic adaptations.

With respect to mitochondrial content and function, more recent research has started to directly address the significance of exercise intensity versus volume. These studies employed young, moderately trained men and all three exercise protocols (LSD, HIIT, and SIT), matching volume in the HIIT and traditional groups. Following a 4-week training period, the SIT group alone showed a 25% increase in maximal mitochondrial respiration; the LSD and HIIT groups did not exhibit any changes in this regard. PGC-1α, p53, and PHF20 protein content all changed in the SIT group along with an increase in mitochondrial respiration. While p53 is involved in the regulation of mitochondrial function and acts as a tumor suppressor, PHF20 is crucial for both upregulating and stabilizing p53. HIIT on its own has been demonstrated to affect respiration and mitochondrial content, in contrast to the Granata study. After just two weeks of HIIT training, mitochondrial respiration and changes in content (as determined by cytochrome c oxidase [COX] activity) lead to an increase in exercise capacity. An additional piece of evidence for HIIT-induced mitochondrial adaptations comes from a within-subject study that demonstrated increased respiration and mitochondrial volume density after just two weeks of training. The variations in subject training status, experimental design, and methodological measures used to evaluate mitochondrial adaptations could be the cause of the discrepancies observed between these studies. Using a within-subject crossover design and all three training models would be the best approach to definitively resolve this question.

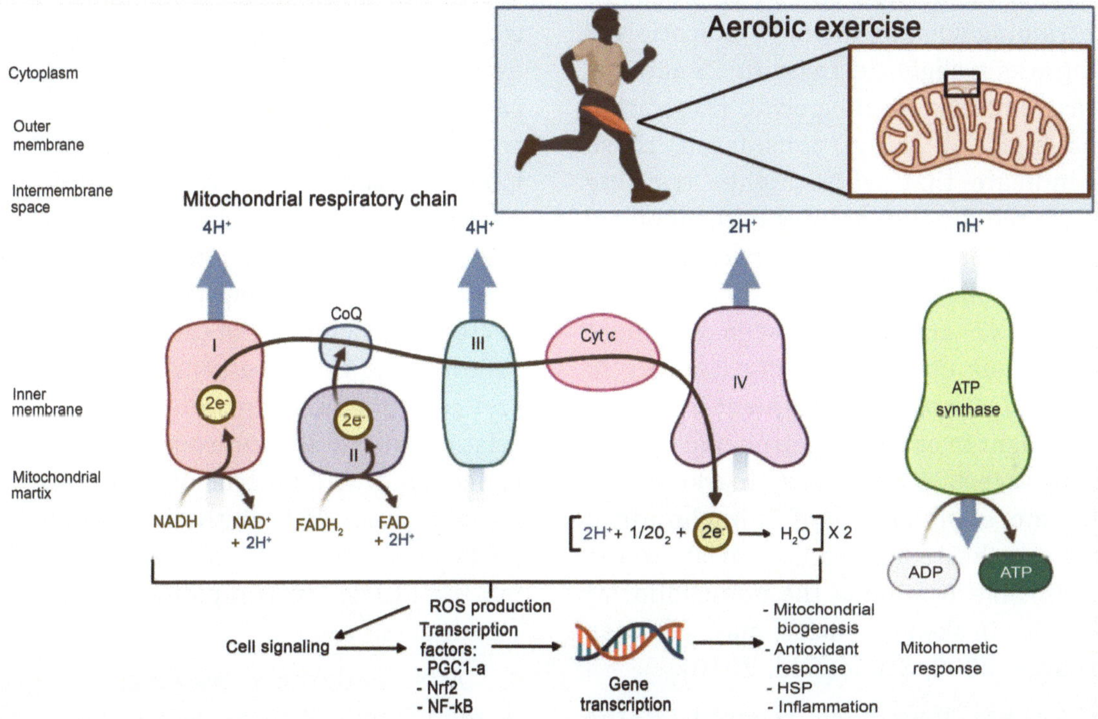

Figure 8.1. *Exercise-induced oxidative stress and the development of the mithormetic response.*

Created with BioRender.com (accessed on 10 November 2021). NADH: reduced nicotinamide adenine dinucleotide; NAD: nicotinamide adenine dinucleotide; FADH: reduced flavin adenine dinucleotide; FAD: flavin adenine dinucleotide; CoQ: coenzyme Q; Cyt C: cytochrome C: PGC1-α: peroxisome proliferator-activated receptor gamma coactivator-1 alpha; Nrf2: nuclear factor erythroid 2-related factor; NF-κB: nuclear factor-kappa beta.

Source: Vargas-Mendoza N, Angeles-Valencia M, Morales-González Á, Madrigal-Santillán EO, Morales-Martínez M, Madrigal-Bujaidar E, Álvarez-González I, Gutiérrez-Salinas J, Esquivel-Chirino C, Chamorro-Cevallos G, et al. Oxidative Stress, Mitochondrial Function and Adaptation to Exercise: New Perspectives in Nutrition. Life. 2021; 11(11):1269. https://doi.org/10.3390/life11111269.

With a design where 10 subjects performed HIIT once a day, three times a week, twice a day, and once a day, two times a week, the mitochondrial adaptation differs once more when the training intensity is maintained and only the volume is changed. Granata et al. demonstrated that only during the high-volume training phase did mitochondrial respiration and citrate synthase (CS) activity increase (by approximately 50%). PGC-1α, p53, and PHF20 were among the regulatory proteins and ETS that increased in tandem with the increase in mitochondrial respiration. After two weeks of reduced training volume, the only indication of detraining was a slight decrease in CS activity. In contrast, mitochondrial-specific respiration remained high. All things considered, these studies indicate that while higher training volumes are required to increase mitochondrial mass, high-intensity training is crucial for raising mitochondrial activity (Figure. 8 1). Nevertheless, CS activity has been the most common marker used to identify changes in mitochondrial content. Subsequent research endeavors ought to employ electron microscopy in order to ascertain alternative markers that could be more indicative of mitochondrial activity (e.g., subsarcolemma in contrast to the intermyofibrillar location of the mitochondria) and variations in skeletal muscle mass (Hawley & Hargreaves, 2008; Schoenfeld, 2010).

PGC-1α has long been revered as the "master regulator of mitochondrial biogenesis" and a key player in the adaptations that exercise causes in endurance training. Another protein that has gained importance recently is p53, which is essential for mitochondrial biogenesis and substrate metabolism. The first known tumor suppressor protein was p53. In this capacity, p53 controls apoptosis, angiogenesis, DNA repair, cell senescence, and cell cycle arrest. Early research employing p53-deficient mouse knockout (KO) models revealed an additional function of this protein in regulating mitochondrial content. KO mice showed fewer mitochondria in the subsarcolemmal and intermyofibrillar compartments, along with lower COX activity and PGC-1α in comparison to animals of the wild type. Moreover, diminished exercise capacity and performance were a consequence of the loss of p53 and the ensuing decline in mitochondrial content and function. According to current theories, p53 may control mitochondrial biogenesis by interacting with mitochondrial transcription factor A (Tfam) and specifically targeting the mitochondrial genome. On the other hand, Granata and associates demonstrated that maximal sprint training raises p53 levels, while continuous endurance training or HIIT has no impact on p53 levels. It is noteworthy that the regulation of p53 could be impacted by factors other than exercise intensity, such as the nutritional state of the working muscle during training sessions (e.g., decreased availability of carbohydrates). To fully comprehend the time course of p53 activation and its role in mitochondrial biogenesis in relation to endurance exercise, more research is needed. It will be crucial to comprehend this signaling cascade from the standpoint of human performance as well as health, since exercise may be utilized to complement cancer therapy treatments.

After endurance training, changes occur in mitochondrial mass, substrate metabolism, and oxygen delivery within skeletal muscle. These changes, along with other factors, lead to improved running economy and increased exercise performance. The muscle-extracellular matrix (ECM)-tendon unit's stiffness is one of these factors, as modifications to this system will improve the body's capacity to store and utilize elastic energy more effectively. Reduced ground contact time and energy cost are the outcomes of increased elastic energy storage and recoil. In fact, when running at submaximal velocities, runners who exhibit and/or develop a longer and stiffer musculotendonous system seem to have a lower oxygen uptake (VO2). Neural adaptation is a second factor that improves running and cycling economy. The patterns of muscle recruitment in highly trained people and their less experienced counterparts differ significantly. More eccentric to concentric muscle activity, leg stiffness, and increased muscle coactivation may be elicited by highly trained individuals. This enables more effective use of elastic energy stores, reducing the metabolic cost of exercise. On the other hand, although the results are conflicting, stretching interventions meant to increase flexibility typically result in a decrease in economy. A few potential explanations for the contradictory data regarding stretching could be the duration of the intervention program (acute vs. chronic), methodological designs, treadmill familiarization, and the impact of gender in pooled studies.

Classic endurance training is very different from training to improve neuromuscular components and connective tissue stiffness. In this case, the focus of training is on plyometric and strength/power exercises to enhance the neuromuscular adaptations (e.g., muscle contraction, recruitment of motor units) and the rigidity of the tendon-muscle complex. The researchers observed a 3% improvement in the 5-kilometer time trial with a tendency to lower VO_{2max} after 9 weeks of training. Much of the improved performance was attributable to running economy improvements. Further studies have demonstrated the beneficial effects of adding a strength-training program to the preseason and in-season training of athletes who are primarily endurance-trained. Improved neural function (maximal voluntary contraction, rate of force development [RFD]), an increase in type IIA muscle fibers (less fatigable), and an increase in muscle-ECM-tendon stiffness are the suggested mechanisms for these gains in endurance performance. Furthermore, it has been shown that adding strength training improves exercise economy more than just adding endurance training, and adding strength training may improve performance in the later stages of competition. Doing strength/plyometric training on one leg and observing whether cross-limb transfer has led to improved performance in the other leg, suggestive of a neural adaptation, is one method to differentiate between muscle-ECM-stiffness and neural adaptations (see below). These studies haven't yet been done with endurance-style exercise, though. Furthermore, there is evidence to suggest that increasing the volume of both strength and endurance training together may impair both adaptations and performance, so caution is advised when using strength training to improve endurance performance.

Muscle hypertrophy and growth are the final adaptations to endurance exercise training that we would like to discuss. It has been reported that during a 12-week endurance training program, muscle mass can increase by 7–11%. This increase in muscle mass is equivalent to training in resistance exercises over the same amount of time. The quadriceps muscle exhibited the majority of these reported increases in muscle mass with endurance training; cycling was the chosen exercise modality; and the participants had either little to no prior experience with exercise or led sedentary lifestyles. However, it seems that if the frequency and load of classical motor endurance training are high enough, hypertrophy in the quadriceps muscle occurs. Acute studies have shown increases in muscle protein synthesis (MPS) with aerobic exercise, independent of age, from a mechanistic perspective. In particular, hypertrophy has been seen almost exclusively after cycling training. Future research should look into incorporating additional endurance exercise techniques, like running with varying loads and modes (uphill vs. flat) at the same volume to see if there is an acute effect on MPS and muscle size after training. Future research must evaluate the mechanistic contributions of myostatin signaling, feeding, and other mTOR-independent mechanisms to endurance-related muscle hypertrophy (Hawley & Hargreaves, 2008; Schoenfeld, 2010).

8.1.3. Strength Training

Strength training increases muscle CSA, modifies connective tissue stiffness, and produces neuromuscular adaptations that increase muscle strength and power. As a person learns an exercise, the outcome is a quick initial increase in strength (Figure. 8.2), then a slower rate of increase as the muscle mass increases. In order to improve the neuromuscular drive or muscle CSA, strength training has traditionally varied the external load and volume. Typically, training involves a load of between 1RM (repetition maximum) and 10RM and a volume of four to twelve repetitions. After eight to twelve weeks, resistance training adaptations are usually noticeable. However, after just two to four weeks, some studies have shown increases in CSA and muscle strength. While the early increases in muscle CSA size could be the consequence of edema, this early increase in strength is most likely the result of neuromuscular and connective tissue adaptations.

The majority of the early research in this field concentrated on these responses due to the quick nature of the neuromuscular adaptations and the capacity to measure changes in CSA. Increases in skill acquisition via the nervous system and increased maximal muscle activation through motor unit synchronization, muscle recruitment, and increased neural activation have been the main adaptations seen in the neuromuscular system.

When it comes to hypertrophy, the primary adaptation strategy has been to boost the CSA of individual muscle fibers while concurrently adding sarcomeres. Early mechanistic research concentrated on changes that occurred in the hormone milieu following acute resistance exercise as a possible cause of hypertrophy. Recent data, however, seems to challenge the theory that hormones play a role in the hypertrophy and growth of muscles brought on by exercise. The strongest evidence for the role of the central neural component in strength adaptations comes from training one limb while leaving the other untrained.

In this case, training the contralateral limb results in a notable increase in strength while the muscle CSA in the untrained leg remains unchanged. According to a meta-analysis on the benefits of contralateral strength training, after 15 to 48 sessions of training, strength increases by 7 points 6% in the nonexercised limb (56% in the exercised limb). Spinal cord excitability modifications, cross-limb cortical interaction, and localized muscle adaptations are a few of the hypothesized mechanisms for this phenomenon. In the end, unilateral strength training may result in neural drive adaptations that "spill over" into the untrained limb.

Additionally, this kind of training may allow the untrained limb to access the neuromuscular adaptations that take place within the control system. The mechanism underlying the effect has been proposed to be a larger increase in corticospinal excitability, which could account for part of the observed greater effect with eccentric loading. Though it was first noted in 1894, our knowledge of the contralateral strength-training effect and the part played by the systemic environment in this phenomenon is still quite limited.

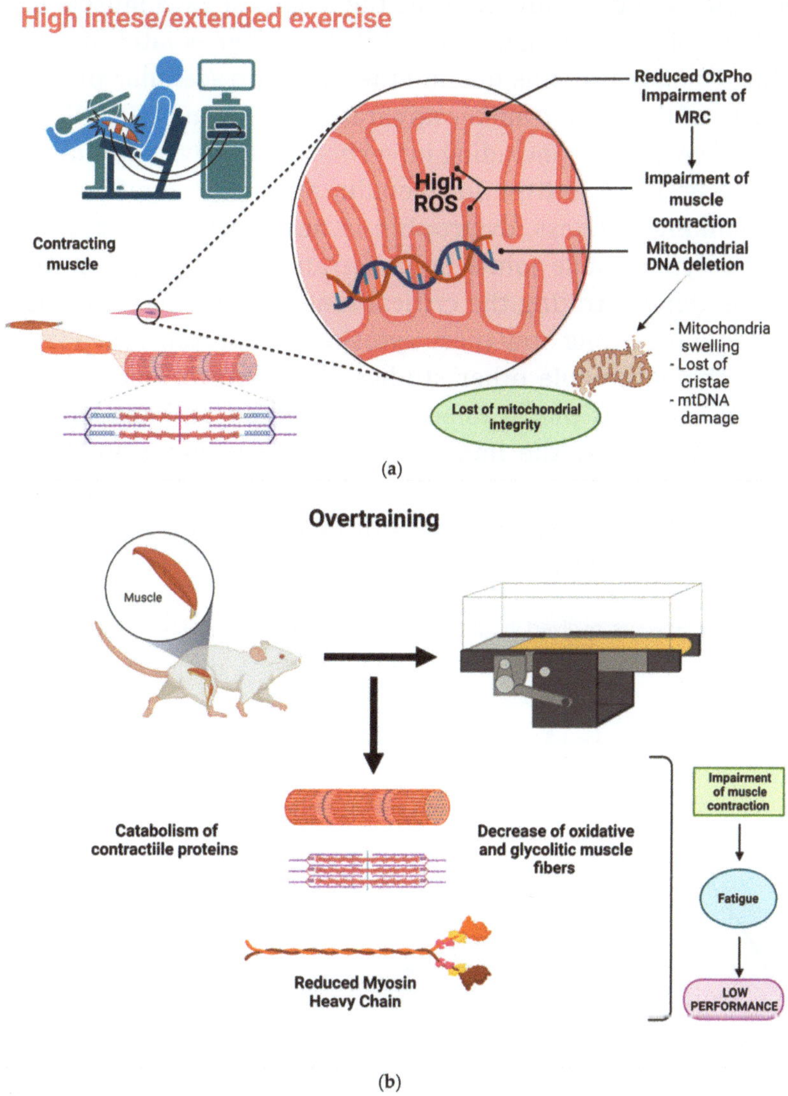

Figure 8.2. *Impact of mitochondrial damage in exercise performance. (a) Graphical representation of mitochondrial reduced function and impairment of muscle contraction in intense or exhausting exercise. (b) Description of overtraining and the impact on muscle catabolism.*

ROS: reactive oxygen species; OxPho: oxidative phosphorylation; MRC: mitochondrial respiratory chain

Source: Vargas-Mendoza N, Angeles-Valencia M, Morales-González Á, Madrigal-Santillán EO, Morales-Martínez M, Madrigal-Bujaidar E, Álvarez-González I, Gutiérrez-Salinas J, Esquivel-Chirino C, Chamorro-Cevallos G, et al. Oxidative Stress, Mitochondrial Function and Adaptation to Exercise: New Perspectives in Nutrition. Life. 2021; 11(11):1269. https://doi.org/10.3390/life11111269 .

An increase in RFD is another adaptation linked to strength training. The slope of the force–time curve, or the rate of force increase at the beginning of contraction, is referred to as the RFD. Force is transmitted by the cytoskeletal network in muscle both laterally, or from the center to the periphery of the fiber, and longitudinally, or along the length of each muscle fiber. It's significant to note that more than 80% of the force generated within a fiber is lateralized from proteins inside the fiber to extracellular matrix proteins outside the fiber. Intracellular proteins (titin, dystrophin, etc.) are important parts of the force transfer apparatus. Collagens I, III, IV, V, and VI; extracellular proteins; and transitional complexes, including integrins and the dystrophin-associated glycoprotein complex (DAGC) (Figure 8.3). While titin and nebulin are more significant for transmitting force longitudinally and sarcomere stiffness, dystrophin is necessary for lateral force transmission. In this study, women with hypermobile joints demonstrated a 15% slower RFD while maintaining the same maximal force, demonstrating the critical function of connective tissue in RFD. There is little information available regarding how these cytoskeleton proteins respond to strength training; some studies show no changes, while other studies show improvements. It's interesting to note that cross-sectional data suggests that trained and untrained athletes have different amounts of force transfer proteins. To address the impact of strength training on the cytoskeleton protein network and force transmission, more research is necessary. This is particularly true because these protein groups seem to be important for both mechanotransduction and protecting against muscle damage brought on by contractions.

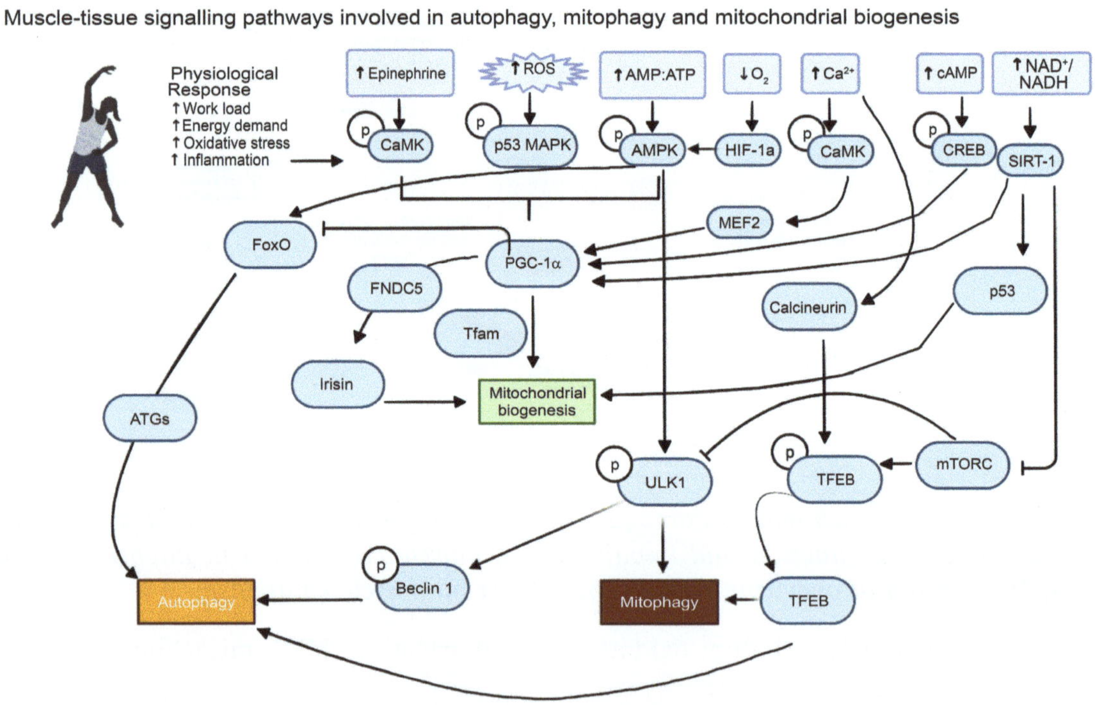

Figure 8.3. *Exercise-induced muscle tissue specific molecular signaling pathways involved in autophagy, mitophagy and mitochondrial biogenesis.*

Source: Roberts FL, Markby GR. New Insights into Molecular Mechanisms Mediating Adaptation to Exercise; A Review Focusing on Mitochondrial Biogenesis, Mitochondrial Function, Mitophagy and Autophagy. Cells. 2021; 10(10):2639. https://doi.org/10.3390/cells10102639.

Similar to endurance training, new research indicates that the increase in CSA that results from strength training is not dependent on load, which appears to be leading to a change in the current paradigm of muscle hypertrophy. According to these studies, using a high load and fewer repetitions to reach failure results in less hypertrophy than lifting a low load to positive failure. According to the new paradigm, hypertrophy depends on brief muscular failure. Muscle fiber recruitment is thought to play a key role in the significance of failure; at failure, all motor units, independent of load, are recruited. The "no-load" and "high-load" groups showed comparable increases in muscle thickness, according to the researchers. High loads are necessary to optimize strength gains, even though the increase in CSA with no-, low-, and high-load training is equal. Given that cycling can increase muscle mass (see above), the impact of low-load training on muscle mass should come as no surprise. Nevertheless, the molecular pathways that transform any load into a biochemical signal that causes muscle hypertrophy are still unknown. According to recent research, there may be a load-dependent rise in mTORC1 activity following resistance training, which is correlated with the subsequent gain in muscle mass. A PI3K/Akt-independent RxRxxS/T kinase is responsible for the signaling that leads to an increase in mTORC1 activity. It is yet unknown, though, how exercising to failure affects the mTORC1 response and whether the rise in mTORC1 activity that follows acute resistance exercise is causing muscle hypertrophy or just reflects the degree of injury and ensuing inflammatory response. Similarly, further investigation is needed to fully understand the role of mTORC1-independent mechanisms, such as ribosomal biogenesis and myostatin signaling, in training-induced muscle hypertrophy (Hawley and Hargreaves, 2008; Schoenfeld, 2010).

8.1.3.1. Strength Training Adaptations

Different resistance training modalities, which differ in terms of volume, intensity, and repetition pattern, cause unique adaptations in muscle morphology and strength that are mediated by particular physiological processes. There are two opposing methods for targeting muscle strength and endurance: high-intensity, low-repetition training and moderate-intensity, high-repetition training. Low-repetition, high-intensity exercise that is usually done at or near one's maximal effort (e.g., 1–5 repetitions per set), which increases maximal strength by mainly promoting muscle hypertrophy and neural adaptations. High threshold motor unit recruitment and increased muscle fiber activation are the results of this kind of training, which encourages changes in motor unit recruitment, synchronization, and firing rate. Furthermore, by putting muscle fibers under maximal or nearly maximal loads, high-intensity resistance training creates mechanical tension—a crucial stimulus for muscle hypertrophy—which in turn activates molecular signaling pathways like the mTOR (mechanistic target of rapamycin) pathway that are involved in protein synthesis and muscle growth. As a result, in order to adapt, muscles expand their cross-sectional area, which increases their capacity to produce force. In contrast, high-repetition, moderate-intensity training that is frequently carried out at lower intensities (e.g., 60–70% of the maximum number of repetitions) and more repetitions in each set (e.g., 10–15 repetitions), which focuses mostly on metabolic adaptations and muscle endurance. The total amount of work completed during moderate-intensity, high-repetition training can still cause considerable metabolic stress and fatigue, even though the absolute load lifted is less than in high-intensity training. This is especially true for type I muscle fibers, which are more oxidative and fatigue-resistant. This kind of training enhances the muscle's capacity to withstand fatigue and maintain extended submaximal contractions by promoting adaptations like increased mitochondrial biogenesis, capillarization, and oxidative enzyme activity. Furthermore, compared to high-intensity training, moderate-intensity, high-repetition training can promote muscle hypertrophy to a lesser degree. This is mainly due to metabolic stress-induced mechanisms like lactate accumulation and hormonal reactions (e.g., insulin-like growth factor 1 and growth hormone).

Generally, the choice of resistance training modality is based on personal preferences and particular training objectives. For athletes and people looking to increase their power and muscular size, high-intensity, low-repetition training is preferred as it maximizes maximal strength gains and muscle hypertrophy. On the other hand, training that is moderately intense but involves a high repetition count is better at improving both muscular endurance and metabolic adaptations. For this reason, individuals who aim to improve their cardiovascular health or endurance as well as endurance athletes can benefit from this type of training. It's important to remember that both modalities can be included in a comprehensive resistance training program. Periodization and changes in volume, intensity, and repetition pattern are essential for maximizing muscle adaptations and avoiding performance plateaus. The response to various resistance training modalities is also influenced by individual factors, including age, genetic predisposition, and training status. This emphasizes the significance of individualized program design and progressive overload for ongoing gains in muscle strength and performance.

8.1.4. Concurrent Training

When compared to strength training alone, concurrent participation in endurance and strength training programs leads to a comparable increase in VO_{2max} but impaired strength adaptations. Concurrent training appears to prevent muscle hypertrophy in certain cases, but normal muscle growth can still occur if the frequency or intensity of concurrent training is reduced to less than four days per week and 70% of $_{VO2max.}$ This implies that the concurrent training effect is caused by something related to training volume and/or intensity. One theory is that a larger caloric deficit from increased training volume and intensity leads to a reduction in the protein synthetic response to feeding. Analyzing the Hickson study's calorie cost of training demonstrates that at week five of the study, the concurrent training group was using approximately 6000 kcal per week, while the strength training alone group was using only 2000 kcal per week. This difference grew over the next five weeks of the study. The difference in muscle size and strength could be explained by the 4000 kcal/week difference in energy expenditure. The reduced neural drive associated with strength training resulting from endurance training could also account for the poor strength adaptation. It should be highlighted, though, that these researchers were unable to observe a concurrent training effect on the strength adaptation, suggesting that the training volume or intensity was insufficient. The impact of concurrent training on force transfer has not yet been thoroughly studied, much like other training modalities. It has been proposed by Gross et al. (2009) that endurance training reduces force transfer, but it is unclear if this could have an impact on the concurrent training effect (Figure 8.4).

In terms of molecular mechanisms, the main area of research has been the interaction between mTORC1, which is activated by resistance exercise, and AMP-activated protein kinase (AMPK), which is activated by high-intensity endurance exercise. This focus is the outcome of research using dividing cells in vitro, which demonstrates three different ways in which AMPK can directly inhibit mTORC1. Consistent with the data from cell culture, the activation of mTORC1 is evidently reduced after resistance exercise in rodent models where the animals receive treatment with the AMPK-activating drug AICAR.

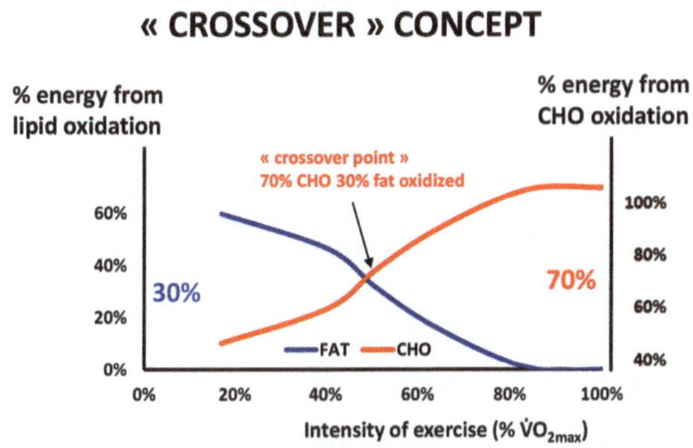

Figure 8.4. *This hypothesis assumes that there is a major shift in the balance of substrates used for oxidation during exercise grossly around 50% of the maximal aerobic capacity, when carbohydrates represent more than 70% of the sources of energy for the exercising body. Oxidative use of fat culminates below this level, and close to it or slightly above it, blood lactate increases and the ventilatory threshold occurs. Note that the ordinates for% of fat oxidation and% of CHO oxidation are not symmetric, in order to better visualize the crossover. In a series of more than 5000 exercise calorimetries, we find that the crossover point is, on average, at 55.1% of VO2max but exhibits a wide variability among individuals.*

Source: *Brun J-F, Myzia J, Varlet-Marie E, Raynaud de Mauverger E, Mercier J. Beyond the Calorie Paradigm: taking into account in practice the balance of fat and carbohydrate oxidation during exercise? Nutrients. 2022; 14(8):1605. https://doi.org/10.3390/nu14081605.*

On the other hand, mTORC1 activation after resistance exercise is not significantly affected by high-intensity endurance exercise-induced AMPK activation in human studies. The discrepancy between the data from rodents and humans may be due to the fact that the α2 isoform is preferentially activated by exercise, while AICAR would activate both the α1 and α2 isoforms. It's interesting to note that the α1 isoform of AMPK is activated to prevent load-induced muscle growth in vivo; greater load-induced muscle hypertrophy results from the knockout of this protein. This shows that the reduced hypertrophy and strength with concurrent training is probably not caused by the inhibition of mTORC1 brought on by the activation of AMPK by endurance exercise (Hawley & Hargreaves, 2008; Schoenfeld, 2010).

8.2. Muscle Adaptations to Aerobic Training

Running or cycling are examples of exercises that require energy utilization within the active muscle, i.e., the rate of energy supply processes (i.e., ATP breakdown) is exactly equal to that of ATP (i.e., resynthesis of ATP). Muscle fatigue results from not meeting the energy demand. When engaging in physical activity that lasts more than a few minutes, aerobic metabolism provides the majority of the energy needed, i.e., the process that uses oxygen to fuel the oxidation of fats and carbohydrates. In response to chemical signals generated during contractions, the mitochondria in muscle fibers use the energy from oxygen consumption to resynthesize ATP from adenosine diphosphate (ADP) plus phosphate, which are byproducts of ATP breakdown. Enough oxygen must be delivered to the active muscle fibers for this process to occur, and the cell must have enough fuel to support oxygen consumption. These fuels come from the circulation or from within the cell and include fatty acids as well as carbohydrates (glycogen and glucose). Adequate blood flow is necessary for the production of oxygen, which then has to diffuse from red blood cells in capillaries to the mitochondria in muscle fibers. Therefore, if the fuel reserves inside the muscle fibers are depleted and/or the circulation isn't supplying enough fuel or oxygen, there may be a disruption in the delivery of energy. Participation in endurance types of exercise training causes muscular adaptations that influence these processes controlling energy provision. Such training adaptations serve to redesign muscle and lead to an improved capacity for oxygen exchange between capillary and tissue and to an improved control of metabolism within the muscle fibers. Both factors provide a better foundation for improved physical performance (Coffey & Hawley, 2007; Bell et al., 2015).

8.2.1. Muscle Design

Muscle becomes more efficient as an energy source through adaptation to aerobic exercise training. The enhanced muscle performance that comes with training is probably due to a better ability to draw oxygen from the blood supply and a change in the cellular regulation of energy metabolism. It goes without saying that adaptations unrelated to biochemical alterations in the muscles and increases in maximal cardiac output also improve performance. Particularly in the muscles that are used actively during the exercise, training adaptations are produced. These adaptations are lost after inactivity and are maintained by continued activity. Exercise training sessions' length and intensity have a significant impact on how muscles adapt. Meaningful adaptations created in non-athletic populations by regular physical activity may also be significant in supporting healthier living, even though the development of optimal muscle adaptations is anticipated to improve performance in competitive sport.

8.2.1.1. Muscle Fiber Type

Adult human skeletal muscle is made up of roughly equal amounts of slow-twitch (type I) and fast-twitch (type II) muscle fibers. Slow-twitch fibers have high blood flow, capillary density, and mitochondrial content, making them highly resistant to fatigue with adequate blood flow. Fast-twitch fibers can be divided into type IIa, with high metabolic capacity and fatigue resistance, and type IIb, with low metabolic capacity and quick fatigue. Exercise intensity is increased by recruiting more muscle fibers, typically in the order of type I, type IIa, and type IIb. While exercise can lead to adaptations in muscle fibers, it does not significantly change the distribution of slow and fast fibers. Elite endurance athletes likely have a high percentage of slow-twitch fibers due to genetics, rather than training-induced adaptations.

8.2.1.2. Mitochondria

An increase in mitochondrial content throughout trained muscle fibers is one basic biochemical adaptation brought on by exercise training. Both slow-twitch and fast-twitch fibers have more mitochondria, which enhances their ability to provide aerobic energy from the oxidation of fatty acids and carbohydrates when the exercise program prompts them to do so. There is now evidence to suggest that an increase in mitochondrial content is required to realize the increased potential for aerobic ATP provision induced in muscle by training. Additionally, it is likely that the increase in mitochondrial content improves the control of energy metabolism, influences the muscle fibers to oxidize more fatty acids and less glycogen, and improves muscle performance. Previously, it was believed that this increased enzymatic capacity was not utilized because the mitochondrial content was considered over maximal needs even in normal untrained muscle.

8.2.1.3. Muscle Capillarity

The number of capillaries surrounding individual muscle fibers increases with exercise training. Essentially, a recruited fiber is better 'bathed' in the blood flow that is supplied to the muscle. An increase in the number of capillaries surrounding each fiber should improve the oxygen exchange between capillary and fiber by presenting a greater surface area for the diffusion of oxygen, by shortening the average distance required for oxygen to diffuse into the muscle, and/or by increasing the length of time for diffusion to occur (i.e., increased capillarity, even though it is most easily observed in the low-oxidative (type IIb) fiber regions where the capillary density is normally the least). Red blood cells remain in the capillaries for longer periods of time. These effects of increased capillarity would account for a portion of the increase in whole-body maximal oxygen consumption observed in endurance-trained individuals, as well as the increased oxygen extraction that occurs in trained muscles of humans and laboratory animals.

8.2.1.4. Blood Flow Capacity

Normal skeletal muscle has an extraordinarily high blood flow capacity; in fact, it is so high that, even if the blood vessels in our muscle mass were to dilate to their maximum extent, cardiac output would not be able to perfuse all of them. Because of this cardiac output limitation, only a portion of an individual's total muscle mass can be active, and even then, only a portion of its blood flow capacity can be achieved during intense exercise requiring maximal oxygen consumption. However, there is proof that endurance training raises muscle's peak flow capacity though it's unclear how beneficial this adaptation is in terms of increasing the muscle's "unused" flow reserve. Likely, the exchange of nutrients between capillaries and fibers and the best use of the flow supplied to the muscle are the key components of vascular adaptations to training. This emphasizes the importance of the diffusion exchange properties of the vessels surrounding the muscle fibers and the vasomotor control of the artery supply/resistance vessels.

8.2.1.5. Metabolism

At least during extended exercise, trained muscles' increased mitochondrial content should have a variety of metabolic benefits that enhance performance. First, even in situations where the muscle's access to circulating fatty acid concentration is not increased, the increase in mitochondria should enable a higher rate of fatty acid oxidation following exercise. Second, during submaximal exercise, an increase in a muscle fiber's mitochondrial content modifies the biochemical signals governing energy metabolism. The signals within trained muscle fibers that speed up metabolism during exercise are, in effect, attenuated when compared to the untrained state. This lowers the rate of carbohydrate breakdown and likely accounts for the sparing of muscle glycogen seen in trained subjects. As a result, the biochemical modifications in muscle serve as the basis for metabolic alterations that improve endurance performance in athletes.

8.2.2. Training Stimulus

8.2.2.1. Duration and Intensity of Exercise

Currently, it is unknown what underlying mechanisms cause the muscle to adapt to training. It is evident, though, that for the muscles to adjust to the training regimen, they must be recruited during the exercise task. Muscles (or individual muscle fibers) that are not used during the exercise task do not change. As a result, the essential stimulus for adaptation is probably very particular to the active fibers and is not likely to be a blood-circulating, general factor that affects all muscles. Additionally, training for a particular exercise program needs to be done for a long enough period of time—days or weeks—to allow the biochemical adaptations unique to each muscle to stabilize. For example, after about 4–5 weeks of training, muscle mitochondrial content seems to reach a steady state. The length of the daily exercise session also affects the size of the mitochondrial content increase brought on by training. Greater increases in mitochondrial content are generally produced by longer exercise bouts. The impact of exercise bout duration is not linear, though, and as training sessions get longer, the extra time spent exercising seems to have less of an effect on the amount of mitochondria present. Additionally, the duration of the exercise bout and exercise intensity interact to enhance the effectiveness of the first few minutes of exercise in creating a stimulus for adaptation. Long training sessions may improve performance, but the benefit may come from changes in fluid balance, substrate availability, cardiovascular function, or other factors unrelated to muscle-specific adaptations.

The impact of exercise intensity on muscle fiber recruitment can be responsible for a portion of the positive effects of increasing exercise intensity on training-induced adaptations in muscles. Once maximum efficiency is responsible for force development and/or power output; recruiting more muscle fibers results in higher power output. The significant adaptation that the low-oxidative fibers show as they are called upon to meet the demands of the more demanding exercise task serves as an example of this.

8.2.2.2. Short-Term Training

Long-term biochemical adaptations cannot explain all of the training-induced improvement in exercise performance. For instance, there is evidence of improved muscle and metabolic performance even days after starting an exercise program. This may be because the brief training induces an initial change in neuromuscular and/or cardiovascular control that enhances blood flow distribution, muscle fiber utilization, and metabolism. This illustrates the range of training times and the intricacy of modifications needed to accomplish specific adaptations that arise during the shift from a comparatively inactive state to one that is optimally trained. The muscle adaptations described in this summary cannot account for all of the improvement in exercise performance following training. Additional alterations (e.g., after training for several weeks or months, several factors (neuromuscular, cardiovascular, and endocrine) may play a significant role in improving exercise performance.

8.2.2.3. Detraining

In the same way that physical activity causes meaningful adaptations, inactivity causes people to gradually lose these adaptations. For many variables, the extent and time course of regression are unknown and are probably related to the particular process being studied. For instance, as shown in Figure 8.5, within one week of detraining, approximately half of the increased muscle mitochondrial content resulting from training can be lost. Muscle adaptations can be recovered by returning to training, but it may take longer than the detraining interval to return to the steady-state trained condition. As an illustration, consider the comparatively long recovery period in Figure 8.5 from the shortened detraining period (a) that resulted in the decrease in mitochondrial content (Tablle 8.1).

Table 8.1. *Summary of Studies Exploring the Effects of Pre-Exercise CHO Food Ingestion on Endurance Exercise Performanc*

Study	Subjects	Exercise Test	Treatments	Timing	Performance
Thomas et al.	8 trained male cyclists (VO_{2max}: 62.5 ± 3.7 $mL·kg^{-1}·min^{-1}$)	Cycling to exhaustion at 65–70% VO_{2max}	L: 1 $g·kg^{-1}$ CHO from lentils (LGI) P: 1 $g·kg^{-1}$ CHO potato (HGI) G:1 $g·kg^{-1}$ CHO glucose W: Water	1 h before exercise	↑L vs. G ↑L vs. P ↑L vs. W
Paul et al.	12 healthy adults (six women VO_{2peak}: 50.6 ± 4.3; six men VO_{2peak}:58.3 ± 5.1 $mL·kg^{-1}·min^{-1}$	90 min of steady state cycling at 60% VO_{2peak} followed by a 6.4 km TT	Oats (O): 41.5 g CHO, 5.7 g fiber, 3.8 g fat, 10 g protein Wheat (W): 53.9 g CHO, 7.2 g fiber, 1.4 g fat, 7.2 g protein Corn (C): 54.7 g CHO, 0.7 g fiber, 0 g fat, 4.5 g protein Fasted (F)	90 min before cycling	↔O vs. W vs. C
Chryssanth-opoulos et al.	10 male recreational runners (VO_2max: 58.6 ± 1.9 $mL·kg^{-1}·min^{-1}$)	Treadmill running at 70% VO_{2max} to exhaustion	M + C: Pre-exercise 2.5 $g·kg^{-1}$ BM CHO [white bread, jam, cornflakes, sugar, skimmed milk, orange juice], and CHO drinks during exercise [6.9% CHO: dextrose, maltodextrin, and glucose syrup] P + C: Pre-exercise PL and CHO ingestion during exercise P + P: Pre-exercise PL and PL drink during exercise	3 h before exercise and during exercise	↑M + C vs. P + C ↑M + C vs. P + P ↑P + C vs. P + P

Jones et al.	8 endurance trained males	60 min self-paced cycle	(Combo): Semi-liquid oat-based CHO/ fat/protein combination (77% CHO, 7% protein and 5% fat) [Oatmeal, sugar, whole wheat, brown sugar, dried bananas, barley flakes, wheat farina, almonds, and guar gum] (O): Semi-liquid, oat-based CHO (68% CHO,14% protein and 1.7% fat) [Whole-grained rolled oats, calcium carbonate, and guar gum] (W): Semi-liquid wheat-based CHO (75% CHO, 11% protein) [Wheat farina, wheat germ, salt, guar gum (460 kcal] (Bar): Dense solid, fructose-based CHO/ protein/ vitamin (69% CHO, 14% protein, 3% fat) [High fructose corn syrup, fruit juice concentrate, oat bran, malto-dextrins, milk protein, banana, cashew butter, rice]	2 h before the test	↔Combo vs. O vs. W vs. Bar

Kirwan et al.	6 recreationally active women ($\dot{V}O_2max$: 48.3 ± 3.0 mL·kg^{-1}·min^{-1})	TTE at 60% $\dot{V}O_2max$	(R): 75 g CHO [sweetened whole-grain rolled oats with 7 g fiber + 300 mL water] (F): 75 g CHO [sweetened whole-oat flour with 3 g fiber + 300 mL water] (C): Control [Water]	45 min before exercise	↑R vs. C ↑F vs. C
Mitchell et al.	10 trained runners ($\dot{V}O_2max$: 59.35 ± 2.46 mL·kg^{-1}·min^{-1})	10 km treadmill run	HGF: 72 g CHO high fructose corn syrup solution LFG: 54 g CHO low volume glucose/fructose GLU: 54 g CHO glucose solution SUG: 54 g CHO sucrose/glucose mixture BAN: 54 g CHO banana with water (900 mL) WP: Water PL	1 h before exercise	↔HGF vs. LFG vs. GLU vs. SUG vs. BAN vs. WP
Kirwan et al.	6 males ($\dot{V}O_{2peak}$: 54.3 ± 1.2 mL·kg^{-1}·min^{-1})	Cycling to exhaustion at 60% $\dot{V}O_{2peak}$	(O): 75 g CHO [rolled oats as a moderate GI meal (~61) + 300 mL water] (P): 75 g CHO [Puffed rice as a HGI meal (~82) + 300 mL of water] (C): Control [Water]	45 min before exercise	↑O vs. C ↔P vs. C

Chryssant-hopoulos et al.	10 male recreational runners (VO2max: 63.5 ± 2.3 mL·kg^{-1}·min^{-1})	Treadmill running at 70% VO_2max to exhaustion	M + C: Pre-exercise 2.5 g·kg^{-1} BM CHO [white bread, jam, cornflakes, sugar, skimmed milk, orange juice], and CHO drinks during exercise [6.9% CHO: dextrose, maltodextrin, and glucose syrup] M + W: Pre-exercise 2.5 g·kg^{-1} BM CHO [white bread, jam, cornflakes, sugar, skimmed milk, orange juice], and water during exercise P + W: Pre-exercise PL and water during exercise	3 h before exercise and during exercise	↑M + C vs. P + W ↑M + W vs. P + W
Kern et al.	8 endurance-trained cyclists 4 males (VO_{2max}: 64.1 ± 3.4 mL·kg^{-1}·min^{-1}) and 4 females (VO_{2max}: 47.5 ± 10.6 mL·kg^{-1}·min^{-1})	Cycling for 45 min at 70% VO_{2max} followed by 15 min performance trial	R: 1 g·kg^{-1} BW CHO raisin S: 1 g·kg^{-1} BW CHO sport gel	45 min before exercise	↔R vs. S
Chen et al.	8 endurance-trained male runners ($VO_{2max:}$ 58.5 ± 1.6 mL·kg^{-1}·min^{-1})	21 km performance run on a level treadmill	HGI meal: [92 g jasmine rice, 90 g parsnips, 265 g orange soda, 55 g canned lychees, 40 g ham, 35 g fish sticks, 80 g egg, 573 g water] LGI meal: [290 g clear chicken broth, 251 g soymilk, 54 g hard boiled egg,	2 h before the test meal was consumed and 2 mL·kg^{-1} BM of 6.6% CHO solution was consumed immediately before exercise and every 2.5 km afterward	↔LGI vs. HGI: ↑HGI vs. CON

			38 g fish sticks, 46 g green peas, 81 g mung bean thread noodles, 467 g water] CON: Control [9 g low-energy sugar-free jelly]		
Aandahl et al.	11 well-trained (VO_{2max}: 71.9 ± 5.1 mL·kg^{-1}·min^{-1}) and 10 recreationally trained (VO_{2max}: 46.9 ± 2.5 mL·kg^{-1}·min^{-1}) men	Five submaximal 5 min constant-velocity bouts of increasing intensity and a graded exercise test to measure TTE (running on a tread-mill)	High CHO meal: 3 g·kg^{-1} BM CHO [white bread, jam, skimmed milk, oats, banana, and raisins] Low CHO meal: 0.5 g·kg^{-1} BM [yogurt, almonds, and avocado] Fasted state	3.5 h before the exercise	↑High CHO meal vs. low CHO meal ↑High CHO vs. fasted state

CHO carbohydrate, VO_{2max} maximal oxygen consumption, VO_{2peak} peak oxygen consumption, TT time-trial, TTE time to exhaustion, VA voluntary activation, CAR central activation ratio, MVC maximum voluntary contraction, sMVC sustained MVC, WE work economy, HGI high-glycemic index, LGI low-glycemic index.

Source: Naderi A, Gobbi N, Ali A, Berjisian E, Hamidvand A, Forbes SC, Koozehchian MS, Karayigit R, Saunders B. carbohydrates and endurance exercise: a narrative review of a food first approach. Nutrients. 2023; 15(6):1367. https://doi.org/10.3390/nu15061367.

8.3. Neuromuscular Adaptations to Exercise

Neuromuscular adaptations probably occur at all levels of the motor pathway, following changes in muscular activity. Adaptations have been mostly investigated in muscle fibers after heavy-resistance and endurance training. In strength training, the rapid improvement is due to poorly understood neural factors, with muscle fiber hypertrophy occurring rather later; fiber hyperplasia is probably unimportant. In contrast to other mammals, muscle fibers in humans do not readily change from "slow" to "fast" and vice versa, although there may be a period of plasticity in infancy especially responsive to weightbearing. A proportion of the changes in the fibers, following training, is probably brought about by stretch-activated mechanisms, in which second messengers express immediate early genes and the latter, in turn, promote the transcription of "muscle" genes; other cellular adaptations occur at the level of mRNA translation. In the spinal cord, adaptations following hemiparesis include a loss of functioning motor units. Impaired motor drive occurs not only in organic brain lesions but also after periods of disuse. In persons with amputations, the peripheral nerve stump undergoes degenerative changes; somatosensory cortical evoked responses, following stimulation of the stump, are diminished. It is possible that both sensory and motor cortical representations are increased for neighboring regions of the body.

8.3.1. Strength Training and Neuromuscular Adaptations

The body adapts, or undergoes structural and functional changes, as a result of systematic strength training. The size and strength of the muscles show the degree of adaptation. The demands that training's volume, frequency, and intensity (load) place on the body, as well as the body's capacity to adapt to those demands, determine how much of these adaptations occur. Training sensibly adjusts to the strain of more demanding physical labor. Stated differently, the body grows stronger in response to a stressor if it receives a reasonable demand that exceeds its capacity and it is allowed adequate time to recover from the training. Up until a few years ago, we thought that the cross-sectional area (CSA) of the muscles was the primary factor in determining strength. Weight training was therefore used to induce muscular hypertrophy, or an increase in engine size. The focus of strength training research has shifted to the neural component of strength expression since the 1980s, even though CSA is still the single best predictor of an individual's strength. In actuality, a 2001 review by Broughton thoroughly documented the central role of the nervous system in the expression of strength. Strength training causes changes in intra- and intermuscular coordination as well as the disinhibition of inhibitory pathways in the brain.

8.3.1.1. Disinhibition affects the following mechanisms:

- Ø Golgi tendon organs – sensory receptors, located near the myotendinous junction, that elicit a reflex inhibition of the muscle they supply when it undergoes excessive tension, either by shortening or passive stretching
- Ø Renshaw cells – inhibitory connecting neurons (interneurons) found in the spinal cord, whose role is to dampen the rate of discharge of alpha motor neurons, thus preventing the muscular damage derived from tetanic contraction.
- Ø Supraspinal inhibitory signals – conscious or unconscious inhibitory signals that come from the brain

The components of intramuscular coordination are as follows:

- Synchronization – the capacity to contract motor units simultaneously or with a minimum latency (that is, with a delay less than five milliseconds)
- Recruitment – the capacity to recruit motor units simultaneously
- Rate coding – the capacity to increase firing rate (motor unit discharge rate) to express more strength

As long as the particular motor pattern (intermuscular coordination) is established, adaptations in intramuscular coordination transfer well from one exercise to the next. For instance, if an athlete knows the technique for an exercise skill specific to their sport, they can apply the maximum voluntary recruitment of motor units developed through maximum strength training to that particular exercise skill. While power macrocycles primarily focus on rate coding, maximum strength macrocycles aim to enhance the motor unit recruitment of the prime movers. Contrary to popular assumption, synchronization is not as important in determining the production of muscular force as these two aspects of intramuscular coordination: recruitment and rate coding. On the other hand, intermuscular coordination refers to the nervous system's ability to synchronize the kinetic chain's rings, improving the efficiency of the motion. As the nervous system becomes more adept at the gesture, fewer motor units are activated by the same weight over time, freeing up more motor units to be activated by heavier weights. Therefore, intermuscular coordination training, or technique training, is the key to increasing the weight lifted in a given exercise over time. However, because intermuscular coordination is highly exercise-specific, there is very little chance that it will transfer to other exercises, including ones that are sport-specific. It still serves as the cornerstone for the athlete's overall strength development, though.

Even though training causes an instantaneous hypertrophic response, it takes at least six weeks for muscular protein to accumulate. The acquired neural adaptations are stabilized by these proteins, which stand for the particular adaptive response to the imposed training. This is how the well-known research by Moritani and deVries should be interpreted because, once they occur, brain adaptations are neither fully developed nor completely stable. Therefore, one needs to continue training the factors covered here in order to gradually increase strength. This is especially true for intermuscular coordination, which permits specific hypertrophy and an increase in load in the medium and long terms due to constantly rising system efficiency.

Strength training programs have been designed and analyzed by Eastern European coaches and training methodologists using training intensity zones as brackets of 1RM for many years. Zones 2 and 1 (loads from 85% and up) were the best training zones to elicit maximum strength gains, according to the majority of the strength training methodology literature. Zone 3 loads—those between 70 and 80%—have taken center stage in recent years, replacing zone 1 loads—those exceeding 90%. This change has been based on the experiences of Russian and Italian powerlifters as well as weightlifters (with the exception of the Greek and Bulgarian schools and their North American clones, who have frequently used very high intensities and, not coincidentally, have a tragic history of positive doping tests). In other words, research on the most successful weightlifting and powerlifting programs has revealed a concentration of training loads in zone 3. Once more, almost all of the classic literature on strength training has suggested that training loads for maximum strength development should be 85% of 1RM or higher. Therefore, identifying zone 3 as the most crucial zone for maximum strength development is a fundamental shift.

The field has shown us that

1. the majority of adaptations of the neuromuscular system necessary to increase maximum strength involve loads lower than 90% of 1RM and
2. the time of exposure to loads of 90% or higher (necessary in order to elicit adaptations specific to that intensity range) should be very short.

From these values, we learn that

- the majority of intramuscular coordination gains involve loads over 80%;
- the majority of intermuscular coordination gains involve loads under 80%; and
- we need to use the full spectrum of intensities to maximize neuromuscular adaptations and, consequently, maximum strength.

The average intensities used in the maximum strength macrocycles will be higher (80–85% of 1RM) during a preparation phase with limited time for maximum strength development, or when coaching of the same group of athletes will likely last only one season. This method is typically applied in team sports. Intermuscular coordination will be the primary focus of the periodized strength plan during the phase of preparation for an individual sport where there is enough time for the development of maximum strength. This is especially true when a multiyear perspective indicates continuous progression in the midterm and long term. Therefore, in maximum strength macrocycles, the average intensity—rather than the peak—will be lower (70–80% of 1RM). However, in order to maximize strength, every periodized plan begins with lower intensities, longer times under tension per set (which support anatomical adaptations), and an emphasis on technique in order to eventually induce high muscular tension from higher intensities.

Periodization of strength provides an approach that is seven phases in length and tracks the physiological rhythm of the response of the neuromuscular system to strength training, which is useful because different types of adaptation can happen. The seven stages of the process are as follows: anatomical adaptation, hypertrophy, maximal strength, conversion, maintenance, reduction, and compensation. Anatomical adaptation, maximal strength, conversion to specific strength, and maintenance are the minimum number of phases that are combined in the periodization of the strength process, depending on the physiological demands of the sport. A phase of anatomical adaptation precedes all models for periodization of strength (Coffey & Hawley, 2007; Bell et al., 2015).

8.3.2. Adaptation to Exercise: The Overload Principle

The improvement in exercise as well as the adaptation to exercise are attributed to the overload principle. There are two possible overloads on the muscular system: mechanical and metabolic. These mechanisms lead to distinct and unique adaptations that improve performance.

The magnitude of these adaptations is dependent on:

- The type of exercise
- The intensity of exercise
- The frequency of exercise
- The duration of exercise

There is also emerging evidence for other factors also playing a role such as:

- The initial level of fitness
- Genetic influences that determine the body's responsiveness (responders and non-responders) to given training interventions

The workout style (either strength or endurance) affects the kind and degree of neuromuscular adaptation. For instance, when high repetition, low load contractions are used in endurance training, the muscular system experiences unique alterations that enhance fatigue resistance and aerobic metabolism. On the other hand, muscle adaptations like increased myofibrillar protein synthesis will result from strength training, which combines low repetitions with high load contractions. Muscle growth, strength, and power may consequently improve. Specificity is a further principle to take into account. In the context of training, the kind of exercise that is done is crucial to take into account. According to the specificity principle, only the bodily part or system that is frequently under stress will be able to cope with long-term overload. As a result, different exercises cause different adaptations, which produce different training effects.

8.3.3. Adaptations to High-Resistance Strength Training

Any form of training that tries to increase muscle size, strength, and power through muscular contraction is referred to as progressive resistance training. This type of exercise is based on the overload principle, which states that working a muscle to its maximum force-generating capacity will increase strength and stimulate muscle growth. A standard program might consist of 6–8 sets of lifting and lowering a weight, repeated three to four times, with loads equivalent to about 70–80% of the highest weight that can be lifted once (1-RM).

8.3.3.1. Neural Adaptations

- Increased central drive (from the higher centers of the brain) after resistance training is partly responsible for the increase in strength
- Increased Motor Unit (MU) synchronization (several MU's firing at similar times)
- Decrease in the force threshold at which Motor Units are recruited
- Increased Motor Unit firing rate
- Decrease in the level of co-activation of antagonist's muscles after training

8.3.3.2. Muscular Adaptations

In response to mechanical overload, skeletal muscle will enlarge. Resistance training causes a variety of signaling mechanisms to become active, which in turn causes the synthesis of new proteins, the enlargement of muscle fibers and muscle cell size, and ultimately, hypertrophy. However, there isn't much evidence that this leads to a rise in the number of muscle fibers (hyperplasia). Various adaptations include:

- Increase in the cross-sectional area of the muscle
- Changes in muscle architecture
- Ultrasound studies have shown changes in the angle of fiber pennation (the angle at which fibers are aligned in regards to their insertion to the aponeuroses of the muscle). This will affect force output by determining the physiological cross-sectional area (where the cross-section area is determined perpendicular to the line of pull of the muscle fibers).
- Hypertrophy of fiber types at the cellular level, especially in Type II fibers:
- Research shows a decrease in the number of Type IIb (also known as type IIx) fibers, together with an increase in Type IIa fibers.
- Fast-twitch muscle fibers are inherently stronger (greater force per unit area) and have a high speed of shortening; therefore, "a given enlargement of a fast-twitch fiber should have a proportionately greater effect on strength and power than the same growth of a slow-twitch fiber.""

8.3.4. Muscle Protein Synthesis

Muscle is known to be responsive to training loads. The muscular system undergoes both synthesis and degradation of proteins, making it a dynamic system. The ratio of protein synthesis to degradation must be adjusted for muscle growth. This can happen by accelerating the rate of synthesis, slowing down the rate of degradation, or doing both at once.

Important findings to know about human muscle protein turnover:

- Muscle protein synthesis is ~ 0.04%

per hour in the fasted state

- Exercise and feeding stimulate muscle myofibrillar protein synthesis
  - o Following resistance training muscle protein synthesis increases 2x–5x post exercise
  - o Increases in protein synthesis occur 1–2 hours post-exercise, but in the fed state it can remain increased for 48–72 hours.
  - o An elevated protein breakdown accompanies this increase in protein synthesis post-exercise.
  - o In a fed state, protein synthesis is greater than protein breakdown, resulting in a net gain of protein.
  - o The accumulated effect of this process over multiple exercise bouts leads to a net gain in protein and therefore muscle growth.

The above-mentioned findings clearly show that adaptations to muscle are dependent on nutrition availability. The protein synthesis and breakdown response post-exercise can be adjusted by altering the availability of certain nutrients. Both resistance training and amino acid ingestion increase protein synthesis. When these two factors are combined, it has an even bigger effect. The consumption of protein post-exercise does the following:

- Promotes protein synthesis
- Suppresses protein breakdown

With the suppression of protein breakdown post-exercise in the fed state, there is also an increase in insulin levels which further aids this suppression of protein breakdown. It is therefore important to maintain adequate nutrition to maximize the benefits of resistance training.

8.3.5. Satellite Cells

Situated in a niche between a muscle fiber's sarcolemma and the basal lamina, satellite cells are specialized muscle stem cells. They support the development and repair of every skeletal muscle. Damage to the muscles and/or enough exercise activates these cells. Activation of these cells results in their proliferation, differentiation, and fusion with an existing myofiber, forming new contractile proteins and healing the damage. In four training days, the number of satellite cells increases with resistance training. Satellite cell counts can rise by about 30% with prolonged resistance training, and they can continue to rise even after training is discontinued. Donating their nuclei to serve as post-mitotic nuclei in the developing muscle fiber is one of the satellite cells' other crucial functions (Coffey & Hawley, 2007; Bell et al., 2015).

8.3.6. Adaptations to Endurance Training

The goal of endurance training is to increase resistance to muscle fatigue during longer-duration exercise. The definition of fatigue is a reduction in a muscle's ability to produce force and/or velocity as a result of activity while under load, which can be reversed with rest. Performance in endurance exercises depends on the body's capacity to use aerobic respiration to create enough ATP. Interaction between the neuromuscular, cardiovascular, and respiratory systems is necessary for this process. For the purposes of this page, the emphasis will be more on the local adaptations that take place in skeletal muscle. In essence, skeletal muscle's oxidative capacity and metabolic efficiency are improved by endurance training and exercise. It uses three adaptations—oxygen consumption (mitochondrial adaptations), oxygen delivery (angiogenesis), and local substrate availability—to accomplish this.

8.3.7. Mitochondrial Adaptations (Oxygen Utilization)

Mitochondria are the "powerhouse" of the cell. These organelles generate the majority of the cell's supply of ATP through aerobic respiration. Endurance training can:

- increase the volume and number of mitochondria, and the magnitude of these changes is dependent on the frequency and intensity of training.
- increase oxygen utilization by skeletal muscle.

With the increased number and size of mitochondria, the proportion of pyruvate formed during glycolysis passing into the mitochondria for oxidative phosphorylation is increased, with less use for the production of lactate and its by-products. As a result, the exercise intensity that can be sustained through relying on aerobic metabolism is higher.

8.3.7.1. Angiogenesis (Oxygen Delivery)

The network of capillaries adjacent to the muscle fibers is responsible for the diffusive exchange of gases, substrates, and metabolites between the circulation and the working muscle fibers. Endurance training results in:

- the growth of new capillaries (a process of angiogenesis), with an increase of ~20% being present after 8 weeks of training in both Type I and Type II fibers

8.3.7.2. Substrate Utilization

During submaximal exercise, the main fuel sources are carbohydrates (mainly muscle glycogen) and fats (local and circulating fatty acids). Endurance training leads to a key adaptation in substrate utilization:

- for a given level of submaximal exercise, the contribution of fatty acid oxidation to the total energy requirement increases with a marked increase in the muscle's ability to utilize intramuscular triglycerides as the primary fuel source.
- Training results in more glycogen being stored in muscle fibers, in the form of granules, this leads to a greater number of intramuscular lipid droplets being in contact with the mitochondria.
- Endurance athletes rely on improved fatty acid oxidation as it conserves muscle glycogen stores (these are more needed during exercise of high intensity).

8.3.7.3. Neural Adaptations

With endurance training the following adaptations occur in the neural system:

- Motor unit discharge rate decreases.
- A slower rate of decline in Motor unit conduction velocity during sustained contractions is found after endurance training.
- Decrease in Motor unit recruitment thresholds (Table 8.2).

Table 8.2. Summary of Human Studies Investigating Myokine Secretion Via Resistance Training Protocols

Myokine	**Study**	***n***	**Study Cohort**	**Training Protocol**	**Trial**	**Results**
IL-6	Buford et al.	24	Physically active postmenopausal women	3 × (10 × 80% 1 RM)	1 session	Muscle biopsies: IL-6-mRNA ↑
	Della Gatta et al.	16	Young men n = 8; elderly men n = 8	2 × (8–12 × 50–80% 1 RM), progressive increase	12 weeks	Muscle biopsies: IL-6 ↑; not significant different between the groups
	Mendham et al.	12	Sedentary men	3 × (10 × 60% 1 RM) vs. 3 × (10 × 80% 1 RM) vs. Low intensity aerobic exercise (40 min) vs. Moderate intensity aerobic exercise (40 min)	4 sessions, randomized cross-over	Serum- IL-6 ↑ in the moderate intensity groups (RE and AE)
	Phillips et al.	14	Healthy men	3 × (12 × 65% 1 RM) vs. 3 × (8 × 85% 1 RM)	2 sessions, controlled	Serum-IL-6 ↑, with association to total volume load
	Quiles et al.	15	RE-experienced men	4–5 × (8–12 × 60–70% 1 RM) vs. 8–10 × (2–6 × 75–85% 1 RM)	3 weekly, 6 weeks, randomized	Plasma-IL-6 ↑ in both groups; no significant effect on BDNF
	Tomeleri et al.	38	Obese older women	3 × (10–15 maximum repetitions)	3 × weekly, 8 weeks, randomized controlled	Baseline-Serum-IL-6 ↓
Myostatin	Kazemi et al.	24	Healthy men	3 × (15 × 55% 1 RM)	1 session	Plasma-Myostatin ↓
	Raue et al.	14	Young women n = 8 Old women n = 6	3 × (10 × 70% 1 RM)	1 session	Muscle biopsies: Myostatin mRNA ↓
Decorin	Bugera et al.	10	Physically active young men	4 × (7 × 80% 1 RM) vs. 4 × (15–30 × 30% 1 RM) vs. BFR 3 × (15–30 × 30% 1 RM)	1 session	Plasma-Decorin ↑

	Kanzleiter et al.	10	Young men	3 × (8 × max weight)	Human study I, single bout	Plasma-Decorin ↑
Follistatin	Bagheri et al.	40	Middle aged men	3–4 × (15 > 12 > 10 > 8 × 50–80% 1 RM) Upper body vs. lower body vs. both vs. control	3 × weekly, 8 weeks, 10% increase every 2 weeks, randomized controlled	Serum-Follistatin ↑, serum-Myostatin ↓, depending on the volume of activated muscle mass
	Hofmann et al.	91	Elderly women	1–2 × 15, elastic bands vs. Training + nutritional supplements vs. Cognitive training	Progressive increase of resistance; 6 months; randomized	Serum-Follistatin ↑ only in the training group
	Negaresh et al.	31	Elderly men n = 15 Young men n = 16	4 × (10 × 50%–85% 1 RM)	3 × weekly, 8 weeks, 5% increase per week	Plasma-Follistatin ↑; plasma-Myostatin ↓ in both groups
Irisin	Blizzard Leblanc et al.	11	Obese youth	4 × (12–15 × 60–65% 1 RM)	3 × weekly, 6 weeks	Plasma-Irisin → after a single bout of RE, but ↑ after a single bout of AE; with greater ↑↑ after 6 weeks of RE
	Ellefsen et al.	18	Untrained women	Progressive full body heavy strength	3 × weekly, 12 weeks	Serum-Irisin →
	Huh et al.	20	Sedentary healthy men n = 14 Men with metabolic syndrome n = 6	3 × (8–12 × 75–80% 1 RM) vs. HIIT (4 ×4 min 90% Vo_2 max) vs. Continuous moderate exercise (36 min 65% Vo2 max)	1 session, randomized cross-over	Serum-Irisin ↑ immediately and ↓ after 1 h back to baseline; no difference between the groups
	Kim et al.	28	Obese adults	3 × (10–12 × 65–80% 1 RM) vs. Aerobic exercise (50 min 65–80% HR max)	5 × weekly, 8 weeks, randomized controlled	Plasma-Irisin ↑ only in the RE group

	Norheim et al.	26	Healthy physically inactive men n = 13 Pre-diabetic men n = 13	Combined strength and endurance training, 2 × weekly 60 min ergometer and 2 × weekly 60 min full body strength workout	4 × weekly, 12 weeks	Plasma-Irisin higher in the prediabetic group; acute ↑ after exercise; baseline ↓ after 12 weeks
	Nygaard et al.	9	Moderately trained, healthy adults	3 × (10–12 × max weight) vs. 6 × 5 min high intensity treadmill, Borg > 18	1 session, randomized cross-over	Plasma-Irisin ↑ in both groups, but remained higher in the RE group
	Pekkala et al.	56	Untrained healthy men	Aerobic exercise (60 min 50% Vo2 max) vs. 5 × 10 repetitions until failure (leg press only) vs. Long term endurance exercise vs. Long term RE and endurance exercise	Single bout vs. 2 × weekly, 21 weeks	Serum-Irisin →
	Tibana et al.	49	Inactive women: Obese n = 26 Non obese n = 23	3 × (6–12 × repetitions maximum)	2 × weekly, 16 weeks	Plasma-Irisin ↓ in the non-obese group after intervention; no change in the obese group
	Tsuchiya et al.	10	Healthy men	3–4 × (12 ×65% 1 RM) vs. Aerobic exercise (60 min 65% Vo2 max) vs. 30 min RE + 30 min AE	3 single bouts of exercise; randomized cross-over	Plasma-Irisin ↑, significant higher in the RE group
	Zhao et al.	17	Older male adults	Class of leg muscle strength and core strength training	2 × weekly, 12 weeks, randomized controlled	Serum-Irisin ↑
BDNF	Church et al.	20	RE-experienced young men	4 × (10–12 × 70% 1 RM) vs. 4 × (3–5 × 90% 1 RM)	4 × weekly, 7 weeks	Plasma-BDNF ↑

	Domínguez-Sanchéz et al.	51	Physically inactive, obese men	(12–15 × 50–70% 1 RM) vs. HIIT vs. HIIT + RE	1 session, randomized controlled	Plasma-BDNF ↑, highest ↑↑ in the combined group
	Figueiredo et al.	21	Physically active men	1 min 100%VO2 max + 8 exercises 8–12 RM	8 weeks, control group	Plasma-BDNF ↑
	Forti et al.	65	Healthy elderly	2 × (10–15 × 80% 1 RM) vs. 1 × (80–100 × 20% 1 RM) vs. 1 × (60 × 20% 1 RM) + 1 × (10–20 × 40% 1 RM)	3 × weekly, 12 weeks, randomized	Serum-BDNF ↑ in male participants, only in the 3rd group
	Lodo et al.	20	Young healthy adolescents	4 × (5 × 70% 1 RM) vs. 4 × (10 × 35% 1 RM)	2 bouts of exercise with equated total load lifted	Serum-BDNF →
	Jørgensen et al.	30	Persons with multiple sclerosis	Progressive high intensity	2 × weekly, 24 weeks, randomized controlled	Plasma-BDNF →
	Marston et al.	45	Healthy adults	5 × (5 × 85% 1 RM) vs. 3 × (10 × 70% 1 RM) vs.	2 × weekly, 12 weeks, randomized controlled	Serum-BDNF (↑) only in the high load group
	Marston et al.	16	Untrained men n = 11 Untrained women n = 5	5 × 5 repetitions to-fatigue vs. 3 × 10 repetitions to fatigue	2 bouts of exercise; cross-over	Greater serum-BDNF ↑ in the second group
	McKay et al.	29	Male adolescents	300 × maximal eccentric contractions	Single bout	Muscle-biopsy: BDNF ↑
	Roh et al.	26	Elderly, obese women	Elastic bands, intensity:10–14 RPE	3 × weekly, 12 weeks, randomized controlled	Serum-BDNF ↑
	Rojas Vega et al.	11	Healthy adults	3 repetitions of maximal effort isokinetic work (knee extension): 40% 1 RM vs. 110% 1 RM	2 single bouts	Serum-BDNF (↑), but no significance
	Urzi et al.	20	Elderly women	Elastic band resistance training	12 weeks, randomized controlled	Plasma-BDNF ↑

	Walsh et al. Alberga et al.	202	Postpubertal adolescent with obesity	HEARTY-Trial: 2–3 × (6–15 × maximum reps) vs. 20–40 min 70–85% HRmax vs. combination	4 × weekly, 22 weeks, randomized controlled	Baseline plasma-BDNF ↑
	Walsh et al.	10	Older adults	4 × (8–10 × 60–80% 1 RM)	3 × weekly, 8 weeks	Serum -BDNF ↑
	Wens et al.	41	Persons with multiple sclerosis n = 22 Healthy persons n = 19	1 × (10 × 12–14 RPE) increased to 4 × (15 x12–14 RPE)	5 sessions per 2 weeks, 24 weeks, randomized controlled	Baseline serum-BDNF were lower in persons with MS; Serum-BDNF ↑ after exercise in both groups
	Yarrow et al.	20	Healthy young adults	4 × (6 × 52,5% 1 RM) trad. vs. 4 × (6 × 40% 1 RM) concentric vs. 3 × (6 × 100% 1 RM) eccentric	5 weeks	Serum BDNF ↑, with higher response at the end of intervention. No baseline change

Abbrevations in order of appearance: RM: repetition maximum; RE: resistance exercise; AE: aerobic exercise; HIIT: high intensity interval training; RPE: rate of perceived exertion; MS: multiple sclerosis.

Source: Zunner BEM, Wachsmuth NB, Eckstein ML, Scherl L, Schierbauer JR, Haupt S, Stumpf C, Reusch L, Moser O. Myokines and resistance training: a narrative review. International Journal of Molecular Sciences. 2022; 23(7):3501. https://doi.org/10.3390/ijms23073501.

A Closer Look

Muscle Development and Growth

The process of muscle development, known as myogenesis, is a complex and highly regulated series of events that begins during embryonic development and continues throughout life. Myogenesis involves the differentiation of mesodermal precursor cells into mature muscle fibers, followed by their growth and maturation into functional muscle tissue. This process is orchestrated by a combination of signaling pathways, transcription factors, and molecular mechanisms that govern cell fate determination, proliferation, migration, and differentiation.

During early embryonic development, mesodermal cells undergo specification to become myogenic progenitor cells, which will give rise to skeletal muscle, smooth muscle, and cardiac muscle. The initial step in myogenesis is the activation of myogenic regulatory factors (MRFs), a family of transcription factors that includes MyoD, Myf5, Myogenin, and MRF4. These MRFs act as master regulators of muscle differentiation and play key roles in initiating the muscle lineage commitment of precursor cells. The myogenic determination process is tightly regulated by various signaling pathways, including the Wnt, Notch, and Hedgehog pathways. Wnt signaling, for example, promotes myogenic differentiation by stabilizing β-catenin and activating the expression of MyoD and Myf5. Notch signaling regulates the balance between myogenic differentiation and proliferation by inhibiting MyoD expression and maintaining precursor cells in an undifferentiated state. Hedgehog signaling also contributes to myogenesis by promoting the proliferation and migration of myogenic progenitor cells. Once committed to the myogenic lineage, precursor cells undergo proliferation and migrate to their final destinations within developing muscle tissues. These migrating precursor cells subsequently withdraw from the cell cycle and undergo terminal differentiation into myoblasts, which fuse together to form multinucleated myotubes. This fusion process is facilitated by cell adhesion molecules such as N-cadherin and integrins, as well as signaling molecules such as neuregulin and hepatocyte growth factor (HGF).

As myotubes mature, they undergo further growth and maturation processes to become functional muscle fibers. This involves the expression of muscle-specific structural proteins, such as myosin heavy chain (MyHC), actin, and troponin, which form the contractile apparatus of the muscle fiber. Additionally, the assembly of sarcomeres, the basic units of muscle contraction, occurs through the coordinated interactions of sarcomeric proteins such as titin, tropomyosin, and troponin.

Throughout adulthood, muscle tissue continues to undergo remodeling in response to various stimuli, such as exercise, injury, and hormonal changes. Satellite cells, a population of quiescent muscle stem cells located beneath the basal lamina of muscle fibers, play a crucial role in muscle maintenance and repair. Upon activation, satellite cells proliferate and differentiate to replenish damaged muscle fibers and contribute to muscle regeneration.

Summary

- Muscle adaptations represent the intricate physiological changes that occur within skeletal muscle in response to repeated bouts of physical activity or exercise training.
- Muscle adaptations to exercise represent the complex physiological changes that occur within skeletal muscle in response to repeated bouts of physical activity or training.
- Muscular hypertrophy refers to an increase in muscle mass. This usually manifests as an increase in muscle size and strength. Typically, muscle hypertrophy occurs as a result of strength training such as weight lifting.
- Strength training can help people build muscle, both from myofibrillar and sarcoplasmic hypertrophy. This involves training against resistance that gradually increases over time. The strain this places on muscles causes damage to muscle fibers, which the body repairs.
- To build muscle through weight lifting, you need to have both mechanical damage and metabolic fatigue. When you lift a heavy weight, the contractile proteins in the muscles must generate force to overturn the resistance provided by the weight.
- Endurance training leads to adaptations in both the cardiovascular and musculoskeletal system that support an overall increase in exercise capacity and performance (Brooks 2011).
- Strength training leads to an increase in muscle strength and power as a result of neuromuscular adaptations, increases in muscle CSA, and alterations in connective tissue stiffness.
- The importance of the central neural component on strength adaptations is most evident when one limb is trained and the other limb goes untrained. In this situation, muscle CSA does not change in the untrained leg, yet a significant increase in strength occurs from training the contralateral limb.
- The ability to sustain an exercise task such as running or cycling requires that the energy utilization within the active muscle (i.e., the rate of adenosine triphosphate or ATP breakdown) is fully matched by energy supply processes (i.e., ATP resynthesis).
- Training adaptations are induced specifically in the muscles actively used in the exercise; these adaptations are sustained by continued activity and lost following inactivity. Both intensity and duration of exercise training sessions are important factors influencing muscle adaptations.
- Exercise training increases the number of capillaries surrounding individual muscle fibers. In effect, when a fiber is recruited it becomes more effectively 'bathed' in the flow of blood delivered to the muscle.

References

1. Bell, K. E., Séguin, C., Parise, G., Baker, S. K., & Phillips, S. M. (2015). Day-to-day changes in muscle protein synthesis in recovery from resistance, aerobic, and high-intensity interval exercise in older men. *The Journals of Gerontology Series A: Biological Sciences and Medical Sciences, 70*(8), 1024–1029.

2. Burd, N. A., Andrews, R. J., West, D. W., Little, J. P., Cochran, A. J., Hector, A. J., & Phillips, S. M. (2012). Muscle time under tension during resistance exercise stimulates differential muscle protein sub-fractional synthetic responses in men. *The Journal of Physiology, 590*(2), 351–362.
3. Coffey, V. G., & Hawley, J. A. (2007). The molecular bases of training adaptation. *Sports Medicine, 37*(9), 737–763.
4. Flück, M. (2006). Functional, structural and molecular plasticity of mammalian skeletal muscle in response to exercise stimuli. *Journal of Experimental Biology, 209*(12), 2239–2248.
5. Hawley, J. A., & Hargreaves, M. (2008). Molecular basis of exercise-induced skeletal muscle mitochondrial biogenesis: historical advances, current knowledge, and future challenges. *Journal of Applied Physiology, 103*(4), 1533–1544.
6. Hyatt, H. W., & Justice, J. N. (2016). Oxygen consumption in aging skeletal muscle: Cross-talk between ROS and NO. *Experimental Gerontology, 86*, 102–107.
7. Petrella, J. K., Kim, J. S., Cross, J. M., Kosek, D. J., & Bamman, M. M. (2006). Efficacy of myonuclear addition may explain differential myofiber growth among resistance-trained young and older men and women. *American Journal of Physiology-Endocrinology and Metabolism, 291*(5), E937–E946.
8. Phillips, S. M. (2012). Nutritional supplements in support of resistance exercise to counter age-related sarcopenia. *Advances in Nutrition, 3*(4), 517S–525S.
9. Schoenfeld, B. J. (2010). The mechanisms of muscle hypertrophy and their application to resistance training. *Journal of Strength and Conditioning Research, 24*(10), 2857–2872.
10. Trappe, T. A., Carroll, C. C., Dickinson, J. M., LeMoine, J. K., Haus, J. M., Sullivan, B. E., & Hollon, C. J. (2011). Influence of acetaminophen and ibuprofen on skeletal muscle adaptations to resistance exercise in older adults. *American Journal of Physiology-Regulatory, Integrative and Comparative Physiology, 300*(3), R655–R662.

Chapter 9

SPINAL MUSCULAR ATROPHY

Contents

Introduction

An autosomal recessive genetic condition called spinal muscular atrophy (SMA) causes paralysis, muscle atrophy, and eventually death. Patients with SMA can now enjoy improvements in numerous aspects of the once devastating natural history of the disease, thanks to significant advancements in antisense oligonucleotide treatment and gene therapy. It is still unclear how the disease-causing gene's product, survival motor neuron (SMN) protein, depletion causes the ensuing pathogenic alterations. Evidence supporting the possibility that gastrointestinal, metabolic, and endocrine abnormalities contribute to disease phenotype has emerged in recent years. These results included abnormalities in the gastrointestinal system, fatty acids, glucose, amino acids, and hormone regulation in addition to altered body composition. When combined, these modifications may have a significant clinical effect on disease characteristics. It's unclear at this time, though, if these results are specific to the SMA phenotype or merely a result of widespread denervation.

Orientation and Directional Terms

Term	Definition	Illustration
Gene therapy	Gene therapy aims to fix a faulty gene or replace it with a healthy gene to try to cure disease or make the body better able to fight disease.	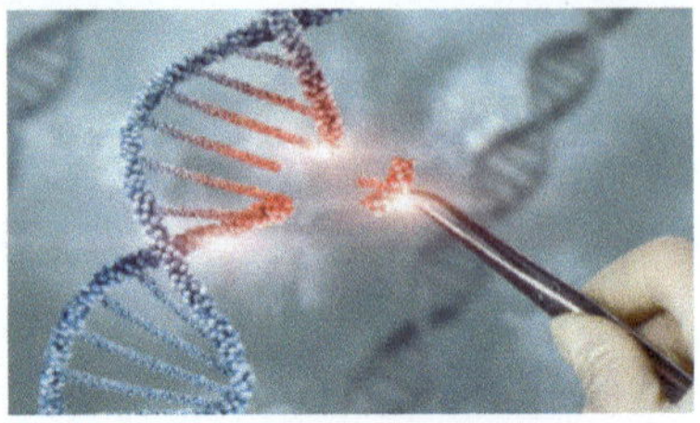
Genetic testing	Genetic testing is a type of medical test that identifies changes in genes, chromosomes, the genome, or proteins.	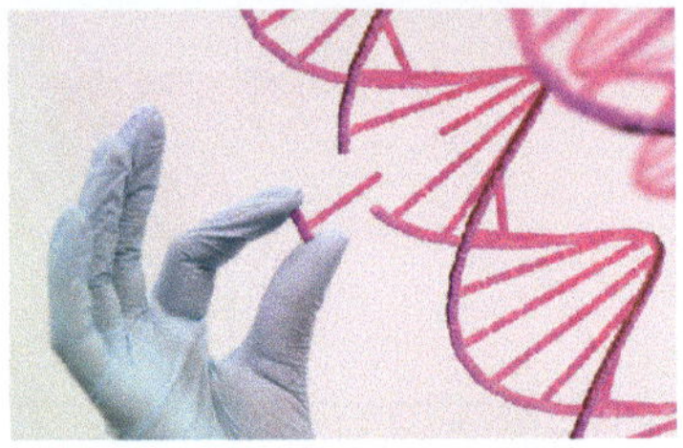
Hypotonia	It can be a condition on its own, called benign congenital hypotonia, or it can be indicative of another problem where there is progressive loss of muscle tone, such as muscular dystrophy or cerebral palsy. It is usually detected during infancy.	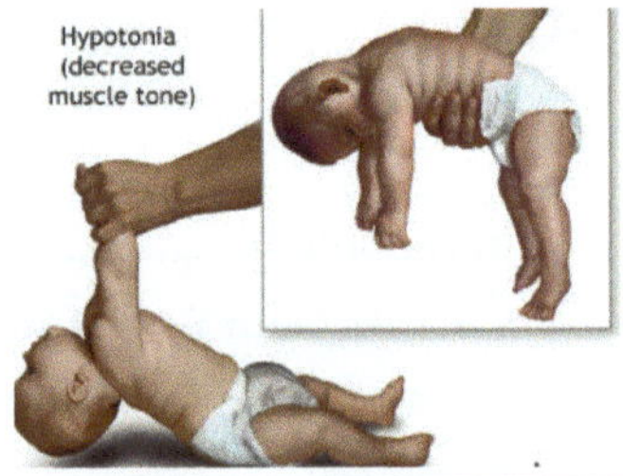
Motor neuron	Motor neurones are cells in the brain and spinal cord that allow us to move, speak, swallow and breathe by sending commands from the brain to the muscles that carry out these functions.	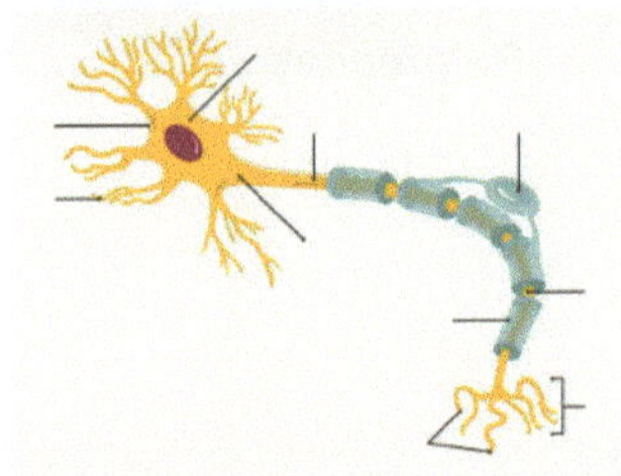
Newborn screening	When your baby is 1 to 2 days old, he has some special tests called newborn screening. Newborn screening checks a baby for serious but rare and mostly treatable health conditions at birth. It includes blood, hearing and heart screening.	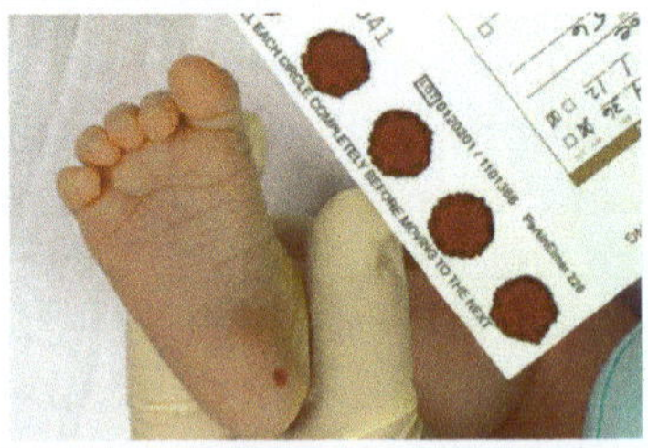

9.1. Basics of Spinal Muscular Atrophy

An autosomal recessive genetic condition, spinal muscular atrophy (SMA), leads to paralysis, muscle atrophy, and eventual death. Recent advancements in antisense oligonucleotide treatment and gene therapy have improved outcomes for SMA patients. The mechanism by which the depletion of the survival motor neuron (SMN) protein, encoded by the disease-causing gene, leads to pathogenic changes remains unclear. Emerging evidence suggests that gastrointestinal, metabolic, and endocrine abnormalities may contribute to the disease phenotype. These abnormalities involve the gastrointestinal system, fatty acids, glucose, amino acids, and hormone regulation, impacting body composition and disease characteristics. It is uncertain whether these findings are specific to SMA or a result of widespread denervation.

In the most severe cases, the disease's natural course results in death within a few weeks of birth, while prolonged SMA forms show normal life expectancy. 2016 saw the implementation of causative treatments, which greatly enhanced the results. Risdiplam, onasemnogene abeparvovec, and nusinersen are among the medications that target the genetic cause of the disease. Physical therapy, occupational therapy, nutritional support, respiratory support, orthopedic interventions, and mobility support are all included in supportive care.

A class of genetic disorders known as spinal muscular atrophy (SMA) can harm or even kill motor neurons, which are specific types of nerve cells found in the brain and spinal cord. Motor neurons regulate skeletal muscle function, including speaking, walking, swallowing, and breathing, as well as movement in the arms, legs, face, chest, throat, and tongue.

9.1.1. Get Spinal Muscular Atrophy

The survival motor neuron gene 1 (SMN1) is the gene responsible for the most prevalent type of SMA. It can be mutated or absent. The survival motor neuron (SMN) protein, which is produced by the SMN1 gene on chromosome 5q, keeps motor neurons healthy and functioning normally. Individuals with SMA have low levels of the SMN protein, which results in the death of motor neurons in the spinal cord, skeletal muscle atrophy, and weakness. The muscles of the upper limbs and arms, as well as the trunk (chest), are frequently weaker than the hands and feet. The same genes can alter in several different forms of spinal muscular atrophy.

Less common SMA forms are caused by changes in other genes including the:

- VAPB gene on chromosome 20
- DYNC1H1 gene on chromosome 14
- BICD2 gene on chromosome 9
- UBA1 gene on the X chromosome

Except in rare cases, SMA is inherited in an autosomal recessive manner, meaning that the affected individual has two mutated genes, often inheriting one from each parent. Those who carry only one mutated gene are carriers of the disease who will not have any symptoms.

9.1.2. Description

A genetic condition called spinal muscular atrophy is characterized by skeletal muscle weakness and atrophy. The loss of specialized nerve cells known as motor neurons, which regulate muscle movement, is the root cause of it. When compared to muscles farther from the body's center (distal), the weakness is typically more severe in the proximal (close to the center) muscles. With aging, muscle weakness typically gets worse. These same gene alterations result in several forms of spinal muscular atrophy. Although there is overlap between the types, the onset age and degree of muscle weakness vary. Mutations in other genes are the cause of other forms of spinal muscular atrophy and related motor neuron diseases, including X-linked infantile spinal muscular atrophy, spinal muscular atrophy with lower extremity predominance, spinal muscular atrophy with progressive myoclonic epilepsy, and spinal muscular atrophy with respiratory distress type 1. Type 0 spinal muscular atrophy is the rarest and most severe form of the condition, exhibiting symptoms prior to birth. Babies affected move less while still in the womb, which frequently results in joint deformities at birth (contractures). When they are born, their muscle tone is incredibly weak, or hypotonia. Because of their extremely weak respiratory muscles, they frequently do not make it past infancy due to respiratory failure. Some infants with congenital (born-with) cardiac defects also have spinal muscular atrophy type 0.

The most prevalent type of spinal muscular atrophy is type I, also known as Werdnig-Hoffmann disease. Muscle weakness is visible from birth or in the first few months of life in this severe form of the disorder. The majority of impacted kids require assistance to sit or to control their head movements. This kind of child may have swallowing issues, which can cause feeding problems and stunted growth. Additionally, they may experience difficulty breathing due to respiratory muscle weakness and an unusually bell-shaped chest that limits the lungs' ability to fully expand. Due to respiratory failure, the majority of children with spinal muscular atrophy type I do not survive into early childhood. Muscle weakness, commonly referred to as Dubowitz disease or spinal muscular atrophy type II, first appears in children between the ages of 6 and 12 months. This type of child can sit unassisted, though they might require assistance sitting up. However, those who are affected may require assistance to sit as their muscle weakness worsens later in childhood. People suffering from type II spinal muscular atrophy are unable to stand or walk independently. They frequently have side-to-side curvature of the spine, involuntary trembling in their fingers, and potentially fatal respiratory muscle weakness. Although the lifespan of people with spinal muscular atrophy type II varies, many of them reach their twenties or thirties.

Known medically as Kugelberg-Welander disease or spinal muscular atrophy type III, this condition usually results in muscle weakness after early childhood. People with this illness are able to stand and walk without assistance, but walking and using stairs may get harder over time. Many of the afflicted people need wheelchair assistance as they age. The life expectancy of a person with type III spinal muscular atrophy is normally normal. Type IV spinal muscular atrophy is uncommon and frequently starts in early adulthood. Those who are affected typically have mild to moderate tremors, mild respiratory issues, and muscle weakness. Individuals with type IV spinal muscular atrophy can expect to live a normal life.

9.1.3. Causes

All of the aforementioned forms of spinal muscular atrophy are brought on by mutations in the SMN1 gene. The quantity of SMN2 copies influences the severity of the illness and influences which kind manifests first. The survival motor neuron (SMN) protein is made by a protein that is encoded by the SMN1 and SMN2 genes. Normally, the SMN1 gene produces the majority of the functional SMN protein, while the SMN2 gene produces a smaller amount. The SMN2 gene produces multiple SMN protein variants, but only one of these variants is functional; the others are smaller and degrade more quickly. One of the proteins in the SMN complex, which is crucial for the upkeep of motor neurons, is the SMN protein. The brain and spinal cord send signals to motor neurons, which cause skeletal muscles to tense or contract, enabling movement of the body. A portion of the SMN1 gene is absent in the majority of cases of spinal muscular atrophy, which reduces the production of SMN proteins. Motor neuron death brought on by a deficiency in SMN protein prevents signals from reaching the muscles of the brain. Since the brain sends signals to muscles in order for them to contract, many skeletal muscles weaken and waste away, resulting in the signs and symptoms of spinal muscular atrophy. Individuals normally have one to two copies of the SMN2 gene and two copies of the SMN1 gene in each cell. But people differ in how many copies of the SMN2 gene they have—some have as many as eight copies. Many copies of the SMN2 gene are typically linked to milder forms of spinal muscular atrophy that manifest later in life in affected individuals. The protein deficit brought on by mutations in the SMN1 gene can be partially compensated for by the SMN protein generated by the SMN2 genes. One copy of the SMN2 gene is typically found in each cell of a person with spinal muscular atrophy type 0; individuals with type I typically have one or two copies; those with type II typically have three copies; those with type III typically have three or four copies; and those with type IV typically have four or more copies. Unknown additional factors also play a role in the varying severity of spinal muscular atrophy.

9.1.4. Diagnosis and Treatment

A blood test is available to look for mutations or deletions of the SMN1 gene. This test identifies at least 95% of SMA Types I, II, and III, and also may reveal if a person is a carrier. If the SMN1 gene is not found to be problematic or the individual's history and examination are not typical of SMA, other diagnostic tests may include:

- Electromyography to record the electrical activity of the muscles during contraction and at rest
- Nerve conduction velocity studies to measure the nerve's ability to send an electrical signal
- Muscle biopsy to diagnose many neuromuscular disorders
- Other blood tests

9.1.4.1. Treating SMA

There is no complete cure for SMA. Treatment consists of managing the symptoms and preventing complications.

9.1.4.2. Medications

- The U.S. Food and Drug Administration (FDA) approved nusinersen (Spinraza™) as the first drug approved to treat children and adults with SMA. The drug is designed to increase the production of the SMN protein, which is critical for the maintenance of motor neurons.
- The FDA approved onasemnogene abeparovec-xioi (Zolgensma™) gene therapy for children less than two years old who have infantile-onset SMA. A safe virus delivers a fully functional human SMN gene to the targeted motor neurons, which in turn improves muscle movement function and survival.
- The FDA approved the orally administered drug risdiplam (Evrysdi) to treat patients aged two months and older with SMA.

Rehabilitation, occupational therapy, and physical therapy can help prevent joint immobility, slow the deterioration of muscles, and improve posture. Exercises that improve range of motion, maintain circulation, and help lessen contractures include stretching and strengthening. Some people need further therapy to address speech and swallowing issues. Enhancing functional independence may benefit from the use of assistive technology such as wheelchairs, orthotics, speech synthesizers, supports, and braces. To maintain strength and weight while avoiding extended fasting, a healthy diet is crucial. For those who are unable to chew or swallow, a feeding tube may need to be inserted. In addition to helping some people breathe better while they sleep, non-invasive ventilation during the night can also be necessary for those who have weakness in their neck, throat, or chest muscles during the day.

9.1.5. Updates on Spinal Muscular Atrophy

The National Institute of Neurological Disorders and Stroke (NINDS), a component of the National Institutes of Health (NIH), conducts basic, translational, and clinical research on SMA in laboratories at the NIH and also supports research through grants to major medical institutions across the country.

Scientists have developed model systems in animals and cells to study disease processes and speed up the testing of potential therapies, including the following:

- Gene therapy and specific drugs have been shown to halt motor neuron destruction and slow disease progression in mouse models and individuals with SMA. NINDS supports research to establish these methods and to provide a path toward clinical tests. Clinical trials for gene therapy in SMA are ongoing.
- Animal models of SMA represent critical tools in discovering and developing new therapies for SMA. Scientists developed zebrafish, mouse, and pig models, including models of less severe SMA types 2 and 3, which may greatly aid the identification of new therapeutic targets and candidate therapies.

Furthermore, pre-symptomatic or recently diagnosed children with SMA types I, II, or III, as well as their healthy siblings, have been the subject of data collection by scientists funded by the NIH. The purpose of this research is to inform and counsel parents regarding potential clinical trial opportunities. In order to expedite the development and execution of clinical trials for neurological disorders affecting adults and/or children, NINDS formed the Neuronxt (NINDS Network for Excellence in Neuroscience Clinical Trials) network. The network's goal is to create early-phase trials that test novel treatments and identify biomarkers, which are typically physical characteristics or substances found in bodily fluids like blood that can be used to measure the presence and severity of a disease. Finding biomarkers for SMA and comprehending the underlying mechanisms and causes of the illness was one of these projects. Information from this study was used to determine whether to approve nusinersen (SpinrazaTM). The design of further clinical trials in SMA has also been improved by the knowledge gained from this study.

9.1.6. Types of Spinal Muscular Atrophy

There are four primary types of SMA:

- Type 1 (severe): Werdnig-Hoffman disease, or type 1, affects about 60% of SMA patients. The onset of symptoms can occur during the first six months of an infant's life. Babies suffering from type 1 SMA have trouble sucking and swallowing. They don't reach common developmental milestones like sitting or holding up their heads. Children are more vulnerable to respiratory infections and collapsed lungs (pneumothorax) as their muscles continue to weaken. The majority of kids with type 1 SMA pass away before turning two.

- Type 2 (intermediate): Type 2 SMA, commonly known as Dubowitz disease, first manifests as symptoms in children between the ages of six and eighteen months. Lower limbs are typically affected by this kind. Type 2 SMA children may be able to sit up, but they are unable to walk. The majority of kids with type 2 SMA grow up to be adults.
- Type 3 (mild): After a child's first 18 months of life, they begin to exhibit symptoms of type 3 SMA, also known as Kugelbert-Welander or juvenile-onset SMA. Some people with type 3 don't show symptoms of the illness until they are young adults. Walking difficulties, recurrent respiratory infections, and mild muscle weakness are examples of type 3 symptoms. Eventually, the symptoms may make it difficult to stand or walk. Life expectancy is not appreciably reduced by Type 3 SMA.
- Type 4 (adult): The rare adult form of SMA doesn't typically appear until the mid-30s. Muscle weakness symptoms progress slowly, so most people with type 4 remain mobile and live full lives.

9.1.7. Symptoms of SMA

There is a wide range of symptoms associated with SMA, from mild to severe. Weakness of the voluntary muscles is the main symptom of chromosome 5-related (SMN-related) SMA. The closest muscles to the center of the body—the shoulders, hips, thighs, and upper back—are the most affected. Deep tendon reflexes are diminished, and the lower limbs appear to be more affected than the upper limbs. If the muscles involved in swallowing and breathing are impacted, abnormalities in these functions arise, leading to additional complications. Scoliosis may arise from a weakening of the back muscles.

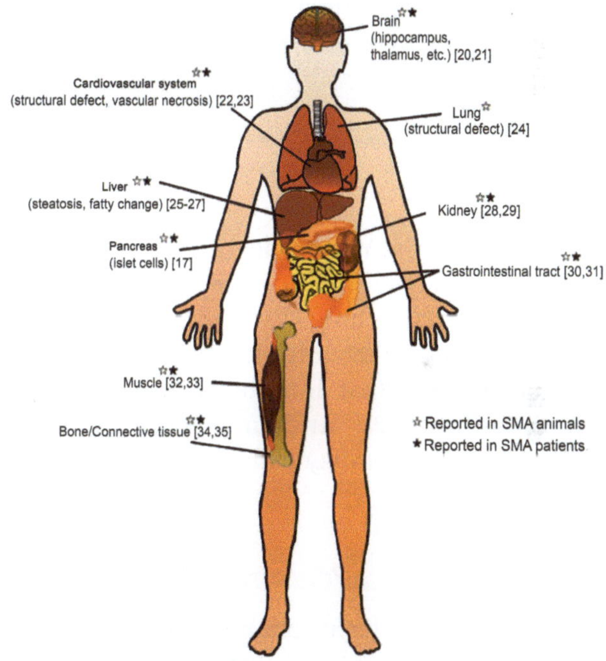

Figure 9.1. *The muscles closer to the center of the body (proximal muscles) are usually more affected in SMA than are the muscles farther from the center (distal muscles).*

Source: *Li Y-J, Chen T-H, Wu Y-Z, Tseng Y-H. Metabolic and nutritional issues associated with spinal muscular atrophy. Nutrients. 2020; 12(12):3842. https://doi.org/10.3390/nu12123842.*

The age of onset and degree of motor function attained in SMA related to chromosome 5 vary greatly. These are roughly correlated with the number of copies of SMN2 genes an individual possesses, which is correlated with the amount of functional SMN protein present in the motor neurons. In chromosome 5 SMA, sensory, mental, and emotional functioning are all perfectly normal. Chromosome 5 or SMN deficiency are unrelated to some forms of SMA. The most affected muscles and degree of severity vary widely between these forms. While the majority of forms, such as the chromosome 5-related form, primarily affect the proximal muscles, there are other forms that, at least initially, primarily affect the distal muscles, or those located further from the center of the body.

9.1.8. Potential Complications of SMA

For those with SMA who only receive supportive care, poor weight gain combined with growth failure, restrictive lung disease, scoliosis, joint contractures, and trouble sleeping are common complications. What long-term issues people who receive early and/or presymptomatic targeted treatment may experience is unknown at this time.

9.1.8.1. Nutrition/Gastrointestinal

- Bulbar dysfunction is universal in individuals with SMA I; the bulbar dysfunction eventually becomes a serious problem for persons with SMA II and only very late in the course of the disease for those with SMA III.
- Gastrointestinal issues may include constipation, delayed gastric emptying, and potentially life-threatening gastroesophageal reflux with aspiration.
- Growth failure can be addressed with gastrostomy tube placement as needed.
- Nonambulatory individuals with SMA II and III are at risk of developing obesity.

Respiratory: Children with SMA I and II (and more rarely, type III) who are treated with supportive care only have a progressive decline in pulmonary function due to a combination of weak respiratory muscles, reduced chest wall and lung compliance, and a reduction in alveolar multiplication.

- Respiratory failure is the most common cause of death in SMA I and II.
- Decreased respiratory function leads to impaired cough with inadequate clearance of lower airway secretions, hypoventilation during sleep, and recurrent pneumonia.
- Noninvasive ventilation, such as BiPAP, and airway clearance techniques are commonly used to improve respiratory insufficiency in those with SMA.

Orthopedic. Scoliosis, hip dislocation, and joint contractures are common complications in individuals with SMA. Scoliosis is a major problem in most persons with SMA II and in half of those with SMA III. With supportive care only:

- Approximately 50% of affected children (especially those who are nonambulatory) develop spinal curvatures of more than 50 degrees (which require surgery) before age ten years;
- Later in the disease course, nonambulatory individuals can develop thoracic kyphosis;

- Progressive scoliosis impairs lung function and if severe can cause decreased cardiac output.

Metabolic. An unexplained potential complication of SMA is severe metabolic acidosis with dicarboxylic aciduria and low serum carnitine concentrations during periods of intercurrent illness or prolonged fasting.

- Whether these metabolic abnormalities are primary or secondary to the underlying defect in SMA is unknown.
- Although the etiology of these metabolic derangements remains unknown, one report suggests that aberrant glucose metabolism may play a role.
- Prolonged fasting should be avoided.

9.1.9. Medical Management

9.1.9.1. Respiratory Muscle Weakness

Respiratory muscle weakness is a major issue in several forms of SMA. While not the only cause, it is the most frequent cause of death in SMA types 1 and 2 with chromosome 5 (related to SMN). Airflow into and out of the lungs is compromised when the respiratory muscles weaken, which has a negative impact on overall health. Headaches, insomnia, yawning or sighing frequently during the day, excessive daytime sleepiness, poor concentration, difficulty lying flat, chest infections, and eventually heart damage and respiratory failure are all indicators of weakening respiratory muscles. When a baby has infantile-onset SMA, the diaphragm muscle usually remains relatively strong, but the muscles between the ribs are often very weak. This makes a child's belly move instead of their chest, giving the impression that they are breathing. The body may also seem to be shaped like a pear. For newborns with SMA, the availability of portable, efficient ventilation devices has expanded options recently and, in certain cases, significantly prolonged life. Additionally beneficial for both adults and children with various forms of SMA is assisted ventilation. Many doctors recommend noninvasive ventilation as a starting point. This type of ventilation typically involves pressurized air delivery through a mask or mouthpiece, with the air being typically ambient and unenriched with oxygen. There are numerous variations of this type of system, and it can be utilized for as long as it's needed, day or night. It is simple to take off when conversing, eating, and drinking. When noninvasive ventilation is insufficient, a tracheostomy—a surgically created opening in the trachea, or windpipe—can be used to provide ventilation support. After that, a tube at the tracheostomy site is used to administer pressurized air. With a tracheostomy tube, people can typically eat, drink, and speak after a period of adjustment.

Preventing infection and clearing respiratory secretions—which can occasionally be done with a mechanical device—are other essential components of respiratory care for people with SMA. One kind of equipment that can help clear the airway of respiratory secretions is an insufflator-exsufflator. In order to simulate a coughing fit, the device quickly switches from applying positive pressure to the airway to negative pressure. Philips Respironics' CoughAssist is an illustration of this kind of equipment. A chest wall oscillation device with a high frequency is another kind of aid for clearing the airways. This apparatus is a vest that quickly inflates and deflates, vibrating the chest and causing tiny coughs to push mucus out of small airways and into larger ones where it can be coughed out more easily. One such product is the Philips Respironics InCourage system. A yearly flu shot is almost a must for individuals with SMA in order to prevent respiratory infections. Other safety measures include avoiding crowded areas and making sure you're getting enough sleep and food. You can get advice from an MDA Care Center team regarding vaccinations, respiratory care, and other related topics.

9.1.9.2. Swallowing Muscle Weakness

Weakness in the mouth and throat muscles can lead to difficulties with swallowing. Infants with SMA of infantile onset typically have difficulty sucking and swallowing. While swallowing weakness can result in respiratory infections and airway obstruction from inhaled food or liquids (aspiration), sucking weakness can cause dehydration and inadequate nutrition. A feeding tube, also known as a gastrostomy tube or g-tube, is one alternative feeding technique for infants who have severe swallowing and weak sucking reflexes. A feeding tube is a tiny, flexible tube with a diameter of about a pencil that passes through the mouth, throat, and esophagus to allow liquid nutrition—whether homemade or purchased—to enter the stomach directly. When not in use, some feeding tube systems are designed to allow the tube to be removed from an abdominal button. Some g-tube users can use the tube in addition to eating and drinking with their mouths. If the primary issue is weak chewing muscles that make eating difficult and time-consuming, then it's acceptable to consume food with your mouth for enjoyment and additional nutrition and use the g-tube for essential calories. In contrast, it's probably not safe to eat or drink by mouth if the tube's primary cause is aspiration of food or liquid. Speech-language pathologists, or SLPs, are trained to treat speech-related issues in addition to swallowing issues. Your MDA Care Center team can provide you with advice on how to manage your weak swallowing muscles, including how to use gastrostomy tubes and prepare meals differently.

This girl with SMA type 2 used a back brace as a toddler. At 9, she underwent surgery to correct a spinal curvature and wore a temporary brace while recovering from surgery.

Weakness of the muscles of the back that normally support the flexible, growing spine is a major problem in childhood-onset SMA. If it's not corrected, the child may develop *scoliosis* — a side-to-side curvature of the spine — or *kyphosis*, a forward curvature of the spine, or both. Some may even end up with "pretzel" types of curvatures that make it impossible to sit or lie down with comfort.

Some physicians believe that severe spinal curvatures may compromise respiratory function in some cases, if the curved spine compresses a lung.

A back brace or corset that supports a child in a certain position is often prescribed to try to direct the spine as it's growing. Braces don't solve the problem, but they may slow the progression of a curve.

The permanent solution to spinal curvature is almost always spine-straightening surgery, which can be done if the child's respiratory status is good enough to withstand the surgery.

The timing of back surgery is tricky. Doctors generally like to wait until maximum spinal growth has been achieved because that allows a simpler surgical technique to be used. On the other hand, if the respiratory status is deteriorating, surgery often can't wait until growth is complete. Here again, an MDA Care Center can help with your decision.

9.1.9.3. Anesthesia Concerns

When an SMA child or adult needs surgery (to correct scoliosis, for example), they must take extra care. The anesthesiologist in particular needs to be well-versed in SMA within the surgical team. Muscle cells that aren't receiving nerve signals occasionally, particularly in the early stages of SMA, develop certain abnormalities in an attempt to connect with nerves. These anomalies may cause harmful reactions to the muscle-relaxing medications that are frequently administered during surgery. If physicians are aware of this issue, they can avoid it by prescribing different medications. Additionally, because patients may have severe spine deformities, anesthesiologists must carefully consider the patient's condition before administering spinal and epidural anesthesia. Although there are currently no rules in place, both vaginal and cesarean sections have been reported to have successful outcomes (Tisdale et al., 2017; Deguise et al., 2021).

9.2. Metabolic Dysfunction in Spinal Muscles

A degenerative neuromuscular disease of the lower motor neurons in the spinal cord's anterior horn is known as spinal muscular atrophy (SMA). The main symptoms are progressive limb, respiratory, and bulbar muscle weakness and wasting. Fasciculations, changed reflexes, joint contractures, and trouble breathing and feeding are examples of clinical hallmarks. SMA is one of the most common inherited neurodegenerative diseases, with an estimated incidence of 1 in 11,000 live births and a reported carrier frequency of 1 in 40. The survival motor neuron 1 (SMN1) gene is involved in SMA. A homozygous deletion or point mutation in this gene results in the loss of SMN production. Nonetheless, SMN2—a paralogous copy of SMN1—is located on the same chromosome. Because of a single nucleotide variation in exon 7, SMN2 undergoes alternative splicing in 85% of transcripts. As a result, only 5–10% of the full-length, functional SMN protein is produced from SMN2. The age of onset and the severity of SMA disease are inversely correlated with the copy number of SMN2. Therefore, mild proximal weakness in ambulatory adults to eventual loss of ambulation comprise the phenotypic spectrum of SMA. The spectrum begins with prenatal symptom onset. Patients are traditionally categorized into types (I to IV) according to the onset and severity of the disease as well as the physical milestones they have reached (walkers, sitters, and non-walkers). The etiology of SMA is still not fully understood. The widely expressed SMN protein is essential for many other cellular functions, including pre-mRNA splicing, as well as for housekeeping. A deficiency in SMN protein appears to preferentially affect α-motor neurons. Nevertheless, mounting data has called into question this established theory. Depletion of SMN also damages other organs and tissues, impacting the physiology of the entire body. The most recent reports of altered function in SMA also included the metabolic and endocrine organs. Early studies concentrated on lipid abnormalities in various types of spinal muscular atrophies. Numerous metabolic changes have been identified in both SMA patients and animal models of the disease, according to a number of recent studies. It should be highlighted, though, that there isn't yet a clear mechanism tying SMN depletion to the different metabolic disorders. However, for SMA patients, these defects may have major clinical ramifications.

Notably, because the STN2 gene is unique to humans, a number of mouse models have been created to study SMA. In summary, the mouse Smn gene was deleted and the human Smn2 gene was introduced to create the "severe model" (Smn−/−; SMN2) and the "delta 7 model" (SmnΔ7 or Smn−/−; SMN2+/+; SmnΔ7+/+), which have a mean survival of 5 and 14 days, respectively. The mouse Smn gene, also known as delta 7, has been knocked out in the "Taiwanese model" ($Smn^{\Delta7/\Delta7}$; $SMN2^{+/+}$), and the human Smn2 transgene has varying copy numbers. With a median survival of 28 days, the "2B/- model" (Smn2B/−) of the mouse Smn gene has an engineered three-nucleotide substitution mutation within the exon splice enhancer in exon 7. The goal of this thorough analysis is to present the most recent data regarding metabolic dysfunction in SMA. Using a top-down approach, we begin by talking about baseline body composition, intake quantity and quality, possible problems in the gastrointestinal (GI) tract, and how macronutrients are handled at the molecular level. Moreover, we provide a comparative analysis with other pertinent neuromuscular disorders to emphasize the distinctiveness of the metabolic profile detected in SMA. Additionally provided is information on the possible clinical ramifications of altered metabolism in SMA. Finally, we suggest a few possible mechanisms to account for the metabolic presentation of SMA and outline directions for future study in this field.

9.2.1. Baseline Anthropometric Data and Energy Expenditure of SMA Patients

Notably, the SMA gene is exclusive to humans, leading to the creation of multiple mouse models for research purposes. The "severe model" (Smn−/−; SMN2) and the "delta 7 model" (SmnΔ7 or Smn−/−; SMN2+/+; SmnΔ7+/+) were created by introducing the human SMN2 gene and deleting the mouse Smn gene, respectively, and have a mean survival of 5 and 14 days. The human SMN2 transgene is present in different copy numbers in the "Taiwanese model" (SmnΔ7/Δ7; SMN2+/+), which consists of the mouse Smn gene with exon 7 (also known as delta 7) deleted. The mouse Smn gene's exon 7 splice enhancer has an engineered three-nucleotide substitution mutation known as the "2B/- model" (Smn2B/−), which has a median survival of 28 days. Highlighting the most recent data on metabolic dysfunction in SMA is the goal of this thorough review. We start by talking about baseline body composition, the kind and amount of food consumed, possible problems in the gastrointestinal (GI) tract, and how macronutrients are handled at the molecular level. This is a top-down approach. To emphasize the distinctiveness of the metabolic phenotype seen in SMA, we also provide a comparison to other pertinent neuromuscular diseases. There is also a presentation of information about the possible clinical consequences of altered metabolism in SMA. Finally, we propose some theoretical explanations for the metabolic presentation of SMA and outline potential directions for future study in this field.

It can be difficult to assess body composition in children, and the SMA population has additional complexities. Since the BMI undervalues body fat, some patients with acceptable fat mass (FM) may appear underweight on a plot. When compared to healthy children, these patients are more likely to be overweight due to their higher fat mass index (FMI) and lower lean tissue concerning age and sex. The distribution of lean body mass (LBM) and fat-free mass (FFM) varies amongst SMA groups. Compared to children with SMA type II, children with SMA type I have lower FFM and LBM, particularly in the arms and trunk. Patients with SMA type I and type II have substantially less total body water than the reference values for age and sex. Water, protein, minerals, and glycogen are all included in the multi-component measure known as FFM. Therefore, the lower FFM found in these studies may be the consequence of different FFM components compared to healthy peers. There is a lack of precision in the evaluation of metabolic parameters and body composition. As a result, conclusions about overfeeding or underfeeding may result from difficulties interpreting these data. As a result, patients who are said to be underfed may not actually have been, which could result in overfeeding and negative effects like increased FM and worsening conditions. In an attempt to get around these problems, a recent study proposed new energy equations to predict energy expenditure for SMA type I patients while taking into account clinical features (ventilatory status and nusinersen treatment). To guarantee better-tailored support, the authors nevertheless advise indirect calorimetry. Recently, a more thorough examination of a few of these studies was released. To make sure we use these objective measurements to support and improve the nutritional status of the changing SMA population, more work will need to be done.

9.2.2. Feeding Difficulties and Nutritional Intake Issues

All forms of SMA have been linked to feeding and swallowing issues as a result of bulbar dysfunction. At least one feeding-related difficulty is prevalent in both sitters (SMA type II) and non-sitters (SMA type I), accounting for 36% of the cases. The most frequently reported problems are choking, weariness from mastication, and jaw problems. Patients with SMA have also reported difficulty with chewing and opening their mouths. Due to a risk of aspiration, pulmonary infections, and recurrent choking episodes, many SMA patients have modified feeding preparation and gastrostomy tubes to assist with feeding. Without a doubt, these issues make it difficult to consume enough nutrients. In addition to these feeding adjustments and longer mealtimes, patients have decreased their food intake, which has resulted in growth failure. Due to lowered demands, dietary and caloric intake in SMA patients may be lower than that of their healthy peers. Therefore, SMA patients are at risk for critical micronutrient deficiencies if they are unable to obtain an adequate micronutrient intake. The recommended ranges for calcium, magnesium, folate, vitamins A, D, E, and K, and other nutrients are often not met. Vitamin D deficiencies are a micronutrient important for bone health and are frequently found to be lower at baseline in SMA patients. Fifty percent of the children had low bone density, and vitamin D levels were below normal. In addition to these inadequacies, SMA patients' decreased muscle mass, activity, and mobility affect bone mass and architecture, increasing their risk of osteopenia, osteoporosis, and fractures. Children with type II and III SMA are susceptible to both symptomatic and non-symptomatic fractures. The SMA population has a suboptimal intake of micronutrients, but there also seems to be an abnormal metabolism of these substrates. Compared to wild-type mice, mice with severe Smn−/−; SMN2 exhibit a significantly higher rate of osteoclast formation and bone resorption. On the other hand, anomalies in the calcium pathways (muscle, astrocytes, motor neurons, kidney) and aberrant calcium levels have been sporadically found in SMA patients. This review is not intended to address the particular mechanism or specifics of these studies. For this population to maintain bone density and health, adequate but cautious vitamin D and calcium supplementation is required, especially in light of any potential intrinsic abnormalities to those pathways.

9.2.3. Gastrointestinal Dysfunction

Constipation, bloating, and gastroesophageal reflux disease are some of the symptoms of gastroesophageal motility problems that can occur in patients with SMA. It is significant to note that many SMA patients become dependent on the use of ventilators, such as Bilevel Positive Airway Pressure (BiPAP), as the disease progresses, which increases the risk of gastric insufflation. This may make stomach emptying worse. Studies have demonstrated that SMN deficiency in mice is associated with enteric nervous system abnormalities that result in problems with intestinal and esophageal motility. Constipation was evident in the fecal pellets of Nestin-F7 ($SMN2^{+/+}$; $Smn\Delta7^{+/+}$; $SmnF^{7/-}$; nestin-cre) and SmnΔ7 mice, which were drier and less frequent. Without changes to the GI tract's morphology, they also experienced problems with prolonged intestinal transit, irregular colonic motility, and slower stomach emptying. On the other hand, Taiwanese ($Smn^{\Delta7/\Delta7}$; $SMN2^{+/+}$) mice showed histopathological defects in the GI tract. In addition to diffuse edema and macrophage infiltration in the small intestine's lamina propria, they also had disproportionately long intestines and altered intestinal crypt size, shape, and distribution. Gut bacteria may translocate into the blood of SMA mice as a result of intestinal barrier damage. Therefore, it seems that in mouse models of SMA, SMN may be crucial for maintaining the integrity of the GI tract. Although these results could account for some of the slow gastric motility observed in SMA patients, they also probably play a role in the disturbance of optimal nutrient absorption. These results have not yet been verified in human pathology. Probiotics and a high-fiber diet are advised as part of the standard of care for SMA patients to help manage constipation and related symptoms of GI dysmotility. Given the mounting data that connects gut microbiota to neurodegenerative illnesses and movement disorders, improving this aspect of the SMA phenotype through probiotic use may be possible.

9.2.4. Intermediary Metabolism in SMA

Thus far, it appears evident that poor nutrition, altered body composition, and suboptimal calorie intake are risks associated with SMA patients. Further evidence indicates that the GI tract's mucosal barrier is also impacted, which could result in deficiencies in the absorption of macro- and micronutrients. These collectively promote a state of modified micro- and macronutrient homeostasis. The majority of research to date has concentrated on the intriguingly obvious disruption in the handling of macronutrients (fat, glucose, protein/amino acids). Below is a comparison to other diseases involving denervation (Figure 9.2).

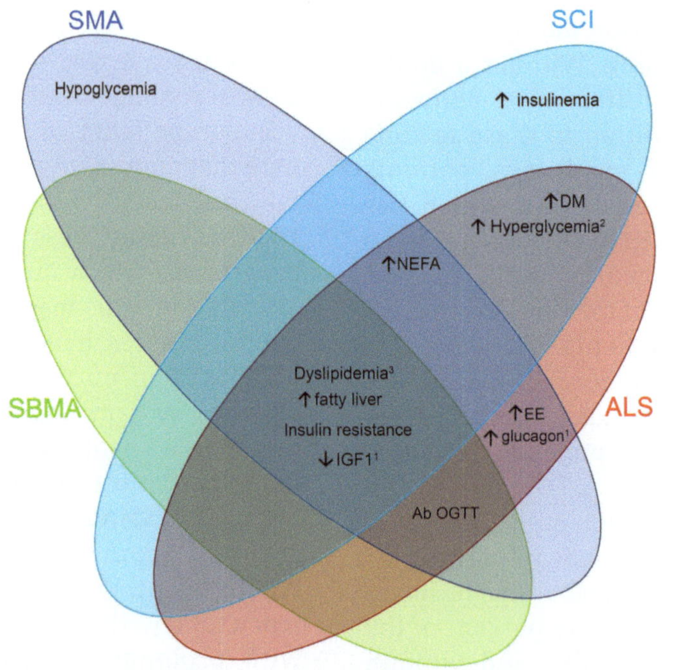

Figure 9.2. *Common metabolic findings within neuromuscular disorders.*

Source: Deguise M-O, Chehade L, Kothary R. Metabolic dysfunction in spinal muscular atrophy. International Journal of Molecular Sciences. 2021; 22(11):5913. https://doi.org/10.3390/ijms22115913

Venn diagram showing similarities and differences in metabolic changes among different neuromuscular disorders with a denervating/loss of motor nerve input component. Note that studies with mixed results in the current literature will be seen as unchanged within this diagram, given lack of consensus. (1) Some features may only be seen in mouse models of the disease, and (2) in the fasting state. (3) Dyslipidemia describes various changes and may not actually be similar between different diseases. For example, it may be hypolipidemia, hyperlipidemia, or differences in frequency or absolute mean of various readouts. DM—Diabetes mellitus, EE—energy expenditure, Ab—abnormal, OGTT—oral glucose tolerance test, HDL—high-density lipoprotein, LDL—low-density lipoprotein, TC—total cholesterol, NEFA—non-esterified fatty acids, black arrow pointing up (↑)—increase, black arrow pointing down (↓)—decrease.

9.2.4.1. Fat Metabolism

Before the identification of the disease's genetic basis, metabolic abnormalities were discovered in SMA patients. In a small case series, the first suggestive feature was observed in some, but not all, SMA patients who were fasting. It was dicarboxylic aciduria. Additional noteworthy discoveries included decreased activity of several enzymes (including 3-ketoacyl-CoA thiolase, acetoacetyl-CoA thiolase, long-chain l-3-hydroxyacyl-CoA dehydrogenase, and short-chain l-3-hydroxyacyl-CoA dehydrogenase), an increase in the ratio of dodecanoic to tetradecanoic acid, normal ketone production, and a variable acylcarnitine profile. Additionally, a higher esterified: free carnitine ratio was noted, which supported previous research connecting lower carnitine levels in SMA muscle with carnitine palmityl transferase activity. Given that denervated controls did not exhibit the same degree of change in certain measures, the authors hypothesized that this might not be related to denervation. Comparable to known mitochondrial defects, the pattern of anomalies in serum fatty acid suggested a distinct defect. In patients with severe SMA, the results were typically more noticeable. A few SMA patients in these three reports also had liver steatosis, a condition that has been reported recently. In a different study, six out of ten patients showed a comparable decline in muscle carnitine, consistent with earlier findings, while ten out of the fourteen patients had a serum carnitine deficiency. A recent review included a thorough analysis of the early reports. It is still unknown what pathogenic mechanism underlies these defects.

A study was conducted to update our knowledge of changes in fat metabolism. Compared to published pediatric data sets, one measure of dyslipidemia was present in SMA patients roughly twice as frequently. Similarly, in the cohort of 72 SMA patients, nearly 13% had three or more dyslipidemia measures; in the average pediatric population, however, there are currently no baseline epidemiological data available. It should be mentioned that after just one blood draw, abnormal lipid levels were found. These anomalies are not persistent for a single person. These results showed no discernible dependence on severity and were evenly distributed across all SMA types. About thirty percent of older SMA type II and type III patients had at least one abnormal lipid level reading, according to a recent study. These findings also bear similarities to earlier research. Lipid abnormalities were present in 11 out of 12 patients from a previous cohort of clinically diagnosed SMA patients. On the other hand, the patient's mean age was 41.5%. Another study, conducted in 1970, involved elderly patients who also had concurrent hyperlipoproteinemia and SMA-like symptoms. Since there was no genetic diagnosis available at the time of the studies, it was challenging to accurately define and link the phenotype to the underlying genetic condition in those specific patients. As such, these older data sets should be interpreted cautiously.

Interestingly, microvesicular steatosis was discovered in three of the eight autopsies of SMA patients (the majority of whom were younger than 14 months old), bringing the total number of patients with fatty livers to five. In children aged 2 to 4 who are not afflicted with SMA, the prevalence of liver steatosis is only 0.7%. This is a significant divergence, particularly in light of the even younger population. More recently, non-invasive imaging techniques like ultrasound revealed steatosis in 11% of SMA type II and III cohorts. It's also intriguing that there were aberrant liver fat contents in four distinct mouse models, ranging in severity. More specifically, mice with higher severity showed decreased liver fat, whereas mice with lower severity showed an accumulation of triglycerides (TGs) in the liver. Of these models, while fed normal chow, the Smn2B/− mice consistently developed dyslipidemia and non-alcoholic fatty liver disease (NAFLD). Remarkably, in pre-clinical models, only slight alterations in fat classes and chain length were found in tissues relevant to SMA disease, such as the muscle and spinal cord. This suggests that the changes might be limited to the liver or other metabolic organs. Nevertheless, metabolism and gene expression were identified as one of the clusters in the Gene Ontology (GO) analysis in the CSF of SMA patients by a recent proteomic analysis study. Additionally, it was found that Apolipoprotein E and Apolipoprotein A1 were dysregulated and that nusinersen might have a beneficial impact. Regretfully, no CSF studies using animal models exist to enable comparable analysis. However, ultrastructural analysis of Smn2B/− muscle, another disease-relevant tissue, revealed increased fat droplets as well as widespread alterations in a fatty acid-specific gene expression PCR array. It should be noted that it is unclear if this is an aftereffect of muscle atrophy and denervation (Tisdale et al., 2017; Deguise et al., 2021).

It is still unknown what causes dyslipidemia and fatty liver in SMA. The isolated hepatic mitochondria from $Smn^2B/-$ mice function better than control, indicating that although there are broad proteomic changes in mitochondrial health and function, mitochondrial dysfunction is unlikely.

This was proposed as a compensatory measure to improve clearance and return homeostasis due to the high TG content in the $Smn^{2B/-}$ livers. Remarkably, a recent investigation revealed that Taiwanese mice ($Smn^{\Delta7/\Delta7}$; $SMN^{2+/+}$) rely more on β-oxidation due to a global shift in their respiratory exchange ratio. More reactive oxygen species are produced by the $Smn^{2B/-}$ hepatic mitochondria, which results in liver damage and functional deficits (iron metabolism, hemostasis, complement, protein synthesis, and insulin-like growth factor 1 (IGF1) pathway).

Notably, dicarboxylic acids are produced by microsomal oxidation, an alternate oxidative pathway activated upon β-oxidation overload. Cytochrome P450 4A (Cyp4A), its primary enzyme, was induced in the $Smn^{2B/-}$ liver. Dicarboxylic aciduria in SMA patients may have a suitable explanation given the confirmation of microsomal induction in $Smn^{2B/-}$ liver. Patients and preclinical models of SMA may be more susceptible to NAFLD due to liver intrinsic defects. Remarkably, the results mentioned above suggest that SMN-depleted mice may have a new function in the modeling of NAFLD. Insulin resistance, fatty liver, dyslipidemia, and functional deficits are all well-established components of the pathophysiology of nonalcoholic fatty liver disease. According to a recent study, the organ with the most disrupted transcriptome in SMA was the liver. However, the pathophysiology of NAFLD in SMA is most likely influenced by pressures from other metabolic organs, including the pancreas, skeletal muscle, adipose tissue, and GI tract. Interestingly, the Smn2B/−;SMN2+/− mouse, a recently described very mild model of SMA (similar to SMA type IV), does not exhibit a fatty liver phenotype over the course of its lifetime. This highlights the fact that the fatty liver phenotype can be reversed by reaching a specific SMN threshold.

While very little work has focused on brown adipose tissue (BAT) and white adipose tissue (WAT), molecular changes are present in these tissues. As part of a broader study, KLF15 mRNA is misregulated in both BAT and WAT. A few clock genes (controlling circadian rhythm) showed abnormal expression in these two tissues as well. Using a microarray screen, symptomatic BAT tissue in Taiwanese ($Smn^{\Delta7/\Delta7}$;$SMN2^{+/+}$) mice displayed a wide array of molecular changes that appeared modulated by light therapy. Additionally, Smn expression in early life may be dependent on circadian rhythm in BAT, WAT, and liver tissues. On the other hand, WAT appears to have increased levels of lipogenic genes in sedentary Taiwanese *(SmnΔ7/Δ7;SMN2+/+)* mice, which was reversed by exercise (Tisdale et al., 2017; Deguise et al., 2021).

9.2.4.2. Glucose Metabolism

The first case series involving two patients who were repeatedly admitted to the hospital due to hypoglycemia raised concerns about glucose metabolism in SMA. These people's glucose levels dropped by half in a day without any changes to the hormones that control blood sugar, but their levels of ketones increased. Despite a 30-hour fast, this was not observed in muscle diseases like Duchenne muscular dystrophy. Low blood sugar, however, seems more common in patients with muscle wasting, defined as muscle mass less than 10% of body mass. It was therefore highly advised that SMA patients and their families optimize the feeding schedule in order to shorten the duration of fasting. The SmnΔ7 mice demonstrated hypoglycemia and elevated β-hydroxybutyrate (BHB) on two distinct diets in preclinical investigations. The $Smn^{2B/-}$ mice had sustained glucose levels after fasting, but at later stages they displayed hypoglycemia. It was suggested that $Smn^{2B/-}$ mice gradually develop glucose intolerance through the administration of an intraperitoneal glucose tolerance test (IPGTT). This may have resulted from the pancreas's α-cells, which produce glucagon, outnumbering β-cells, which produce insulin. As a result, the $Smn^{2B/-}$ mice showed normal insulin levels but hyperglucagonemia. In this study, patient blood sugar values were not easily interpreted; however, pancreatic islet phenotypes from autopsies were found to be similar. The development of NAFLD in $Smn^{2B/-}$ mice is thought to be facilitated by these pancreatic alterations, as hyperglucagonemia and increased phosphorylation of CREB (cAMP response element-binding protein) may be causing an increase in energetic substrates in the blood. Chronically low blood sugar may be the cause of hyperglucagonemia. Alternatively, the α-cells' intrinsic pancreatic defects might be the reason. Additionally, Smn2B/− mice exhibit hepatic insulin resistance. Taiwanese ($Smn^{\Delta7/\Delta7}$; $SMN2^{+/+}$) mice showed decreased plasma glucose levels as early as P4, and following glucose loading, they also showed signs of glucose intolerance, which was alleviated by exercise. In the longer-living model, fasting hyperglycemia was seen as the aging process occurred rather than hypoglycemia or changes in insulin sensitivity or levels. Regrettably, no measurements of glucagon levels were made.

It's interesting to note that animals who are heterozygous for SMA (carrier), although asymptomatic neurologically, are vulnerable to metabolic abnormalities when they age and are exposed to dietary challenges (HFD). The metabolic alterations observed in these circumstances did, however, reveal some distinctions with young SMA mice. Although there were comparable elevations in the phosphorylation of protein kinase B, or Akt, the Smn+/− animals did not exhibit hyperglucagonemia. Rather, they showed signs of hyperinsulinemia along with similar histological alterations in the pancreas. Additionally, increased CREB phosphorylation was observed in various mouse models and environments, which may indicate a shared characteristic of increased pathological sensitivity to glucagon. A tiny subset of patients showed normal glucagon levels. It would be difficult to demonstrate glucagon sensitivity in human subjects, though. Therefore, it's still possible that CREB activity could be affected without reference to glucagon levels.

Since CREB activity is low in SMN-depleted neural stem cell (NSC)-34 cells, a cell line that resembles a mouse motor neuron, CREB activity may also be specific to a given cell type. It is currently unknown if this might make heterozygous SMA carriers more susceptible to metabolic abnormalities. To the best of the available knowledge, no association between diabetes and the SMN gene has been found in studies. Nonetheless, it has been linked to a possible part in diabetic polyneuropathy, one of the effects of diabetes (Tisdale et al., 2017; Deguise et al., 2021).

Whether treated or not, SMA patients may experience metabolic consequences from a state of altered blood glucose. A small number of case reports demonstrate ketoacidosis both with and without coexisting diabetes. There have been several reports of untreated SMA patients exhibiting irregular blood sugar levels. Six children with SMA type II were included in the small pilot study; three of them had impaired glucose tolerance, and five of them had insulin resistance, which was found in 53% of patients in a more recent study. Seven out of the fifteen SMA type II and III patients showed similar results in the glucose tolerance test, and 29.7% of their cohort satisfied the laboratory criteria for prediabetes. In SMA, glucose levels appear to vary a lot. During the oral glucose tolerance test (OGTT), one patient experienced hypoglycemia, but fasting glucose levels did not change in any other study participants.

Upon reviewing their charts, 10 of the 12 SMA type I patients who regrettably passed had at least one glucose reading that was higher than normal. In contrast, a study of 45 SMA type I patients revealed that 17 of them experienced hypoglycemia following a 4- to 6-hour fast, whether as a result of an acute illness or a scheduled procedure. This didn't seem to depend on how bad their illness was or how well they were breathing. In two investigations, the median glycated hemoglobin subunit alpha 1 (HbA1C) of patients with SMA was approximately 4 points.

In a different study, the HbA1C was measured in fifteen patients; however, aside from being largely qualitatively normal, no objective values were given. It's crucial to remember that HbA1C only shows blood glucose levels from the previous three months and might not accurately reflect variations in acute glucose management. Furthermore, higher ranges of HbA1C are associated with significant changes in diabetes diagnosis and monitoring. Conversely, low HbA1C values have been linked to disability in non-diabetic individuals, liver disease (HbA1C < 4%), cancer (HbA1C < 5.0%), and all-cause mortality (HbA1C < 4%, HbA1C < 5%, HbA1C < 5%) in various settings. Nevertheless, there has been discussion surrounding this idea, and the majority of the research has been done on adult populations. Therefore, it's unclear if this would hold true for people with SMA. Furthermore, there could be confounding factors due to the wide range of causes of low HbA1C, which include liver disease, anemia, and related conditions. In a newly treated population where most patients may live well into adulthood, the possibility of glucose abnormalities in SMA patients should continue to be taken into account. The problems, if any, with glucose metabolism are still mainly unknown. This results from variations in the anomalies noted in various patient cohorts and model systems. Given the extreme variability of the SMA spectrum and the possibility that these abnormalities only affect a small percentage of patients, it may not come as a surprise.

9.2.4.3. Amino Acid Metabolism

The metabolism of amino acids in SMA is poorly understood. Few research has shown that fasting hypoglycemia in SMA type II patients is accompanied by reduced levels of three particular amino acids (alanine, phenylalanine, and branched-chain amino acids). A compelling theoretical explanation for fasting hypoglycemia was proposed, based on the diminished muscle mass in SMA, and the exhaustion of the amino acid required for gluconeogenesis. However, there aren't any objective results at this time to support this theory.

The serum levels of branched-chain amino acids (BCAAs) in a symptomatic SMA mouse model are markedly reduced. The Taiwanese (SmnΔ7/Δ7; SMN2+/+) mice's weight gain and survival were enhanced by dietary supplementation of BCAAs. It's interesting to note that a diet known as "The Amino Acid diet," which was started by an SMA caregiver in the hopes of easing SMA symptoms, has become popular among families raising children with SMA. Their website states that it is believed to supposedly enhance constipation, strength, function, and respiratory health. Because there aren't many studies on the metabolism of amino acids in SMA nutrition, these observations are still subjective. Furthermore, if this diet is not properly followed, it may have negative effects on health. We did not look into comparisons with other neuromuscular diseases because there is so little information available in the SMA field on this subject (Tisdale et al., 2017; Deguise et al., 2021).

9.2.5. Hormonal Regulation

9.2.5.1. Comparison to Models of Denervation and Other Diseases

Very little information has been provided about how hormone regulation may impact metabolism in SMA. Many SMA patients (15 out of 35) had hyperleptinemia, with the majority of these patients being underweight, according to a recent study. It is noteworthy that reduced motor functions were linked to hyperleptinemia. In a preclinical model of SMA, however, leptin levels remained unaltered. Within a cohort of SMA patients, a recent cross-sectional study found that 24% had premature pubarche without corresponding changes in androgen levels. For patients with SMA type I and type II, this was linked to a notable reduction in muscle mass and an appreciable rise in insulin resistance. IGF1 was always low in preclinical models. It was also observed that IGF1 binding proteins were dysregulated, specifically IGFals but not IGFbp3, the latter of which displayed inconsistent findings in one investigation. The small size of SMA mice may be caused in part by low IGF1. In muscle biopsies, patients with SMA type I and type III exhibit different expression levels of IGF1-R. In comparison with the control group, 15 SMA patients had lower levels of IGF1. Comparing IGF1 in SMA patients to standard values, however, revealed normalcy in two additional investigations. Remarkably, early research that overexpressed IGF1 in preclinical models across different settings only slightly improved motor phenotype; metabolic readouts were not evaluated.

9.2.6. Metabolic Crosstalk and Proposed Mechanisms

The field of metabolism research is complex. It has multiple levels of complexity. Although all cell types engage in some level of metabolic activity, their molecular machinery or contribution may vary. The GI tract, liver, pancreas, skeletal muscle, and white and brown adipose tissues are among the organs that play a significant metabolic role. These tissues are separated from one another and interact with one another through a variety of signaling pathways. Numerous hormones that are rapidly induced or repressed and may exhibit circadian rhythmicity can further regulate metabolic function. This complexity is increased in the context of SMA by the theory that each type of cell involved may be specifically impacted by SMN depletion. Because of this, determining a plausible mechanism behind a metabolic phenotype necessitates a comprehensive strategy that takes into account each of these factors. It is difficult to pinpoint the initial event(s) that gave rise to the SMA metabolic phenotype as it exists today. Many results can be unified by starting with the development of the NAFLD phenotype in preclinical models of SMA. As seen in Figure 9.3, NAFLD is characterized by a deficit in the intake and output of fatty acids, which can be made worse by certain mechanisms like insulin resistance.

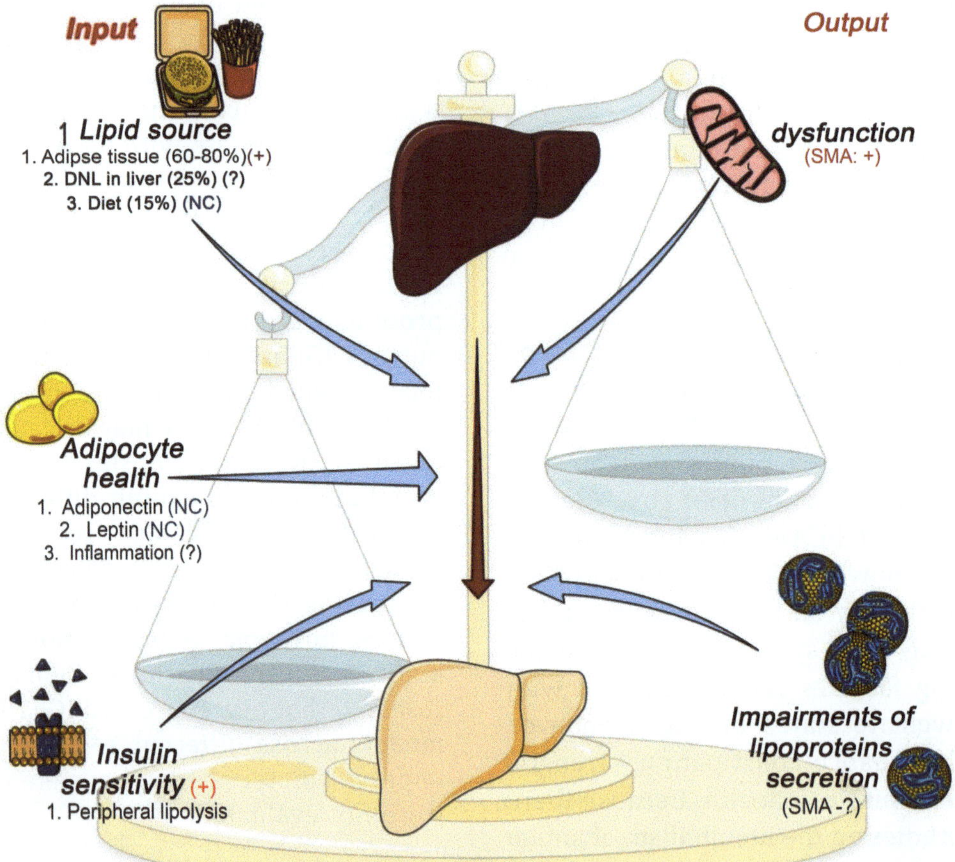

Figure 9.3. *Overview of mechanisms contributing to non-alcoholic fatty liver disease (NAFLD) and their influence in the Spinal Muscular Atrophy (SMA) metabolic phenotype.*

Source: Deguise M-O, Chehade L, Kothary R. Metabolic Dysfunction in spinal muscular atrophy. International Journal of Molecular Sciences. 2021; 22(11):5913. https://doi.org/10.3390/ijms22115913.

NAFLD can be seen at the basic level as an imbalance in input and output of fat substrates. The input of fatty substrates can come from various sources, most of which are generally from non-esterified fatty acids from adipose tissues. The input can be influenced by other factors including adipocyte health as well as insulin resistance. On the other hand, the liver deals with these substrates by either using them during fatty acid oxidation or exporting them out of the liver. The contribution of these findings to SMA is described by (+) as found in SMA, (NC) no change seen in SMA, (?) no data in current literature. DNL—de novo lipogenesis. Black arrow pointing up (↑)—increase.

9.2.6.1. Fatty Acid Overloading

It is crucial to recognize that fatty acid overload is probably possible in the liver that has been depleted of SMN. A recent RNA-seq study revealed a number of splicing alterations brought on by the liver's depletion of SMN. Compared to the brain, spinal cord, and skeletal muscle tissues, the liver is assumed to have the most extensive transcriptomic alterations. Proteomic alterations are also most noticeable in the liver, even in the womb. However, no connection has been found yet between these transcriptomic and proteomic alterations and the hepatic phenotypes that are currently being seen. It seems that intron retention frequently occurs when SMN depletion is present. Seven genes were identified by U12-dependent intron retention that was seen in all tissues tested; however, none of these genes seem to play a significant role in metabolism. The phenotype may also be influenced by additional modifications, possibly liver-specific. In fact, a number of the transcriptome's significantly downregulated pathways—including those related to the lipid metabolic process and cellular lipid metabolic process—and the Kyoto Encyclopedia of Genes and Genomes (KEGG) pathway analysis—which includes pathways related to fatty acid metabolism, fatty acid degradation, and type I diabetes mellitus—point toward a variety of possible culprits that may be the subject of further research. While hepatic proteomic analysis in utero did not clearly identify metabolic pathways, proteomic analysis as early as birth identified multiple pathways involved in metabolism and mitochondrial function.

Apart from the aforementioned intrinsic alterations in the liver, pathogenesis may also be influenced indirectly by stimuli originating from other metabolic organs. We think that pancreatic and WAT contributions are directly related to the fatty acid input to the liver in Smn2B/– mice. Normally, during a fast, glucagon breaks down glycogen, promotes gluconeogenesis, and lipolysis in peripheral WAT to provide constant energy substrate availability. A probable contributing factor to the excess non-esterified fatty acids in the bloodstream from potential WAT lipolysis is the severe hyperglucagonemia and the ensuing molecular activation of CREB during this period. It is interesting to note that free fatty acid levels in SMA patients significantly increase during fasting, though it is unclear if this is the case initially. In the context of NAFLD, this mechanism typically contributes to 60% of the lipid accumulation. A comparable mechanism has been proposed for SBMA, wherein malfunctioning androgen receptors cause an increase in fat mass, which in turn causes an increase in the production of free fatty acids in the bloodstream. Since diet modification had no effect on hepatic lipid accumulation but did affect other measures like ketones, it is unlikely that dietary intake is involved. Although de novo lipogenesis in SMA has not been thoroughly investigated, it is still plausible.

For now, speculation is the main explanation for the nearly 40-fold increase in glucagon. The pathological expression of excess glucagon may result from the idiopathic expansion of α-cells that produce glucagon in the pancreas of Smn2B/− mice. We still don't know why this cellular alteration occurred. The sustained low blood sugar levels observed in Smn2B/− mice may trigger the production of glucagon. The SMA motor phenotype's inability to provide the right nutrition could be another factor contributing to the rise in glucagon levels. While glucagon induction appears to occur prior to motor neuron loss and motor impairment in Smn2B/− mice, fasting or starvation cannot be disregarded because of limitations in the ambulation of SMA patients. Food intake can be modulated by leptin, a general indicator of energy reserve. Thus, its secretion can be used to distinguish between states of fasting and overfeeding. Leptin in Smn2B/− mice did not change. However, in order to analyze the contribution associated with SMA versus severe starvation, future research should compare results in SMA mice with a severe starvation model. Naturally, hyperglucagonemia is most likely explained by a combination of these factors. A wide range of additional substances, such as gut peptides, amino acids, and neural signals, can also alter the expression of glucagon (Tisdale et al., 2017; Deguise et al., 2021).

Though it is up-regulated similarly to glucagon in Smn2B/− mice, GLP1 appears to have a limited effect as a glucagon inhibitor. Interestingly, although amino acids can stimulate glucagon expression, hyperglucagonemia can also cause low levels of amino acids. Nevertheless, α-cells in the context of hyperplasia can also cause glucagon expression. It's interesting to note that during fasting, low amino acid levels are observed in SMA and SMA patients. To complicate matters even more, hyperglucagonemia and NAFLD-related phenotypes are linked, so it's unclear which comes first. It should be noted that during OGTT, a small cohort of six SMA patients did not exhibit hyperglucagonemia. It's unclear if inflammation and/or dysfunction of WAT accelerate the lipolysis, or if glucagon acts alone as the driving force. In Smn2B/− mice, no alterations have been noted in the levels of circulating adipokines, such as leptin. On the other hand, hyperleptinemia is present in a portion of SMA patients, and this may lead to increased lipolysis and, ultimately, liver steatosis. Important genes involved in WAT and BAT tissue physiology have anomalies related to their circadian rhythm, according to a recent study. It is currently unknown how they contribute to the NAFLD phenotype. A recent study suggested that liver steatosis in patients with milder SMA (type II–III) may be established similarly to nonalcoholic fatty liver disease (NAFLD) because the patients in the study cohort with fatty liver were also obese and had dyslipidemia and prediabetes. The increased fatty acid burden in the bloodstream is probably made worse by the denervated muscle in SMA. This is mostly because of its non-functional state and the resulting decreased energy source uptake for maintenance. Furthermore, the atro.

9.2.6.2. Fatty Acid Clearance

There are various levels at which fatty acid clearance can be examined. Reduced use of the denervated and eventually wasted SMA muscles is probably the cause of the increased levels of energy substrates (including fatty acids) in the circulation (as previously described). The circulation's relative availability of substrate increases as a result, and the liver may eventually absorb it. It's also unclear if skeletal muscles or adipose tissue have decreased insulin sensitivity, which would significantly alter their metabolism. It is clear that hepatic insulin resistance plays a role in the current pathogenic progression of NAFLD. In the future, research should concentrate on determining whether insulin resistance is systemic and what effects it has. Lipid overload is likely compensated for by hyperactivation of the hepatic β-oxidation pathway, which is responsible for hepatic lipid clearance at the local level. Nevertheless, an equal quantity of mitochondria was used for this assay. Given that the mitochondrial content appears to be reduced in the Smn2B/– mouse model, it is plausible that overall β-oxidation is decreased. We found evidence of elevated microsomal oxidation, an unusual form of oxidation that the cell usually does not use unless it is compromised by β-oxidation. Dicarboxylic acids, a byproduct of this oxidation process, are seen in SMA patients, which makes this particularly intriguing. Increased lipid storage may also be facilitated by the incapacity to secrete lipoproteins.

Remarkably, a malfunctioning pathway in SMN-depleted cells was found to be endocytosis. Data regarding exocytosis defects are less abundant. In fact, the peripheral tissues' incapacity to absorb lipoproteins would exacerbate the lipids' circulatory density. At the moment, little is known about this field of study. Similarly, for a variety of reasons, including metabolic rate and substrate utilization, exercise is generally considered a protective factor in both metabolic disorders and neuromuscular diseases. The majority of SMA field reports center on the impact of exercise on motor function; little is known about the impact of exercise on metabolic dysfunction in SMA. Following high-intensity swimming and low-intensity running, mice with mild SMA showed improvements in their energy metabolism, according to one study. More precisely, adipocytic deposition, glucose homeostasis, energy production, and mitochondrial enzymatic activity in fast-twitch muscles were all enhanced by the exercise program. It was recently demonstrated that while SMN protein expression in skeletal muscles remained unchanged, exercise could modulate SMN2 exon 7. The precise impact of exercises on metabolic outcomes and the mechanism underlying them—whether SMN-dependent or independent—remain unclear overall. To determine exercise's overall benefits, more research is required in this area (Tisdale et al., 2017; Deguise et al., 2021).

9.2.7. Nutritional Guidelines for SMA Patients

The overwhelming body of research indicates that SMN depletion causes multilevel metabolic disruption and limitations, which most likely make it difficult for SMA patients to receive adequate nutrition. This begins with erratic intake in terms of both quality and quantity, changes in gut motility, and possibly impaired absorption capacity. It then proceeds to the stage of macronutrient processing as a source of energy. This results in pancreatic abnormalities in preclinical models and the metabolic ramifications of non-alcoholic fatty liver disease; these findings have been replicated in some SMA patients, but not in all of them. It is likely that only a subset of SMA patients will be vulnerable to more significant metabolic problems, in contrast to mouse models, which are typically highly homogeneous in their genetic makeup and surroundings. Figure 9.4 shows the metabolic alterations that are similar and different between SMA mouse models and findings in human patients.

Position statements on the standard of care have consistently called for more research to improve our understanding of nutrition and metabolism. There are numerous studies that use questionnaires. Overall, a large number of potential flaws have been reported; the majority were compiled in a recent systematic review. The optimal nutritional standards for SMA are unknown due to a lack of prospective studies. Research in this area is crucial because, according to a study, over one-third of caregivers supported modifying the feeding schedule on their own, without assistance from the medical care team. Furthermore, a great deal of families use elemental formulas, about which no research has been done to date. Malnutrition still exists in cohorts receiving nusinersen treatment, but different nutrition measures improved more when adequate nutritional intervention was given prior to nusinersen treatment.

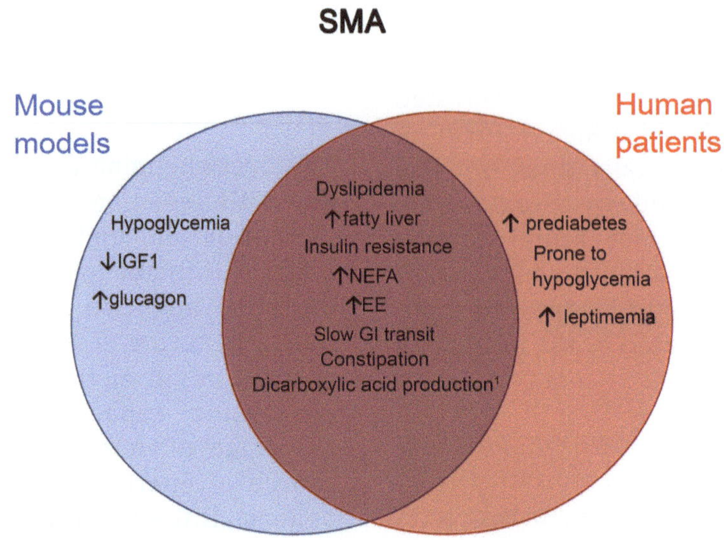

Figure 9.4. *Commonalities between SMA mouse models and human patients. Note that findings in SMA patients may represent a subgroup rather than something found in all patients. (1) Dicarboxylic acid production is inferred by evidence of microsomal oxidation in Smn2B/– mouse model. EE—energy expenditure; NEFA—non-esterified fatty acids, black arrow pointing up (↑)—increase, black arrow pointing down (↓)—decrease.*

Source: Deguise M-O, Chehade L, Kothary R. Metabolic dysfunction in spinal muscular atrophy. International Journal of Molecular Sciences. 2021; 22(11):5913. https://doi.org/10.3390/ijms22115913–.

Remarkably, a recent investigation into the metabolomes of SMA patients revealed little change following nusinersen therapy, suggesting that centrally delivered (i.e., intrathecal) SMA treatments might not have an impact on this aspect of the SMA phenotype. As far as we are aware, research on metabolism during treatment is not yet available for other options like risdiplam or Zolgensma. In a phase 3 trial (STR1VE), 68% of patients were able to maintain weight that was appropriate for their age and did not require feeding assistance. Nutrition has not yet been thoroughly studied. Consequently, it is evident that additional research is necessary to fill in these gaps. Authors of metabolic studies have conjectured and offered ideas based on their findings over the years. The majority support diets high in proteins and carbohydrates. This is partially consistent with a recent preclinical study showing that in the Smn2B/– mouse model, a low-fat diet doubles lifespan. The best diets for normalizing abnormal readouts (like ketones) were low-fat and high-sucrose, indicating a reduced dependence on fat as an energy source. There are, however, some contradictory studies that have been covered in greater detail elsewhere. A small study that looked at a low-fat/high-carb diet in the past claimed positive results, but its validity was questioned because it was conducted before genetic testing and it wasn't clear how the patients were classified. A low-fat, high-sucrose diet may be beneficial for SMA patients. Foods high in fat do cause the stomach to empty more slowly and take longer to transit, which can exacerbate constipation and reflux disease. In the SMA population, these two characteristics are already well-known. These routines might, however, also have negative effects on the person. Elevated carbohydrate intake might facilitate the development of insulin resistance. Low fat can exacerbate a deficiency in fat-soluble vitamins. To guarantee the best possible use of energy sources, the macronutrient content should be adjusted and optimized to the metabolic functions, whether they are normal or changed in SMA. It is still unknown whether SMN-depleted cells have preferred energy sources based on enzyme level and function, despite the preliminary data discussed here. Furthermore, this might only apply to a portion of SMA patients who also have a genetic program (polymorphism in other genes) that predisposes them to metabolic changes. It is necessary to look into different nutritional options for this set of patients. Whether this should be applied to all patients or just those who exhibit metabolic abnormalities like dyslipidemia and fatty liver would be an intriguing question to research. However, if a metabolic phenotype is suspected in a population with a longer life expectancy, the tests that screen for these changes in metabolism should be taken into consideration even though they are not currently considered standard of care. As SMA patients age, long-term dyslipidemia may have secondary effects on cardiovascular disease, among other conditions (Tisdale et al., 2017; Deguise et al., 2021).

A Closer Look

Genetics of Spinal Muscular Atrophy

The genetic basis of Spinal Muscular Atrophy (SMA) revolves around mutations in the Survival Motor Neuron 1 (SMN1) gene, located on chromosome 5q13. SMN1 encodes the survival motor neuron (SMN) protein, which plays a crucial role in the assembly of small nuclear ribonucleoproteins (snRNPs) involved in RNA splicing. Mutations or deletions in the SMN1 gene result in a deficiency of functional SMN protein, leading to the progressive degeneration of motor neurons in the spinal cord and subsequent muscle weakness and atrophy characteristic of SMA.

The severity of the SMA phenotype is largely determined by the copy number of the SMN2 gene, a nearly identical copy of SMN1 with a single nucleotide difference that renders it less efficient at producing functional SMN protein. Individuals with SMA typically have at least one copy of SMN2, which partially compensates for the loss of SMN1-derived protein. However, the number of SMN2 copies varies among individuals and correlates inversely with disease severity: fewer copies of SMN2 are associated with more severe forms of SMA, while higher copy numbers may mitigate disease severity.

SMA is inherited in an autosomal recessive manner, meaning that affected individuals inherit two mutated copies of the SMN1 gene, one from each parent. Carriers of a single SMN1 mutation are typically asymptomatic but have a 25% chance of having an affected child with SMA in each pregnancy. Genetic testing, including SMN1 gene deletion analysis and determination of SMN2 copy number, plays a crucial role in diagnosing SMA, identifying carriers, and predicting disease severity in affected individuals and their families.

Genetic counseling is essential for individuals and families affected by SMA to understand the inheritance pattern, recurrence risks, and available reproductive options. Carrier screening, prenatal testing, and preimplantation genetic diagnosis (PGD) are options available to families to inform reproductive decisions and reduce the risk of having a child affected by SMA. Additionally, advances in newborn screening programs have enabled early detection of SMA, allowing for prompt intervention and improved outcomes for affected individuals through early initiation of disease-modifying therapies.

Summary

- Spinal muscular atrophy (SMA) is a rare neuromuscular disorder that results in the loss of motor neurons and progressive muscle wasting.
- The most common form of SMA is caused by a mutated or missing gene known as the survival motor neuron gene 1 (SMN1). The SMN1 gene is located on chromosome 5q and produces the survival motor neuron (SMN) protein which maintains the health and normal function of motor neurons.
- Physical therapy, occupational therapy, and rehabilitation may help to improve posture, prevent joint immobility, and slow muscle weakness and atrophy. Stretching and strengthening exercises may help reduce contractures, increase range of motion, and keep circulation flowing.
- Poor weight gain with growth failure, restrictive lung disease, scoliosis, joint contractures, and sleep difficulties are common complications of SMA in those who receive supportive care only.
- Swallowing problems occur when the muscles of the mouth and throat are weak. Babies with infantile-onset SMA usually have trouble swallowing and sucking. Sucking weakness can lead to dehydration and poor nutrition, while swallowing weakness can lead to obstruction of the airway and respiratory infections from inhaled food or liquids (aspiration).
- A child or adult with SMA who must undergo surgery (e.g., to correct scoliosis) needs to take special precautions. The surgical team, particularly the anesthesiologist, must thoroughly understand SMA.
- Spinal muscular atrophy (SMA) is a degenerative neuromuscular disease of the lower motor neurons in the anterior horn of the spinal cord. It is primarily characterized by progressive weakness and wasting in the limb, respiratory, and bulbar muscles.
- Body composition and nutritional status are significantly altered in SMA patients. Across all types, both under- and overnutrition are reported. Thus, prescribing tailored energy requirements for SMA patients is challenging due to various possible nutritional phenotypes.

References

1. Arnold, A.-S., Gueye, M., Guettier-Sigrist, S., Courdier-Fruh, I., Coupin, G., Poindron, P., & Gies, J.-P. (2004). Reduced expression of nicotinic AChRs in myotubes from spinal muscular atrophy I patients. *Laboratory Investigation, 84*(10), 1271–1278. doi:10.1038/labinvest.3700163.
2. Bevan, A. K., Hutchinson, K. R., Foust, K. D., Braun, L., McGovern, V. L., Schmelzer, L., Ward, J. G., Petruska, J. C., Lucchesi, P. A., Burghes, A. H., & et al. (2010). Early heart failure in the SMNΔ7 model of spinal muscular atrophy and correction by postnatal scAAV9-SMN delivery. *Human Molecular Genetics, 19*(20), 3895–3905. doi:10.1093/hmg/ddq300.
3. Boyer, J. G., Deguise, M. O., Murray, L. M., Yazdani, A., De Repentigny, Y., Boudreau-Larivière, C., & Kothary, R. (2014). Myogenic program dysregulation is contributory to disease pathogenesis in spinal muscular atrophy. *Human Molecular Genetics, 23*(15), 4249–4259. doi: 10.1093/hmg/ddu142.

4. Bricceno, K. V., Martinez, T., Leikina, E., Duguez, S., Partridge, T. A., Chernomordik, L. V., Fischbeck, K. H., Sumner, C. J., & Burnett, B. G. (2014). Survival motor neuron protein deficiency impairs myotube formation by altering myogenic gene expression and focal adhesion dynamics. *Human Molecular Genetics, 23*(17), 4745–4757. doi: 10.1093/hmg/ddu189.

5. Chang, H., Dimlich, D. N., Yokokura, T., Mukherjee, A., Kankel, M. W., Sen, A., Sridhar, V., Fulga, T. A., Hart, A. C., & Van Vactor, D., et al. (2008). Modeling Spinal Muscular Atrophy in Drosophila. *PLoS ONE*. doi: 10.1371/journal.pone.0003209.

6. Chaytow, H., Huang, Y. T., Gillingwater, T. H., & Faller, K. M. E. (2018). The role of survival motor neuron protein (SMN) in protein homeostasis. *Cellular and Molecular Life Sciences, 75*(21), 3877–3894. doi:10.1007/s00018-018-2849-1.

7. Cifuentes-Diaz, C., Frugier, T., Tiziano, F. D., Lacène, E., Roblot, N., Joshi, V., Moreau, M. H., & Melki, J. (2001). Deletion of murine SMN exon 7 directed to skeletal muscle leads to severe muscular dystrophy. *Journal of Cell Biology, 152*(5), 1107–1114. doi:10.1083/jcb.152.5.1107.

8. Deguise, M. O., Pileggi, C., De Repentigny, Y., Beauvais, A., Tierney, A., Chehade, L., Michaud, J., Llavero-Hurtado, M., Lamont, D., Atrih, A., & et al. (2021). SMN depleted mice offer a robust and rapid onset model of nonalcoholic fatty liver disease. *Cellular and Molecular Gastroenterology and Hepatology, 12(1), 354–377.* doi: 10.1016/j.jcmgh.2021.01.019.

9. Deguise, M.-O., Chehade, L., & Kothary, R. (2021). Metabolic dysfunction in spinal muscular atrophy. *International Journal of Molecular Sciences, 22*(11), 5913. doi: 10.3390/ijms22115913.

10. Feldkötter, M., Schwarzer, V., Wirth, R., Wienker, T. F., & Wirth, B. (2002). Quantitative analyses of SMN1 and SMN2 based on real-time Light Cycler PCR: Fast and highly reliable carrier testing and prediction of severity of spinal muscular atrophy. *American Journal of Human Genetics, 70*(2), 358–368. doi:10.1086/338627.

11. Gabanella, F., Carissimi, C., Usiello, A., & Pellizzoni, L. (2005). The activity of the spinal muscular atrophy protein is regulated during development and cellular differentiation. *Human Molecular Genetics, 14*(24), 3629–3642. doi:10.1093/hmg/ddi390.

12. Guettier-Sigrist, S., Hugel, B., Coupin, G., Freyssinet, J.-M., Poindron, P., & Warter, J.-M. (2002). Possible pathogenic role of muscle cell dysfunction in motor neuron death in spinal muscular atrophy. *Muscle & Nerve, 25*(5), 700–708. doi:10.1002/mus.10081.

13. Heier, C. R., Satta, R., Lutz, C., & DiDonato, C. J. (2010). Arrhythmia and cardiac defects are a feature of spinal muscular atrophy model mice. *Human Molecular Genetics, 19*(20), 3906–3918. doi:10.1093/hmg/ddq330.

14. Hua, Y., Sahashi, K., Rigo, F., Hung, G., Horev, G., Bennett, C. F., & Krainer, A. R. (2011). Peripheral SMN restoration is essential for long-term rescue of a severe spinal muscular atrophy mouse model. *Nature, 478*(7367), 123–126. doi:10.1038/nature10485.

15. Kolb, S. J., & Kissel, J. T. (2015). Spinal muscular atrophy. *Neurologic Clinics, 33*(4), 831–846. doi: 10.1016/j.ncl.2015.07.004.

16. Lefebvre, S., Bürglen, L., Reboullet, S., Clermont, O., Burlet, P., Viollet, L., Benichou, B., Cruaud, C., Millasseau, P., & Zeviani, M. (1995). Identification and characterization of a spinal muscular atrophy-determining gene. *Cell, 80*(1), 155–165. doi:10.1016/0092-8674(95)90460-3.

17. Lorson, C. L., Hahnen, E., Androphy, E. J., & Wirth, B. (1999). A single nucleotide in the SMN gene regulates splicing and is responsible for spinal muscular atrophy. *Proceedings*

of the National Academy of Sciences of the United States of America, 96(11), 6307–6311. doi:10.1073/pnas.96.11.6307.

18. Martínez-Hernández, R., Soler-Botija, C., Also, E., Alias, L., Caselles, L., Gich, I., Bernal, S., & Tizzano, E. F. (2009). The developmental pattern of myotubes in spinal muscular atrophy indicates prenatal delay of muscle maturation. *Journal of Neuropathology and Experimental Neurology, 68*(5), 474–481. doi: 10.1097/NEN.0b013e3181a10ea1.
19. Rindt, H., Feng, Z., Mazzasette, C., Glascock, J. J., Valdivia, D., Pyles, N., Crawford, T. O., Swoboda, K. J., Patitucci, T. N., Ebert, A. D., & et al. (2015). Astrocytes influence the severity of spinal muscular atrophy. *Human Molecular Genetics, 24*(13), 4094–4102. doi: 10.1093/hmg/ddv148.
20. Rudnik-Schöneborn, S., Heller, R., Berg, C., Betzler, C., Grimm, T., Eggermann, T., Eggermann, K., Wirth, R., Wirth, B., & Zerres, K. (2008). Congenital heart disease is a feature of severe infantile spinal muscular atrophy. *Journal of Medical Genetics, 45*(10), 635–639. doi:10.1136/jmg.2008.057950.
21. Shababi, M., Habibi, J., Ma, L., Glascock, J. J., Sowers, J. R., & Lorson, C. L. (2012). Partial restoration of cardiovascular defects in a rescued severe model of spinal muscular atrophy. *Journal of Molecular and Cellular Cardiology, 52*(5), 1074–1082. doi: 10.1016/j.yjmcc.2012.01.005.
22. Shababi, M., Habibi, J., Yang, H. T., Vale, S. M., Sewell, W. A., & Lorson, C. L. (2010). Cardiac defects contribute to the pathology of spinal muscular atrophy models. *Human Molecular Genetics, 19*(21), 4059–4071. doi: 10.1093/hmg/ddq329.
23. Shafey, D., Côté, P. D., & Kothary, R. (2005). Hypomorphic Smn knockdown C2C12 myoblasts reveal intrinsic defects in myoblast fusion and myotube morphology. *Experimental Cell Research, 311*(1), 49–61. doi: 10.1016/j.yexcr.2005.08.019.
24. Sugarman, E. A., Nagan, N., Zhu, H., Akmaev, V. R., Zhou, Z., Rohlfs, E. M., Flynn, K., Hendrickson, B. C., Scholl, T., Sirko-Osadsa, D. A., & et al. (2012). Pan-ethnic carrier screening and prenatal diagnosis for spinal muscular atrophy: Clinical laboratory analysis of >72,400 specimens. *European Journal of Human Genetics, 20*(1), 27–32. doi:10.1038/ejhg.2011.134.
25. Tisdale, S., & Pellizzoni, L. (2017). RNA-Processing Dysfunction in Spinal Muscular Atrophy. In Sumner, C. J., Paushkin, S., & Ko, C. P. (Eds.), *Spinal Muscular Atrophy: Disease Mechanisms and Therapy* (pp. 75–97). Elsevier.
26. Verhaart, I. E. C., Robertson, A., Wilson, I. J., Aartsma-Rus, A., Cameron, S., Jones, C. C., Cook, S. F., & Lochmüller, H. (2017). Prevalence, incidence and carrier frequency of 5q-linked spinal muscular atrophy—A literature review. *Orphanet Journal of Rare Diseases, 12*(1), 124. doi: 10.1186/s13023-017-0671-8.
27. Walker, M. P., Rajendra, T. K., Saieva, L., Fuentes, J. L., Pellizzoni, L., & Matera, A. G. (2008). SMN complex localizes to the sarcomeric Z-disc and is a proteolytic target of calpain. *Human Molecular Genetics, 17*(21), 3399–3410. doi:10.1093/hmg/ddn234.
28. Wijngaarde, C. A., Blank, A. C., Stam, M., Wadman, R. I., van den Berg, L. H., & van der Pol, W. L. (2017). Cardiac pathology in spinal muscular atrophy: A systematic review. *Orphanet Journal of Rare Diseases, 12*(1), 67. doi: 10.1186/s13023-017-0613-5.
29. Wijngaarde, C. A., Huisman, A., Wadman, R. I., Cuppen, I., Stam, M., Heitink-Polle, K. M. J., Groen, E. J. N., Schutgens, R. E. G., & van der Pol, W. L. (2019). Abnormal coagulation parameters

are a common non-neuromuscular feature in patients with spinal muscular atrophy. *Journal of Neurology, Neurosurgery & Psychiatry, 90*(10), 1075–1080. doi:10.1136/jnnp-2019-321506.

30. Zhang, Z., Lotti, F., Dittmar, K., Younis, I., Wan, L., Kasim, M., & Dreyfuss, G. (2008). SMN deficiency causes tissue-specific perturbations in the repertoire of snRNAs and widespread defects in splicing. *Cell, 133*(4), 585–600. doi: 10.1016/j.cell.2008.03.031

31. Zhou, C., Feng, Z., & Ko, C. P. (2016). Defects in motoneuron-astrocyte interactions in spinal muscular atrophy. *Journal of Neuroscience, 36*(10), 2543–2553. doi:10.1523/JNEUROSCI.3534-15.2016.

Chapter

MUSCLE DISORDERS AND DISEASES

10

Contents

Introduction

Skeletal muscle weakness is the primary symptom of diseases and disorders that affect the human muscle system, known as muscle disorders. The phrase "muscle disorders" encompasses the terms "muscular dystrophy," "neuromuscular conditions," and "neuromuscular disorders." These disorders comprise a broad range of conditions that impact either the nerves that control the muscles (e.g., arms, legs, heart, lungs) or the muscles themselves. When the nervous system is intact, disorders of the muscles can result in weakness or paralysis. An electromyogram (EMG), patterns of weakness, loss of muscle tissue, or results from a biopsy that point to a muscle issue are all indicative of a muscle disorder. Muscular disorders can be acquired (like alcoholic or steroid myopathy) or inherited (like muscular dystrophy). Proximal muscles are typically more affected by myopathic weakness than distal muscles, and the face may also be affected. However, in peripheral neuropathies, reflexes may be compromised prior to clinical manifestations of weakness because the affected afferent limb of the reflex arc is compromised. In contrast, muscle tone and deep tendon reflexes are reduced in direct proportion to muscle weakness. Another way that myopathies and peripheral neuropathies differ from one another is that the latter do not exhibit sensory abnormalities.

Orientation and Directional Terms:

Term	Definition	Illustration
Rheumatism	Rheumatism or rheumatic disorders are conditions causing chronic, often intermittent pain affecting the joints or connective tissue.	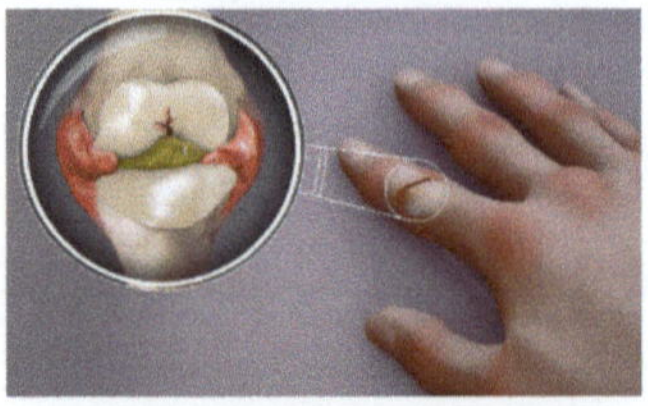
Brucellosis	Brucellosis is an infectious disease caused by bacteria. People can get the disease when they are in contact with infected animals or animal products contaminated with the bacteria.	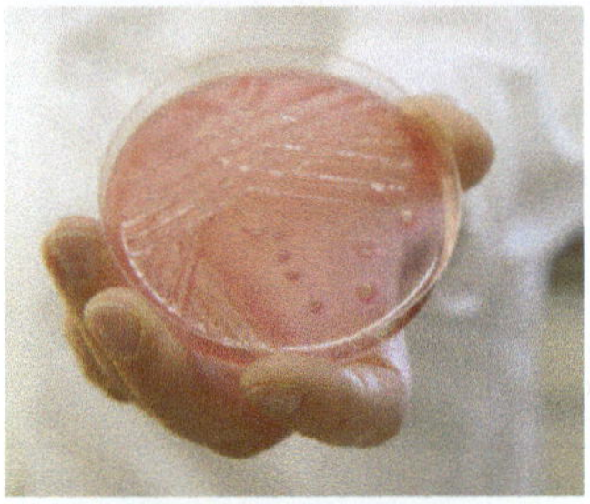
Microorganisms	An organism of microscopic size, which may exist in its single-celled form or as a colony of cells.	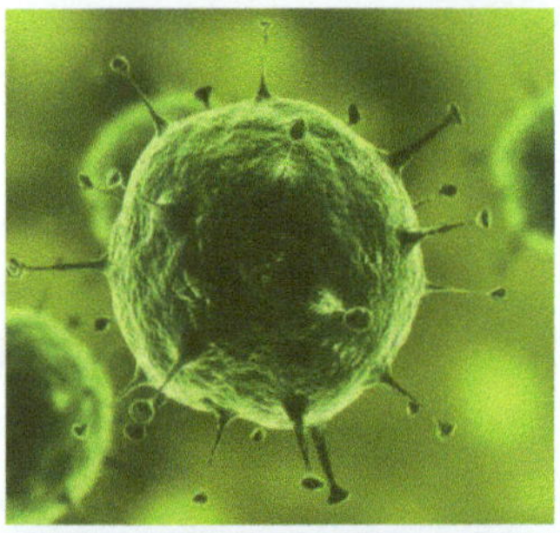
Osteomyelitis	A serious infection of the bone that can be either acute or chronic. It is an inflammatory process involving the bone and its structures caused by pyogenic organisms that spread through the bloodstream, fractures, or surgery.	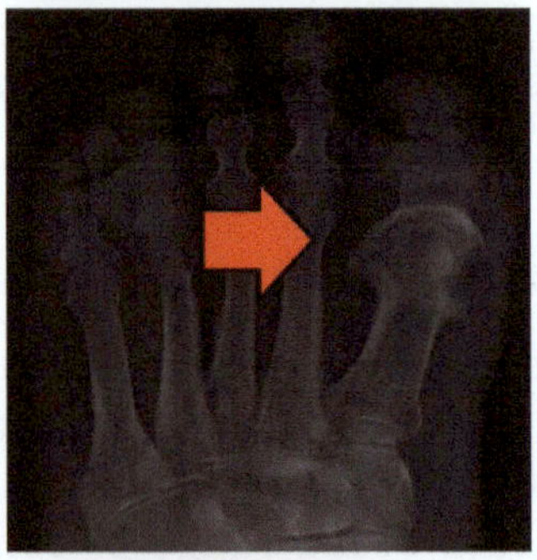
Staphylococci	A genus of Gram-positive bacteria in the family Staphylococcaceae from the order Bacillales. Under the microscope, they appear spherical, and form in grape-like clusters. Staphylococcus species are facultative anaerobic organisms.	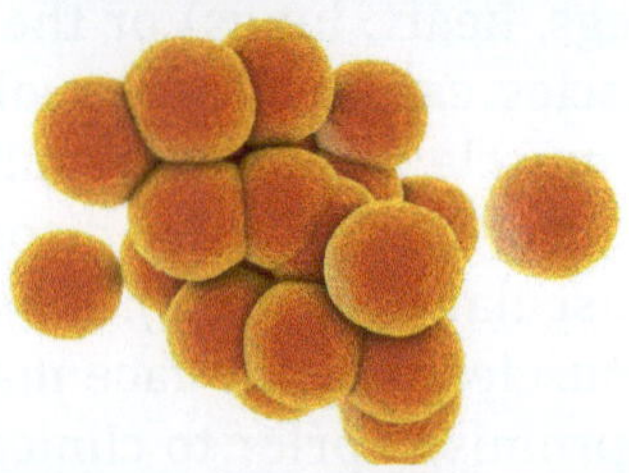

10.1. Basics of Muscle Disorders

A diverse range of inherited and acquired diseases are collectively referred to as muscle disorders. Although these can manifest in many different ways, weakness is the most typical symptom linked to primary muscle disease. In recent years, there has been a significant surge in the number of diagnostic tests available for the examination of muscle disorders, especially genetic myopathies. A greater number of disease genes can now be sequenced, and new genetic methods like whole exome and whole genome screening, high-throughput sequencing of specialized gene panels, and others are increasing the success rate of identifying causative mutations when compared to standard candidate gene sequencing. But before starting a long and sometimes expensive list of investigations, a complete history and physical examination are crucial to help identify conditions for which a particular treatment is available and to help choose the investigations that are most likely to produce results.

10.1.1. Overview of the Clinical Presentations of Muscle Disorders

The initial step in diagnosing a patient with muscle weakness is identifying the neuroaxis segment that is primarily compromised. Subsequently, investigations are focused on identifying the underlying pathology. Although there are many different causes of weak muscles, a history and physical examination can typically distinguish between myopathy, neuromuscular junction syndrome, and peripheral neuropathy. Clinically, these conditions can coexist.

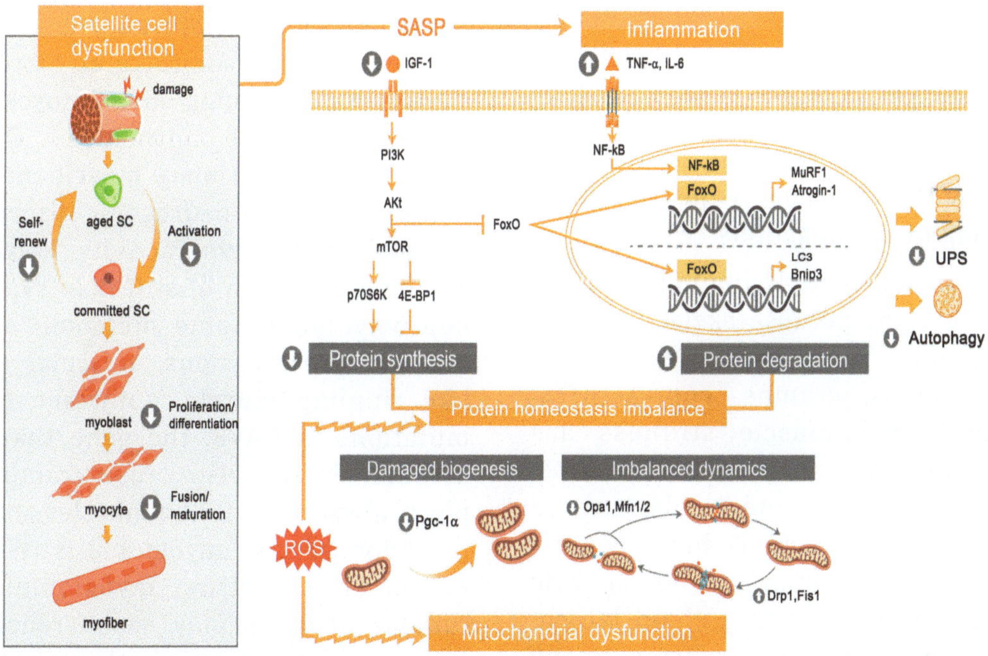

Figure 10.1. *Overview of sarcopenia pathophysiology.*

Source: Kim J, Lee J-Y, Kim CY. A comprehensive review of pathological mechanisms and natural dietary ingredients for the management and prevention of sarcopenia. Nutrients. 2023; 15(11):2625. https://doi.org/10.3390/nu15112625

Abbreviations: Akt, protein kinase B; Bnip3, Bcl-2 interacting protein 3; Drp1, dynamin-related protein 1; Fis1, fission 1 homolog protein; FoxO, forkhead box O; IGF-1, insulin-like growth factor-1; LC3, light chain 3; Mfn, mitofusin; mTOR, mammalian target of rapamycin; MuRF1, muscle RING-finger protein-1; NF-κB, nuclear factor kappa B; Opa1; optic atrophy-1; PI3K, phosphatidylinositol 3-kinase; Pgc-1α, proliferator-activated receptor γ coactivator-1 alpha; p70S6K, ribosomal protein S6 kinase; ROS, reactive oxygen species; SC, satellite cell; SASP, senescence-associated secretory phenotype; UPS, ubiquitin-proteasome system; 4E-BP1, 4E-binding protein 1.

Therefore, additional research is frequently necessary, such as nerve conduction studies and electromyography (EMG). After the pathology has been identified as affecting the muscle, the doctor needs to determine whether the symptoms are exclusive to the affected muscle or if they are a symptom of another, more widespread illness. An example involving muscles can be found in Figure 10.1. The likelihood that the disorder is inherited or acquired must also be determined by the clinician, as this can affect the sequencing of investigations.

Patients present with a limited range of symptoms and signs because skeletal muscle can only respond to a limited number of damages. Myalgias, cramps, contractures, myoglobinuria, and muscle stiffness are examples of positive symptoms. Weakness, fatigue, muscle atrophy, and intolerance to exercise are negative symptoms. In the context of a typical physical examination, non-specific symptoms like myalgias, cramps, and fatigue are common among patients referred to the neuromuscular clinic and do not always signify a primary muscle disease. Certain combinations of symptoms in the medical history and physical examination indicators may point to a specific muscle ailment.

Clues to specific diseases with particular symptoms and signs

Myotonic dystrophy type 1 is indicated by a history of muscle "stiffness" in the presence of myotonia (such as grip myotonia) and distal weakness on examination. Myotonia congenita is suggested by myotonia that deteriorates with rest, such as when trying to get out of a chair or start walking. This myotonia is frequently accompanied by muscle hypertrophy. Paramyotonia congenita is indicated by myotonia that is made worse by physical activity, especially in the cold and most severe in the face and forearms. When contractures appear on a clinical examination and occur early in the course of the disease, they may indicate either a collagen VI disorder like Bethlem myopathy or Emery-Dreifuss muscular dystrophy, which includes early elbow contractures. Collagen VI, SEPN1-, and MYH7-myopathies cause prominent spinal rigidity and/or scoliosis due to paraspinal muscle contractures. Fibrosis, muscle shortening, and antagonistic muscle weakness are the causes of contractures. Cramping is less common in primary muscle disorders and more common in neurogenic disorders linked to motor nerve hyperactivity. Muscle cramps can be a symptom of stiff-man syndrome and neuromyotonia. Some metabolic myopathies and, on rare occasions, muscular dystrophies like rippling muscle syndrome (caused by mutations in CAV3, the gene that codes for caveolin 3) can also cause cramping during physical exertion. When muscles are destroyed (rhabdomyolysis), myoglobin is released from the muscles, causing myoglobinuria. Acute tubular necrosis may cause renal failure if this is severe. A myopathy such as RHR1-myopathy, muscular dystrophy, or metabolic myopathy is frequently indicated by recurrent myoglobinuria. When children experience life-threatening episodes of rhabdomyolysis during concurrent illnesses, recessive mutations in

LPIN1 are linked to normal muscle function in between episodes (Table 10.1) (Engel, 2004; Lane, 2012; Dalakas, 2015; Schapira, 2015; Merlini and Wang, 2018).

Table 10.1. *Examples of Causes of Muscle Damage*

Acquired	Genetic
Consumption of alcohol and illegal substances	Metabolic myopathies
Prescription medications such as antipsychotics	Channelopathies
Electrolyte and metabolic disturbances	Muscular dystrophies
Pesticide and toxin ingestion	Mitochondrial disorders Disorders of lipid metabolism or glycolysis/glycogenolysis
Injury including crush syndrome Exposure to extreme temperatures e.g., malignant neuroleptic syndrome, heat stroke	
Exertion including intense physical exertion, seizures, epileptic status	
Viral/bacterial infections	

Source: Młynarska E, Krzemińska J, Wronka M, Franczyk B, Rysz J. Rhabdomyolysis-induced aki (riaki) including the role of COVID-19. International Journal of Molecular Sciences. 2022; 23(15):8215. https://doi.org/10.3390/ijms23158215.

Muscle pain alone, without any other clinical symptoms, is a common complaint for which there is frequently little return on investigation. It could be a sign of a systemic illness like fibromyalgia, chronic fatigue syndrome, drug use (such as amiodarone, fibrates, statins, alcohol, or heroin), infection, or inflammation (such as sarcoidosis, myositis, amiodarone-myalgia syndrome, or amiodarone withdrawal). Exercise-induced myalgia, however, may indicate an ischemia (claudication), muscular dystrophy, lipid storage disorder, or glycogen-storage disorder. In addition to neuromuscular junction disorders, certain metabolic and mitochondrial myopathies can cause abnormal fatigue following exercise, although muscle fatigue can also be non-specific (Table 10.2).

Table 10.2. *Neuromuscular Diseases Associated With Fatigue*

Neuromuscular Diseases Associated with Fatigue
Neuromuscular junction diseases (Myasthenia Gravis, Congenital Myasthenic Syndromes)
Muscle Channelopathies
Charcot–Marie–Tooth disease (CMT)
Guillain–Barre' syndrome (GBS)
Infectious diseases (poliomyelitis, Lyme disease, viral infections)

Chronic inflammatory demyelinating polyneuropathy (CIDP)
Muscular Dystrophies
Metabolic (glycogenoses, lipid storage myopathies)
Primary mitochondrial diseases
Inflammatory Myopathies
Motor neuron disease (Amyotrophic Lateral Sclerosis—ALS, Spinal Muscular Atrophy—SMA, Spino-bulbar Muscular Atrophy—SBMA)

Source: Torri F, Lopriore P, Montano V, Siciliano G, Mancuso M, Ricci G. Pathophysiology and management of fatigue in neuromuscular diseases. International Journal of Molecular Sciences. 2023; 24(5):5005. https://doi.org/10.3390/ijms24055005.

10.1.1.1. Clues on Examination From the Pattern of Muscle Involvement

Certain patterns of weakness are pathognomonic of specific muscle conditions, so clinical signs—in particular, the pattern of muscle weakness—provide crucial hints for the diagnosis. For example, severe weakness in the knee extensors and long forearm flexors is a characteristic of sporadic inclusion body myositis (sIBM). The biceps, tibialis anterior, serratus anterior, humeral head of the pectoralis major, and facial muscles are asymmetrically involved in facioscapulohumeral muscular dystrophy (FSHD). Scleroderma is usually associated with scapulospinal myopathy, which causes head drop or camptocormia. Myasthenia gravis, myotonic dystrophy, thyroid conditions, mitochondrial myopathies, oculopharyngeal muscular dystrophies, and certain congenital myopathies all affect the extraocular muscles. Unlike the large proximal girdle muscles (with the notable exception of sIBM), which are typically affected by non-selective acquired myopathies, the presence of a selective pattern of muscle involvement frequently indicates an inherited muscle condition. Furthermore, a variety of muscle disorders, including myotonia congenita, neuromyotonia, and muscular dystrophies (especially the dystrophinopathies and some limb girdle muscular dystrophies), can present with hypertrophy or pseudohypertrophy.

10.1.1.2. Other Organ Involvement

The diagnostic process can be aided by determining the involvement of other organs, such as the heart, lungs, and central nervous system. For instance, myotonic dystrophy, dystrophinopathies, mitochondrial myopathies, dermatomyositis, lipid storage disorders, and certain muscular dystrophies are among the muscle disorders linked to cardiac involvement. Furthermore, early in the course of some muscle disorders—most notably Pompe disease—the respiratory muscles are involved. Respiratory dysfunction usually starts as nocturnal hypoventilation, which can manifest as excessive daytime sleepiness or headaches in the morning. In addition to myopathy, mitochondrial myopathies can affect many different systems and cause a wide range of symptoms such as encephalopathy, seizures, diabetes, peripheral neuropathy, multiple lipomas, gastrointestinal issues, deafness, and stroke-like episodes. Until a clinical examination or other investigations are conducted, these might go unnoticed. To identify cardiorespiratory involvement, various diagnostic tests such as an electrocardiogram, Holter monitor, echocardiogram, respiratory function tests (erect and supine forced vital capacity, maximal inspiratory and expiratory pressures, and nasal pressures), and occasionally formal sleep studies are recommended.

10.1.1.3. Importance of Family History

Establishing a three-generation pedigree and having a complete family history are important. In certain cases, this shows compelling evidence supporting a specific inheritance pattern and offers a crucial diagnostic hint. Yet, due to recessive inheritance, the occurrence of a novel dominant mutation (20–30% of probands with FSHD and dystrophinopathies), or the fact that the disease was mild or subclinical in earlier generations—a trait common to trinucleotide repeat disorders due to anticipation—many patients with genetic neuromuscular disorders lack a family history. Gene testing is now the standard procedure when the typical clinical presentation for a genetic muscle disorder is discovered during history or examination (as is frequently the case in FSHD or myotonic dystrophy). Still, additional research is needed if the answer remains unclear following the preliminary assessment (Engel, 2004; Lane, 2012; Dalakas, 2015; Schapira, 2015; Merlini & Wang, 2018).

10.1.2. Initial Investigations

10.1.2.1. Blood Tests

Establishing a three-generation pedigree and having a complete family history are important. In certain cases, this shows compelling evidence supporting a specific inheritance pattern and offers a crucial diagnostic hint. Yet, due to recessive inheritance, the occurrence of a novel dominant mutation (20–30 percent of probands with FSHD and dystrophinopathies), or the fact that the disease was mild or subclinical in earlier generations—a trait common to trinucleotide repeat disorders due to anticipation—many patients with genetic neuromuscular disorders lack a family history. Gene testing is now the standard procedure when the typical clinical presentation for a genetic muscle disorder is discovered during history or examination (as is frequently the case in FSHD or myotonic dystrophy). Still, additional research is needed if the answer remains unclear following the preliminary assessment.

Making the distinction between primary genetic myopathies, such as muscular dystrophies, and inflammatory, metabolic, and other myopathies come next. The anticyclic citrullinated peptide antibodies, C-reactive protein, erythrocyte sedimentation rate, rheumatoid factor, antinuclear antibody assay (ANA), and myositis-specific antibodies should be taken into consideration when ordering blood tests for immune-mediated myopathies that may be suspected. Traditional immunofluorescence assays for ANA can identify auto-antibodies present in a large number of myositis patients. These auto-antibodies bind to elements of the cell's cytoplasm or nucleus. Whereas some are linked to multisystem autoimmune disorders that may involve myositis, others are unique to myositis. The antibodies that attach to the transfer RNA synthetases are particularly noteworthy among those specific to myositis. These are indicators of the "antisynthetase syndrome," which also involves calloused hands, myositis, fever, polyarthritis, interstitial lung disease, and arthritis.

Anti-signal recognition particle is another significant marker of severe myositis, which is currently known as necrotizing autoimmune myositis (NAM). This entity has also been linked to the use of statins, tumors, and viral infections such as hepatitis C and the human immunodeficiency virus. After years of statin use, statin-related NAM can appear and resemble polymyositis, which persists or even gets worse even after statin use is stopped. It was discovered that there was a strong correlation between the use of statins in the past and antibodies against the 3-hydroxy-3-methylglutaryl-coenzyme A reductase (HMGCR) protein. It is now possible to test for HMGCR antibodies, which are very specific for NAM linked to statins. This test's sensitivity is still being determined. Patients with sIBM have recently been found to have cytosolic 5?-nucleotidase IA autoantibodies, which are specific to myositis. Thirty-three percent of sIBM patients had these antibodies in their sera, compared to less than five percent of patients with polymyositis and dermatomyositis. This is the first serological biomarker for synthetic intelligence. In the early stages, when the biopsy may appear inflammatory, it may help distinguish this type of myositis from polymyositis and aid in its diagnosis. Furthermore, some have been found to indicate a higher chance of cancer in individuals with dermatomyositis. Autoantibodies specific to myositis can help confirm the diagnosis of autoimmune myositis, but their primary function is to subclassify, which helps with prognosis and treatment selection.

10.1.2.2. Aerobic Forearm Exercise Testing

Testing with forearm exercises can also be helpful when looking into a possible disorder related to the storage of glycogen. To lessen the chance of compartment syndrome, the test should be carried out aerobically without the use of a tourniquet. Using a handgrip dynamometer, the patient is instructed to execute isometric contractions for 4 seconds, followed by a 1-minute release period for 1 second, at 80 percent of maximal grip strength with maximum effort. Ammonia, lactate, and venous oxygen are measured at baseline as well as at 1, 2, 5, and 10 minutes. A myophosphorylase or phosphofructokinase deficiency will not cause a change in the lactate level, but an acid maltase deficiency (Pompe disease) is indicated by a blunted rise in lactate. An indication of myoadenylate deaminase deficiency is a normal rise in lactate accompanied by little to no rise in ammonia levels.

10.1.2.3. Role of EMG

When separating myopathies from motor neuropathies, anterior horn cell, and neuromuscular junction disorders, EMG is the most useful method. The character of each individual motor unit's action potential, the muscle's spontaneous activity, its response to the insertion of a probe, and the speed at which new motor units are recruited in response to an electrical signal are all evaluated by electromyography (EMG). An inflammatory myopathy, for instance, is characterized by increased spontaneous activity, complex repetitive discharges, positive sharp waves, and fibrillations. The insertion of the electrode may cause an extended series of repetitive discharges that last up to 30 seconds, and electromyography (EMG) can also be useful in identifying myotonic disorders.

10.1.3. More Specialized Investigations

10.1.3.1. Muscle Ultrasound

When diagnosing skeletal muscle disorders in children, ultrasound muscle imaging has primarily been utilized as a non-invasive technique. Different muscles may be involved in different patterns in different neuromuscular disorders, and this can be seen in the way different muscles appear on ultrasonography. For example, in many muscular dystrophies, the biceps and quadriceps exhibit a homogeneously increased echo intensity; in spinal muscular atrophy, on the other hand, the muscle changes are usually inhomogeneous, exhibiting both atrophic and hypertrophic regions (Figure 10.2).

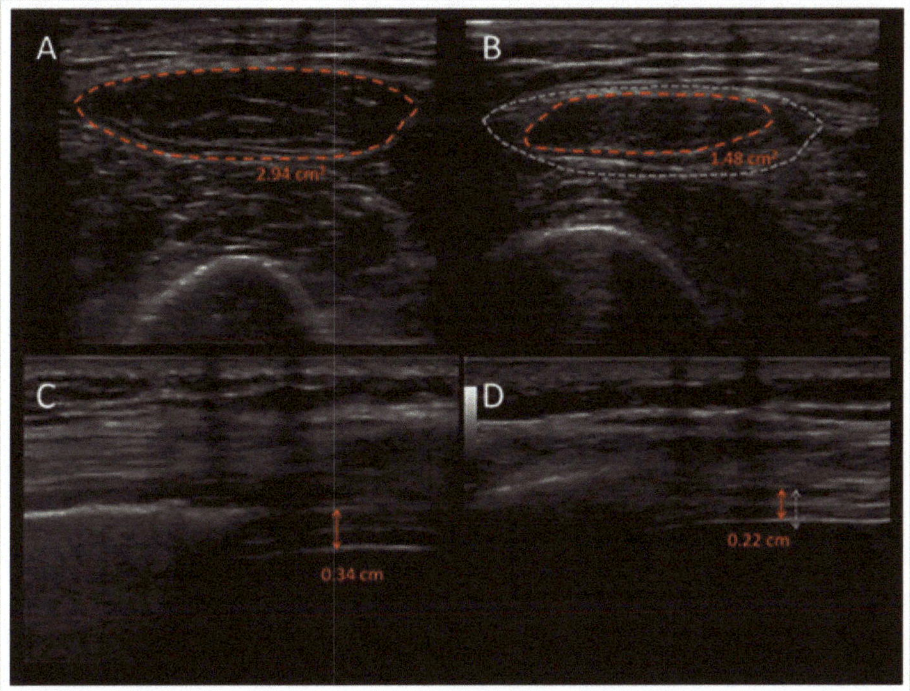

Figure 10.2. *Ultrasonographic images of the quadriceps muscle and the diaphragm during the first week of ICU stay of a critically ill patient. The figure shows the images of the quadriceps muscle (upper panels (A,B)) and the diaphragm (lower panels (C,D)) of a critically ill patient during the first (left panels) and seventh day of ICU stay (right panels) and highlights the loss in muscle mass. Upper panels: The red, shaded line represents the cross-sectional area of the rectus femoris muscle; the gray, shaded area in panel (B) is the cross-sectional area of the first ICU day, and highlights the reduction in mass of the muscle. Lower panels: the red arrows show the diaphragm end-expiratory thickness; the gray, shaded line in panel (D) is the end-expiratory diaphragm thickness of the first ICU day.*

Source: Umbrello M, Brogi E, Formenti P, Corradi F, Forfori F. Ultrasonographic features of muscular weakness and muscle wasting in critically ill patients. Journal of clinical medicine. 2024; 13(1):26. https://doi.org/10.3390/jcm13010026.

10.1.3.2. Muscle Magnetic Resonance Imaging

To evaluate deep muscles that are difficult to assess with electromyography (EMG), magnetic resonance imaging (MRI) can be a helpful tool. It can also be used to detect subclinical muscle involvement, which can help with diagnosis. Different patterns of muscle involvement (fatty infiltration and muscle atrophy) of the thighs and lower legs in different types of inherited myopathy have been reported in a number of earlier studies. Among the myopathies, sIBM (Figure. 10.1) and those resulting from RHR1 and DNM2 mutations have unique patterns that can help focus genetic testing on those genes. For adults and children over five who can handle the procedure without general anesthesia, it offers a multiplanar, non-invasive, radiation-free examination of the muscles. T2-weighted fat-suppressed and T2-weighted images are useful in myositis diagnosis as they can identify edema and consequent inflammation. Dystrophic processes are frequently accompanied by fatty infiltration, which can be identified using T1-weighted images. Muscle MRI also serves as a secondary tool for identifying the muscles involved in the myopathic process, which helps determine the optimal location for a muscle biopsy (Figure 10.3).

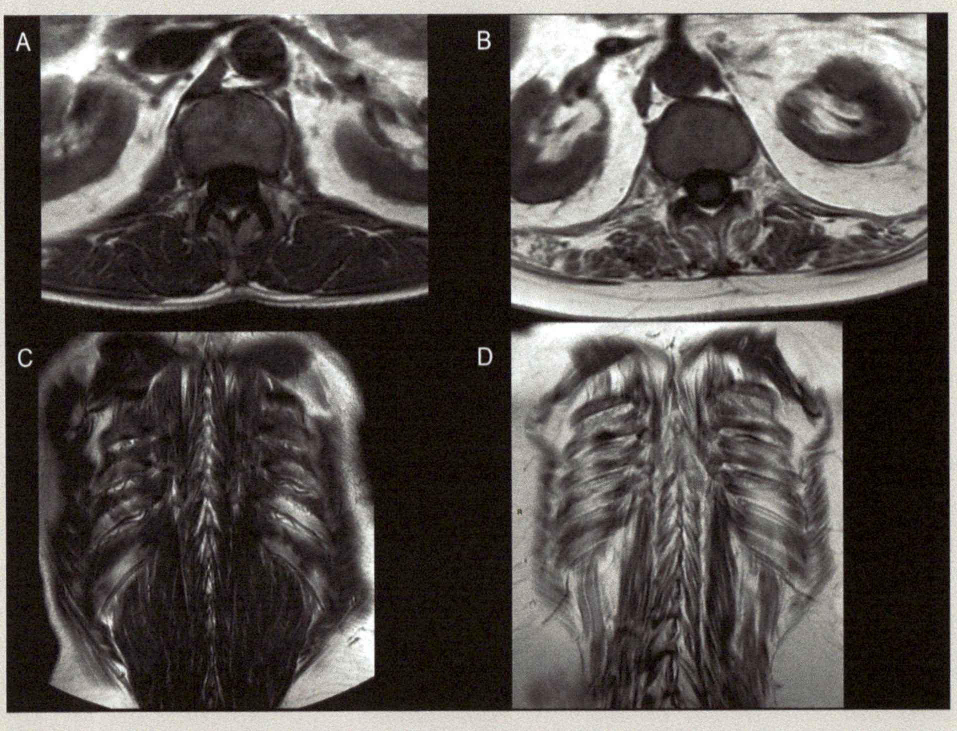

Figure 10.3. *MRI scans of a healthy control (A,C—Healthy control (HC) #4) and an ALS patient (B,D—patient #10). Paraspinal axial (A—HC #4, B—patient #10), and coronal T1 (C—HC #4, D—patient #10) images show an extensive degree of fat replacement in the ALS patient compared to the HC.*

Source: Diamanti L, Paoletti M, Di Vita U, Muzic SI, Cereda C, Ballante E, Pichiecchio A. mri study of paraspinal muscles in patients with amyotrophic lateral sclerosis (ALS). Journal of clinical medicine. 2020; 9(4):934. https://doi.org/10.3390/jcm9040934–.

10.1.3.3. Muscle Biopsy

When non-invasive investigations have been exhausted and the diagnosis is still unclear, patients typically decide to have a muscle biopsy. The muscles that are not severely atrophy-prone but are only mildly impacted by the disease process are the best candidates for biopsy. Avoiding trauma, EMG exams, and injection sites in the past is advised. The deltoid, biceps, and vastus lateralis are the most frequently used biopsy sites. An in vitro contracture test, typically carried out by an anesthetist, can be carried out concurrently with the muscle biopsy if vulnerability to malignant hyperthermia is suspected. When analyzing the biopsy, the pathologist should have access to the patient's clinical history because it affects the type of stains that should be used and whether electron microscopy (EM) is necessary. Even though the presence of "dystrophic features" can help narrow the diagnosis to muscular dystrophy, more testing is typically necessary because the features are rarely specific to a particular subtype. Sometimes presumptive or conclusive diagnoses can be obtained using immunostaining and Western blotting, which employ particular antibodies to identify the presence and concentrations of different proteins in frozen muscle biopsies (e.g., dystrophinopathies, sarcoglycanopathies, and merosin-deficient congenital muscular dystrophy). More precise observations that can be proved include amyloid deposits (in amyloidosis or sIBM), ragged red fibers (in mitochondrial myopathies), lipid accumulation (in lipid storage myopathy), and glycogen accumulation (in glycogen storage diseases). Major Histocompatibility Classes I and II (MHC-I/II) immunostaining is upregulated in myofibers in inflammatory myopathies, while MHC-I immunostaining on its own is non-specific. Note that certain muscular dystrophies can be extremely inflammatory, which can occasionally lead to confusion. There are specific roles for other non-standard histochemical stains in the diagnosis of specific myopathies, which highlights the importance of communication between the pathologist and the clinician.

Electron microscopy (EM) provides visualization of the ultrastructural elements of muscle fibers and can reveal anomalies not visible with light microscopy stains. It is employed in suspected mitochondrial myopathies to characterize accumulations of aberrant material, such as those seen in amyloid and myofibrillar myopathies, and to detect paracrystalline inclusions in suspected sIBM. Not every biopsy needs to be evaluated by EM.

10.1.4. Exome Sequencing

Until now, efforts to pinpoint the genes responsible for hereditary myopathies have been made using candidate gene sequencing or linkage analysis in large families. We can now identify genetic variations at base pair resolution throughout the human genome in a single experiment thanks to advancements in computing power and genetic techniques such as next-generation sequencing (NGS). NGS techniques include whole exome and whole genome sequencing, custom gene panel sequencing, microarray or "chip" technology, and others. Targeted "capture" or amplification of a particular list of genes—for instance, all genes known to cause neuromuscular disease—is typically required for sequencing custom gene panels. Sequencing 200 genes in a custom panel is frequently less expensive than standard (Sanger) sequencing of a single large gene thanks to new gene sequencing techniques. There are custom panels available overseas for different combinations of neuromuscular genes, and panels specifically for Australia are being established. The goal of whole exome sequencing is to "capture," "sequence," and analyze the Exome, or the approximately 2% of the human genome that codes for proteins. Whole genome sequencing skips the "capture" step and sequences the entire DNA code, including the non-coding regions. This results in a vast amount of data that needs to be carefully filtered and analyzed. The ability to quickly and cheaply check the sequence of multiple genes at once is being revolutionized by new sequencing techniques, but they also present new difficulties for labs and medical professionals. Currently, it is difficult to distinguish the thousands of tiny genetic variations (polymorphisms) that exist between individuals but do not result in disease from the changes in DNA sequence that cause disease. As we gain more knowledge about the range of DNA variations found in healthy individuals, labs and researchers will be better able to differentiate these variations from DNA alterations linked to disease. Our capacity to discover novel disease genes has significantly increased thanks to these novel "genome-wide" methods, even for uncommon illnesses for which there are only a few known families worldwide. The data from whole-genome sequencing can be used to study multigenetic disorders and complex traits as the technique becomes more widely used. The analysis and management of the massive volumes of generated sequencing data will be the main challenge in the coming years. It takes bioinformatic techniques to weed out possible pathogenic variants or genes. Sanger sequencing is currently needed to validate the variations found by exome sequencing (Engel, 2004; Lane, 2012; Dalakas, 2015; Schapira, 2015; Merlini & Wang, 2018).

These new technologies have various limitations as well, which require attention. A constraint concerns the detection of certain classes of mutations and their corresponding sensitivity and specificity. Hoischen et al. discovered, for instance, that sequences rich in guanine and cysteine can be challenging to capture and sequence. Furthermore, the new technologies might not be able to fully sequence a large number of genes. Large deletions and duplications represent a significant class of mutation in numerous neuromuscular diseases, but their detection is difficult to achieve with the current methods. Typical instances are Charcot-Marie-Tooth disease type 1A and Duchenne muscular dystrophy. High-throughput sequencing techniques currently in use have a hard time identifying expansions or contractions in repetitive sequences. To diagnose FSHD and myotonic dystrophy type 1, the two most prevalent adult-onset muscular dystrophies, different techniques are therefore required. There are many additional ethical considerations in light of the emerging genetic technologies. For instance, it is feasible to find genetic information about health risks unrelated to the neuromuscular condition under investigation when hundreds or thousands of genes are analyzed simultaneously. There is a substantial amount of health-related data that could be extracted from whole-genome sequencing; what kind of information should be provided to patients prior to these new tests, what kind of consent should be obtained, and how should "incidental" genetic findings be handled? As more tests become a part of standard clinical care, laboratories and clinics are addressing these issues. How should the health system assist patients in understanding and applying this information in an informed and positive way? A great deal of these issues will require education for all medical personnel, as well as for patients to some extent, so that the exciting opportunities we have to learn about our genetic sides lead to better lives rather than worry or unaffordable demands on our health system.

10.2. Neuromuscular Disorders and Diseases

Neuromuscular diseases impact the nerves responsible for regulating specific muscles in your body. These muscles, which include the ones in your arms, legs, and face, are referred to as your voluntary muscles because you can choose to move them. Voluntary muscle disorders can be inherited genetically (inherited from your parents) or they can develop gradually as a side effect of certain medical conditions, like autoimmune disorders. Nerves or muscles can be impacted by neuromuscular disorders. This group includes a wide range of illnesses with various causes, signs, and therapies. We use the most up-to-date diagnostic techniques to identify your neuromuscular disorder, whether you have muscle weakness, spasms, or persistent pain in your muscles or nerves. Together, we'll identify the best course of action to enhance your life. Specialized nerves allow the brain to regulate the voluntary movements of skeletal muscles. The neuromuscular system is made up of the nervous system and muscles that cooperate to enable movement.

Upper motor neurons are specific types of neurons (nerve cells) that receive a signal when you want to move a particular part of your body. Long tails, or axons, on upper motor neurons extend into the brain, spinal cord, and other parts of the body before joining forces with lower motor neurons. The lower motor neurons in the spinal cord send their axons directly to the muscle they control at the spinal cord through nerves in the arms and legs. Anywhere from 50 to 200 (or more) lower motor neurons supply a typical muscle. Every lower motor neuron has numerous tiny branches that branch off of it. A presynaptic terminal is the point where each branch terminates. The neuromuscular junction is another name for this connection that exists between the muscle and the tip of the nerve. Acetylcholine is released from the presynaptic terminals in response to an electrical signal that originates in the brain and travels down the nerves. In the muscle tissue, this chemical is detected by unique sensors called receptors. Your muscles will contract if acetylcholine stimulates enough receptors (Engel, 2004; Lane, 2012; Dalakas, 2015; Schapira, 2015; Merlini & Wang, 2018).

10.2.1. Classifications of Neuromuscular Disorders

Some of the major diseases that affect the neuromuscular system are classified into four main groups.

Motor neuron diseases. The lower motor neurons (and occasionally the upper ones, too) gradually die for unknown or genetic reasons. Adult spinal muscular atrophy, juvenile spinal muscular atrophy, intermediate spinal muscular atrophy, and infantile progressive spinal muscular atrophy are a few of the various forms of genetic (inherited) motor neuron diseases. Lou Gehrig's disease, also known as amyotrophic lateral sclerosis or motor neuron disease, is the most prevalent type of the condition. Its cause is still unknown and it is typically not inherited.

Neuropathies. Affected nerves are those that are not part of the spinal cord or the peripheral nervous system. The genetic condition Charcot-Marie-Tooth disease, the hormonal disorder diabetes (if poorly controlled), and autoimmune diseases like chronic inflammatory demyelinating neuropathy (CIDP) are a few of the various diseases that affect the peripheral nerve.

Neuromuscular junction disorders. The transmission of the signal to move (contract) a muscle is obstructed in neuromuscular junction disorders as the muscle attempts to bridge the gap between the nerve and muscle. Myasthenia gravis is the most prevalent of these autoimmune diseases. In this condition, the immune system creates antibodies that cling to the neuromuscular junction and stop the nerve impulse from reaching the muscle.

Myopathies including muscular dystrophies. Genetic mutations that impede the upkeep and repair of muscle tissue result in a variety of forms of muscular dystrophy, also known as muscle wastage. Becker muscular dystrophy, congenital muscular dystrophy, Duchenne muscular dystrophy, and facioscapulohumeral muscular dystrophy are a few of the various forms. Other muscle diseases, or myopathies, can be brought on by autoimmune diseases like polymyositis or polymyalgia rheumatica, hormonal disorders like hypothyroidism, or uncommon drug side effects like those associated with statins, which lower cholesterol.

10.2.2. Common Neuromuscular Disorders

Common neuromuscular disorders include:

- Amyotrophic lateral sclerosis (ALS): This condition leads to the loss of nerve cells in the brain and spinal cord. Weakness in the muscles causes trouble with movement and speech. ALS may also eventually lead to issues with swallowing and breathing.
- Charcot-Marie-Tooth disease (CMT disease): This group of disorders is inherited. Early symptoms include weakness in the lower limbs/feet and hands. CMT progresses slowly and may not affect a person's life span.

- Chronic inflammatory demyelinating polyneuropathy (CIDP): This condition leads to weakness in the extremities (arms/legs). It's caused by autoimmune issues that damage the insulation surrounding the peripheral nerves (myelin sheath).
- Guillain-Barré syndrome (GBS): This condition also affects the myelin sheath. Symptoms and progress vary by person, but it typically begins with weakness in the legs and spreads rapidly to the rest of the body. Similar to CIDP, the cause is likely the immune system attacking the peripheral nervous system.
- Lambert-Eaton syndrome: This autoimmune condition leads to weakness and fatigue in the arm and leg muscles. It's caused by antibodies that damage the voltage-gated calcium channels in the neuromuscular junction.
- Multiple sclerosis (MS): This condition is also caused by the immune system attacking the myelin sheath around the peripheral nerves. It affects the brain, spinal cord, and optic nerves. People with MS have attacks that lead to either a progression of symptoms or periods of time where there are no new symptoms (stabilization).
- Myasthenia gravis: This autoimmune condition is caused by damage to muscle receptors. It leads to muscle weakness throughout the body. Symptoms include weakness in the arms/legs, issues with the eyes and vision, and trouble with speaking and eating.
- Peripheral neuropathy: This group of disorders affects nerves beyond the brain and spinal cord. It leads to weakness, pain, and numbness in the extremities (arms, legs, hands, feet, face, mouth, etc.).
- Spinal muscular atrophy (SMA): This group of genetically inherited disorders causes symptoms such as hypotonia (decreased muscle tone) in the arms/legs, feeding issues, and breathing issues. Many forms start in infancy/childhood, but some begin in adulthood as well.

10.2.3. Symptoms of Neuromuscular Disorders

Muscle weakness, rigidity, loss of control, tingling, twitching, spasms, pain in the muscles, and some forms of limb pain are some of the symptoms of muscle disease. Even though muscle atrophy is not painful, the weakness that results can sometimes lead to contracture, which is the tightening and freezing of joints. It can also cause cramping, stiffness, joint deformities, and chronic aches and pains. Depending on the type of neuromuscular disorder you have, you may have different symptoms. The intensity of those symptoms is likewise relevant. It's possible for someone to have extremely minor symptoms while someone else has potentially fatal ones. Similarly, symptoms may appear at any time from early childhood to adulthood. The symptoms may appear slowly, quickly, or even differently over time.

Symptoms may include:

- weakness in the muscles
- wastage of the muscles
- cramps in the muscles
- stiffness (spasticity) in the muscles
- pain in the muscles
- difficulty breathing

- difficulty swallowing
- issues with balance and movement
- trouble with vision

10.2.4. Causes of Neuromuscular Disorders

The cause of neuromuscular disorders depends on the specific disorder. For some, such as ALS, the cause isn't known. Others, such as CIDP and MS, are caused by autoimmune issues and, therefore, by whatever triggers the immune response. Other disorders, such as SMA and CMT, may be inherited or caused by spontaneous gene mutations during reproduction. Additional risk factors may include:

- age;
- family history;
- smoking.

10.2.5. Diagnosis of Neuromuscular Disorders

Various tests are used to diagnose neuromuscular disorders depending on the condition. These tests include muscle biopsies, blood tests, genetic testing, electromyography (EMG) to assess muscle health, and electrical tests called nerve conduction studies to measure the ability of nerves to conduct electricity. The course of treatment varies greatly depending on the specific disorder, and certain conditions are easier to treat than others. To make a diagnosis of a neuromuscular disorder, a physician or other healthcare provider will probably test your reflexes and look for symptoms like atrophy, or loss of muscle tone. From there, the subsequent examinations could aid in the diagnosis:

- blood tests to look for levels of certain enzymes
- electromyography to assess the electrical activity in the muscles
- imaging, such as MRI, to look for issues with the brain and spinal cord
- spinal tap (also known as lumbar puncture) to test the cerebrospinal fluid
- nerve conduction velocity testing to determine how well messages are being sent from the nerves to the muscles
- muscle biopsies to evaluate the muscle tissue
- genetic testing to find any mutations that may have been inherited

10.2.6. Manage and Treat with Neuromuscular Disorders

Neuromuscular disorders can't be cured. Instead, treatment is prescribed to ease symptoms and slow the disease from getting worse.

Medications may include:

- drugs to relieve muscle pain, weakness, cramps, and stiffness
- drugs to address nerve impulses and strength in the muscles
- immunosuppressants if a disorder is caused by autoimmune issues
- high dose immunoglobulin therapy to build antibodies

Other treatments include:

- physical therapy to restore muscle tone and work on motor skills
- occupational therapy to learn new ways to go about daily tasks and save energy
- surgery—with neuropathy—to relieve pressure on the nerves or—with myasthenia gravis—to remove the thymus.

10.2.7. People with Neuromuscular Disorders

Every neuromuscular condition is distinct, as is every individual. Certain illnesses may only cause minor symptoms that don't get worse. Others might advance quickly, becoming crippling or even fatal. The good news is that certain disorders may not progress as quickly with treatment. Therapies can also aid in everyday tasks and motor function. In an effort to enhance outcomes, researchers are also exploring novel therapeutic approaches, such as bone marrow transplantation for the treatment of mitochondrial neurogastrointestinal encephalomyopathy or the use of the medications rasagiline, tirasagiline, and mexiletine (Engel, 2004; Lane, 2012; Dalakas, 2015; Schapira, 2015; Merlini & Wang, 2018).

10.3. Pathology of Muscle Disease

Any illness or condition that affects the human muscle system is considered a muscle disease. Primary muscle diseases are those that originate directly from abnormalities in the muscles; diseases and disorders that are identified as signs or symptoms of problems in the nervous system or other systems are not appropriately categorized as primary muscle diseases. Muscular atrophy (wasting) and paralysis are the outcomes of diseases affecting both the neurological system that supplies the muscles and the muscles themselves. Numerous illnesses and conditions can affect muscles, some of which are lethal to both humans and animals. Accurate diagnosis is essential for their management or treatment. The diagnosis process involves the following procedures: (1) history and clinical examination; (2) blood biochemistry; (3) electromyography; (4) muscle biopsy; (5) nuclear magnetic resonance; (6) measurement of muscle cross-sectional area; (7) tests of muscle function; (8) provocation tests; and (9) studies on protein turnover. It is important to note that no single method can be used to identify all diseases. Even after one or more of these procedures prove useful in the diagnosis process, the disorder may still not be able to be identified. All of these processes, however, can yield valuable data. Muscular dystrophies are among the most prevalent diseases affecting muscles. Both Duchenne and Becker's muscular dystrophy are caused by the newly discovered muscle protein dystrophin, which is either absent or present in lower than normal amounts. Even though dystrophin's identification marks a significant advancement, treatment has not advanced to the experimental stage. Neuropathies and inflammatory myopathies are two more serious muscle diseases. Our understanding of the behavior of normal and abnormal muscle is enhanced by the study of muscle atrophy and hypertrophy as well as the relationship between aging, exercise, and fatigue. Myasthenia gravis, muscular dysgenesis, and myoclonus are a few other intriguing diseases and disorders of the muscle.

10.3.1. Muscular System Disease Symptoms

One of the first signs of muscle problems is muscle weakness. This means the muscle lacks strength and cannot do its job. Many different diseases can cause muscles to become weak.

Muscle pain that improves with home therapies is usually nothing to worry about. Pain from severe injuries or a serious illness that affects the whole body often requires medical care.

Seek immediate medical attention if you have any of the following symptoms:

- Muscle pain with breathing issues
- Dizziness
- Muscle weakness

- High fever
- Stiff neck

People with muscle disease may also experience muscle spasms, cramping, or twitching. Other symptoms of muscle diseases include:

- Muscle wasting or muscle loss
- Problems with movement and balance
- Numbness, tingling, or painful sensations
- Double vision
- Droopy eyelids
- Dysphagia, problems with swallowing
- Breathing troubles, especially dyspnea, which is a shortness of breath

10.3.2. Causes of Muscle Diseases

There are many different causes of muscle diseases. Some muscle diseases are genetic. Genetic conditions may be inherited, or they may be the result of a new genetic mutation in the affected person. Some muscle diseases are autoimmune diseases, which occur when the immune system attacks its own healthy muscle tissues.

Sometimes, the cause of the muscle disease is unknown. Additional causes of muscle diseases include:

- Overuse or injury of muscles
- Some cancers
- Infections
- Nerve diseases
- Medications

10.3.3. Diagnosis of Muscle Diseases

Muscle diseases are often diagnosed with electromyography (EMG). An EMG measures electrical activity in the muscles. This can help identify neuromuscular abnormalities.

EMG can diagnose several problems, including:

- Muscle disorders
- Nerve and motor problems
- Degenerative diseases (diseases that get worse over time)

An electrode, a tiny needle, is inserted into the skin and muscle tissue during an EMG test. The patient is instructed to either contract or relax their muscles after the needle is inserted. Electrical activity is detected by the electrode. An EMG may be used to perform a nerve conduction velocity test. This examination gauges how quickly electrical impulses pass through your nerves. This can assist in identifying whether a nerve or muscle ailment is the source of the symptoms. Your doctor may perform a muscle strength examination if they believe you suffer from a muscle ailment. This aids in identifying any muscle weakness or other issues with the muscles.

Additional testing may include:

- Blood tests for measuring antibodies and muscle enzymes, which may be specific to one disorder or many
- Muscle biopsy, where a small sample of muscle tissue is taken and sent for testing
- Magnetic resonance imaging (MRI) to show areas of abnormal muscle

10.3.4. Treatment of Muscle Diseases

The majority of muscular system disorders are

irreversible. The good news is that they are frequently curable and controllable. Relieving symptoms, postponing the progression of the disease, and enhancing quality of life are possible treatment objectives. Drug therapy is one possible form of treatment. Immunosuppressive medications, which lessen or stop the immune system from being overactive, may fall under this category. Some diseases of the muscles and nerves may be treated with these medications. They can also be applied to ailments affecting the muscles and nerves. Other drugs may be administered to lessen cramping and spasms in the muscles, and corticosteroids may be used to treat inflammation.

10.3.5. Indications of Muscle Disease

One of the most prevalent signs of muscle disease is muscular atrophy and weakness (see below Muscle weakness). Even though the amount of wasting does not always correlate with the degree of weakness, this is typically the case when specific nerve or muscle involvement occurs. The main sign of myasthenia gravis is persistent weakness that gets worse with exercise. Muscle inflammation, injury, or abnormalities in blood circulation can all cause pain in patients with muscle diseases. Pain is uncommon in muscular dystrophy, a genetic illness marked by progressive muscle atrophy, unless it results from weariness or aberrant posture. Cramps can be brought on by illnesses of the motor or sensory neurons, specific metabolic conditions (e.g., hypocalcemia – a condition in which the blood level of calcium is abnormally low), when there is poisoning that affects the muscle tissues, blood vessel disease, and during exercise, especially in the winter.

Athletes naturally experience muscular hypertrophy, or muscle enlargement. Myotonia congenita is a rare form of muscular dystrophy that combines increased muscle size with strength and stiffness. It is characterized by hypertrophy not related to exercise. Other types of muscular dystrophy, especially the Duchenne type, result in pseudohypertrophy, or the enlargement of the muscles through the deposition of fat instead of muscle fiber. Tetany is the occurrence of sporadic spasms, or involuntary contractions, of muscles, especially in the voice box, arms, and legs. It is caused by alkalosis, or an elevated alkalinity of the blood and tissues, and low blood calcium levels. Tetanus, also known as lockjaw, is a condition in which the bacillus Clostridium tetani produces toxins that cause persistent muscle spasm, especially in the jaw muscles. Fasciculation, or the twitching of muscle fibers under the control of a single motor nerve cell, can happen in a healthy individual, but it typically signifies that the disease affecting the motor nerve cells in the spinal cord is the cause of the muscular atrophy. Muscles near to the skin's surface exhibit the greatest degree of fascicle contraction (Figure 10.4).

Energy is produced through the breakdown of glycogen, a type of carbohydrate that is used as storage. Glycogen storage diseases are a rare class of hereditary diseases that cause muscle weakness. These diseases are caused by various enzyme defects that impede the normal breakdown of glycogen in muscles, which releases energy. Consequently, the muscles and other organs store excessive amounts of glycogen. The most well-known muscle glycogen storage illness is McArdle disease, where the lack of the enzyme phosphorylase prevents the muscles from breaking down glycogen into lactic acid during physical activity. Glycogen builds up abnormally in various places within muscle cells. When the condition is exerted, the muscles experience pain, stiffness, and weakness. Usually, McArdle disease starts in childhood. There is no known cure, and those who are impacted must often limit their activity to manageable levels. The illness doesn't seem to get worse over time, but when the muscle protein myoglobin is expelled in the urine, it could lead to dangerous complications. The enzymes phosphofructokinase or acid maltase deficiencies cause other diseases related to glycogen storage. Both the heart and voluntary muscles are impacted by acid maltase deficiency, and death typically happens within a year of birth.

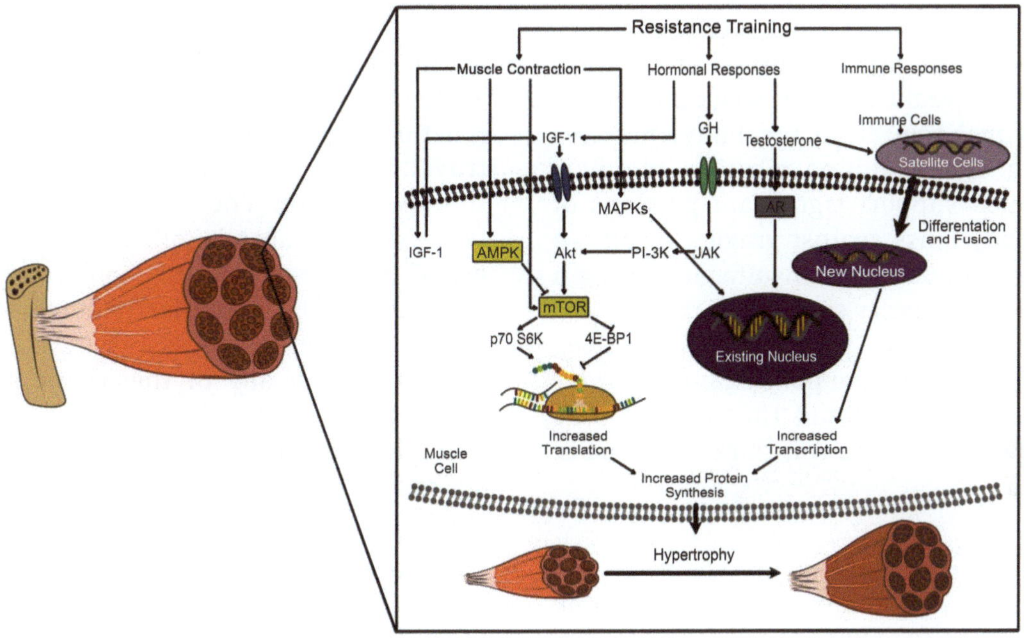

Figure 10.4. *Intracellular adaptions following resistance training and leading to increased protein synthesis. Only the most important steps are pictured, the processes in vivo are much more complex. Abbreviations: Akt = protein kinase B; AMPK = adenosine monophosphate-activated protein kinase; AR = androgen receptor; GH = growth hormone; IGF-1 = insulin-like growth factor 1; JAK = janus kinase; MAPKs = mitogen-activated protein kinase; mTOR = mammalian target of rapamycin; PI-3K = phosphatidylinositol-3 kinase; p70 S6K = 70 kDa ribosomal protein S6 kinase; 4E-BP1 = eukaryotic initiation factor 4 E.*

Source: Zunner BEM, Wachsmuth NB, Eckstein ML, Scherl L, Schierbauer JR, Haupt S, Stumpf C, Reusch L, Moser O. Myokines and resistance training: a narrative review. International Journal of Molecular Sciences. 2022; 23(7):3501. https://doi.org/10.3390/ijms23073501--.

10.3.6. Muscle Weakness

10.3.6.1. Signs and Symptoms

A muscle that is weak fails to produce the anticipated force. The type of muscle disease can be determined by the pattern of muscle weakness, which can affect all or just some of the muscles. The wasting of impacted muscle groups is frequently linked to muscle weakness. When a muscle is weak, it could be due to a defect in the muscle itself, a disease of the brain, spinal cord, or peripheral nerves that prevents the muscle fibers from receiving the right electrical stimulation, or a less-than-maximum voluntary effort. The failure of the contractile machinery can only be linked to weakness after all other factors have been taken into account (e.g., the muscle cell's anatomy). The impact of weakness in a specific muscle group varies according to the muscle's typical function and the extent to which force fails to develop. When muscles close to the extremities weaken, it typically manifests as a tendency to drop objects in the case of upper limb weakness or as "foot drop" in the case of lower limb weakness. The weakness of the more proximal (closer to the body) muscles controlling the shoulder girdles or pelvic girdles, which support significant portions of the total body mass against gravity, results in a greater overall disability. Insufficient strength in the proximal muscles controlling the scapula, for instance, leads to "winging" (i.e., with the arms extended, when the pointed inner border extends rearward). Should the weakness be extreme, there will be no way to raise the arms.

10.3.6.1.1. Assessment

Muscle disease can be identified by evaluating the patient's ability to withstand or outperform the doctor's pull or push, by observing the patient performing isolated voluntary movements against gravity, or by observing the patient engaging in more intricate and coordinated activities like walking. A myometer, which measures force using a hydraulic or electrical principle, can be used to quantify the weakness of individual muscles or groups of muscles. Contraction force recordings over time are useful for assessing whether a weakness is getting better or getting worse. Finding signs of inflammation or damage to the muscles is the goal of evaluating muscle weakness (and wasting). Blood tests or measurements of the electrical characteristics of contracting muscles are used to identify these changes. Muscle biopsies are another investigative tool that can be used for pathological diagnosis and biochemical analysis. Muscle biopsies can be obtained during surgery or with a needle.

10.3.6.1.2. Classification of Muscle Weakness

A nerve impulse that originates in the upper motor neuron and travels from the cerebral cortex of the brain to the spinal cord causes a muscle contraction. The neurotransmitter acetylcholine is released at the neuromuscular junction, which is reached by the nerve impulse traveling via the lower motor neuron from the spinal cord. The neuromuscular junction is crossed by acetylcholine, which stimulates acetylcholine receptors to depolarize the muscle membrane. The muscular fiber contracts as a result. Muscle weakness results from disease or disorder in any of these components, as contraction is dependent on each one of them being healthy.

10.3.6.2. Upper Motor Neuron Disease

One side of the body becomes weak after a stroke due to the muscle weakness typical of upper motor neuron disease. Usually, the leg is extended, the arm is flexed, and the limbs have more tone. While there may be some residual movement, hand function is severely restricted. When it comes to upper motor neuron weakness, the muscle bulk is typically well preserved, in contrast to lower motor neuron or muscle weakness caused by disease. Additional reasons for disorders affecting the upper motor neurons are spinal cord injury, tumors, and multiple sclerosis.

10.3.6.3. Lower Motor Neuron Disease

A flaccid weakness of the muscles is caused by degeneration of the lower neuron. Because denervation of the muscle results from the shrinkage and eventual death of neurons, muscle wasting is a prominent feature. Motor neuron diseases are conditions affecting the motor neurons in the spinal cord. The most prevalent is motor neuron disease, which is also referred to as Lou Gehrig's disease and amyotrophic lateral sclerosis. The affected people typically have upper and lower motor neuron weakness and range in age from 50 to 70. Rapid paralysis progression frequently leads to death in three years. A collection of conditions known as spinal muscular atrophies impact newborns, kids, and young adults and are frequently inherited via an autosomal recessive pattern (i.e., the expression of which requires the gene from both parents). Although older cases of amyotrophic lateral sclerosis typically have less severe symptoms, the infantile form of the disease is fatal within a year. For all these illnesses, there is currently no known cause and no known treatment. Peripheral neuropathies, also known as polyneuropathies, are diseases of the peripheral nerves that can cause symptoms resembling those of motor neuron disorders. Usually, there is also sensory disturbance brought on by involvement of the nerve fibers that carry sensory impulses. Usually, the hands and feet experience symptoms before moving on to other parts of the body. The axons, which make up the core of nerve fibers, can degenerate as a result of peripheral neuropathies. Axon regeneration is possible, but it only occurs at a rate of 1–2 millimeters per day. Thus, the hand will not heal for six to nine months following an injury to a nerve at the elbow. Axonal types of neuropathy are typically brought on by toxins and blood vessel damage. Degeneration of the myelin sheaths, which are the axons' protective sheaths, can also result in peripheral neuropathy. We call these neuropathies demyelinating. The symptoms resemble neuropathies involving axonal degeneration, but the muscles hardly ever atrophy because the axons are still present. Demyelinating neuropathies can heal quickly. Demyelinating neuropathies are brought on by autoimmune illnesses like Guillain-Barré syndrome and diphtheria. Peripheral neuropathy can also be caused by diabetes mellitus, nerve injury, genetics, and long-term renal failure.

10.3.6.4. Neuromuscular Junction Disorders

The production of an end-plate potential that is too low to cause an action potential to propagate through the muscle fiber is a common feature of diseases affecting the neuromuscular junction. Weakness and fatigue with exercise are linked to these diseases. Neuromuscular transmission diseases can be inherited or acquired, and they can be brought on by autoimmune diseases like myasthenia gravis, congenital diseases, toxins like those found in botulism, and certain drug-induced disorders (Engel, 2004; Lane, 2012; Dalakas, 2015; Schapira, 2015; Merlini & Wang, 2018).

10.3.7. Primary Diseases and Disorders

It seems that the use of a muscle determines how much of its mass and function it retains. For instance, the muscle fibers of weightlifters and sprinters have a high capacity for glycolysis, which produces ATP, and rapid force production. After suffering damage, strained muscles can repair themselves and adjust to the weights they support. Therefore, a muscle biopsy from a person with any of the muscular dystrophies is likely to show a combination of the cellular alterations linked to damage and those linked to growth and regeneration (hypertrophy). More damage is done to the muscle cells during eccentric contractions (the resistance to an extending force) than during isometric contractions, or contractions where the muscle shortens (concentric contractions). Even though the metabolic rate during an eccentric contraction may be one-sixth that of an equivalent concentric or isometric contraction, the damage is still greater. When muscles are immobilized, such as after a long bone fracture and placed in a plaster cast, the muscle fibers tend to waste quickly. The reduction of muscle oxidative capacity is a consistent finding. Muscle-strengthening exercises can reverse these changes.

10.3.7.1. The Muscular Dystrophies

A class of inherited diseases known as muscular dystrophies is typified by progressive weakness and atrophy of the muscles. The pelvic and shoulder muscles, which make up the limb girdles, are involved in the majority of varieties. It is commonly established that the primary cause of muscle weakness is muscle degeneration through blood creatine kinase activity measurements, muscle biopsy analysis, and electromyograph recordings. When muscle fibers degenerate, as they do in muscular dystrophies, an enzyme called creatine kinase is released into the bloodstream. Muscle biopsies show the typical degeneration of muscle fibers along with attempts at regeneration. Electromyography demonstrates variations in the electrical patterns of healthy muscle, myopathy, and long-term denervation, including atrophies of the spinal muscles. The Duchenne type of muscular dystrophy, which primarily affects boys, is severe compared to several other varieties that are relatively benign. It results in walking difficulties around the age of four, walking loss around the age of eleven, and death before the age of twenty, usually from pneumonia or respiratory failure. The term pseudohypertrophic muscular dystrophy refers to the paradoxical increase in calf muscle size, which results from the replacement of fat and fibrous tissue instead of the growth of fibers, as in true hypertrophy. An X-linked disorder called Duchenne muscular dystrophy is caused by a gene defect on the X chromosome. While females do not show symptoms of the illness, they are 50% likely to pass on the gene to their sons and daughters, who then become carriers of the gene. The absence of a protein known as dystrophin leads to a rupture in the membrane encasing the muscle fiber, which permits an excessive amount of calcium ions to enter the cell and results in muscle degeneration. Prednisone is one glucocorticoid medicine that may be used to treat the condition and slow its progression.

Similar to Duchenne muscular dystrophy, Becker muscular dystrophy manifests later in life and advances more slowly. Duchenne muscular dystrophy is caused by distinct damage to the same gene on the X chromosome, which results in the production of some functional dystrophin. The face, the muscles surrounding the shoulder blades, and the upper arms are the first areas affected by facioscapulohumeral muscular dystrophy. Compared to Duchenne muscular dystrophy, it progresses more slowly, and most people who have it live normal lives. The weakening of the legs often results in "foot drop" and a waddling gait. Due to the autosomal dominant inheritance pattern of facioscapulohumeral muscular dystrophy, affected individuals inherit the disease from one parent and have a 50% chance of passing it on to their offspring. Similar to facioscapulohumeral muscular dystrophy, but excluding the face, is limb-girdle muscular dystrophy. In most cases, inheritance is autosomal recessive when it is seen; i.e., for the disease to manifest, the impacted gene must be donated by both parents. Other muscular dystrophies exist, and they are all distinguished by a unique pattern of muscle weakness and inheritance. The muscles that move the eyes are primarily affected by ocular muscular dystrophy, also known as myopathy. Oculopharyngeal muscular dystrophy is a condition that primarily affects the muscles of the throat and eyes. It typically manifests in later life and is inherited autosomally dominantly. Distal myopathy mostly affects the hands and feet muscles. Physical therapy, spinal supports, and limb splints are all part of the treatment. Obesity prevention is thought to be important, particularly in cases of Duchenne muscular dystrophy, and infections are treated right away. The best chance of lowering the incidence of this class of diseases is through trait carrier identification, genetic screening, and counseling.

10.3.7.2. Myasthenia Gravis

Muscles with myasthenia gravis are prone to being easily fatigued and exhibit persistent weakness due to a failure in nerve impulse transmission to the muscles. Myasthenia gravis is an acquired autoimmune disorder. Those who are affected have weakness, especially in the neck, limbs, and face. Double vision, trouble breathing and swallowing, and extreme muscle exhaustion during exercise with only a partial recovery following rest are some of the symptoms. Acetylcholine receptors in the neuromuscular junction are destroyed by autoimmune antibodies, which are made against the body's own cells. The disease can be effectively controlled by thymus removal, high doses of corticosteroids (which suppress the immune response), anticholinesterase drugs (which increase nerve impulse transmission), and plasmapheresis (a process that removes autoimmune antibodies from the blood).

10.3.7.3. Toxic Myopathies

Numerous medications and poisons have the potential to harm striated muscle. Certain procedures, like injecting the anesthetic drug bupivacaine intramuscularly, damage muscle fibers by rupturing the membrane, which allows calcium to enter and kill the cell. Certain medications, like the antimalarial drug chloroquine and the cancer treatment drug vincristine, appear to alter the internal biochemistry of the muscle fiber. Some medications, like corticosteroids (which are used to treat inflammation), have an impact on how muscles metabolize. This is especially the case with fluoro-substituted corticosteroids, which increase catabolism and cause proximal muscle weakness, especially in the upper limbs. Lastly, some medications, like the antihypertensive hydralazine, can cause dermatomyositis or polymyositis and lead to an autoimmune disease resembling lupus. Rarely, exposure to anesthetics like halothane and muscle relaxants like succinylcholine can result in malignant hyperthermia, a potentially fatal attack of hyperthermia and muscle rigidity. A rise in body temperature and rigidity occur in the patient during or after the anesthesia is induced. When the core temperature rises above 43 °C (110 °F), sudden death may occur. Such attacks have a high fatality rate; even in the event that the patient survives, exposure to these medications in the future will cause recurrences. The illness may be inherited as an autosomal dominant trait and tends to run in families. Although the exact cause is unknown, it appears to be related to an anomaly in the calcium chemistry of the muscle fiber. When the anesthetic agents are present, extra calcium is released into the sarcoplasm, which encourages the mitochondria to burn glycogen and produce heat. Additionally, too much calcium leads to the contraction and stiffness of the muscle fibers. When taken at the first indication of an attack, medications that stop the release of calcium into the muscle seem to stop the attack. The anesthetic agent should be stopped, and the patient cooled as soon as the attack starts.

10.3.7.4. Inflammatory Myopathies

Following an injury, bacterial myositis—a bacterial infection resulting in muscle tissue inflammation—usually settles into a localized area. Usually, bacteria called Streptococcus and Staphylococcus cause the problem. In addition to localized symptoms of inflammation like reddening, swelling, and warmth, general indicators of infection include fever and elevated white blood cell counts. Except in those who live in tropical areas, abscess formation is uncommon. Antibiotics and minimal surgery are typically used in the treatment of bacterial myositis. Pleurodynia, which is brought on by the Coxsackie virus and is also referred to as Bornholm disease, epidemic myalgia, and devil's grip, is an illustration of viral myositis. After a brief period of intense fever and muscle pain, affected individuals recover fully. Protozoa and helminths, or worms, can also infiltrate the muscles. Eating pork that has been infected and not fully cooked can lead to the roundworm *Trichinella spiralis* infection known as trichinosis. The intestines are the worm's reproductive organ. The larvae migrate out of the walls of the intestine and burrow into the muscle. Fever, aches in the muscles, and occasionally weakness are symptoms. Infection of the heart muscle can cause death, although most trichinosis patients recover in two months or less.

The autoimmune diseases of the muscle, collectively referred to as polymyositis, are oftentimes linked to a characteristic distribution of skin inflammation. Often affected areas include the backs of the hands, elbows, knees, knuckles, cheeks, and eyelids. Dermatomyositis is the term used to describe the joint condition of polymyositis and typical dermatitis. One can have diffuse or proximal muscle weakness. A weak neck and difficulty swallowing are common. The illness may appear suddenly in a few days or gradually over years. A muscle biopsy reveals that white blood cells, primarily lymphocytes, have infiltrated the striated muscle. These seem to harm the muscle fibers as they gather in the spaces between them and around tiny blood vessels. Another important characteristic of dermatomyositis, especially in the pediatric form, is vascular damage. It is unknown what triggers the autoimmune response to the striated muscle. In addition to being commonly linked to other autoimmune disorders like rheumatoid arthritis and progressive systemic sclerosis, the disease has also been linked to cancer in a considerable number of elderly patients, especially those with dermatomyositis. The use of high-dose corticosteroids, frequently in conjunction with cytotoxic immunosuppressants (i.e., cyclophosphamide, which kills cells and weakens the immune system, is often effective in halting the illness and promoting the regeneration of damaged muscles (Engel, 2004; Lane, 2012; Dalakas, 2015; Schapira, 2015; Merlini & Wang, 2018).

10.3.8. Endocrine and Metabolic Myopathies

10.3.8.1. Hormones

In most disorders resulting from either an excess or insufficient production of hormones, striated muscle is either directly or indirectly impacted. This is accurate since there are differences in the rates at which muscle proteins are synthesized or broken down. There is muscle atrophy of both type 1 (oxidatively rich, endurance-producing fibers) and type 2 (glycogen-rich, sprint-type muscle contraction) fibers if the thyroid gland is overactive (thyrotoxicosis, hyperthyroidism). In cases of hypothyroidism or myxedema, which are underactive thyroid conditions, type 1 fibers predominate and type 2 fiber size occasionally decreases. The type 2 fibers selectively atrophy in cases of overactive adrenal gland (Cushing syndrome). This pattern is also observed in patients receiving long-term corticosteroid medication (prednisone for asthma), which can cause significant proximal muscle weakness and wasting.

10.3.8.2. Vitamin D deficiency

The wasting and weakness linked to vitamin D deficiency, which can lead to significant atrophy of type 2 fibers, are caused by a similar mechanism. Although the exact functions of vitamin D in muscle are unknown, it seems that at least one of its metabolites, 25-hydroxycholecalciferol, may have an impact on both the protein turnover and the muscle's resting energy state. Endocrine-related diseases may be highly treatable, in contrast to hereditary muscle diseases.

10.3.8.3. Mitochondrial Myopathies

The parts of cells called mitochondria are responsible for producing energy from the oxidation of fuels like fat and glucose. This energy is then converted into heat and work. There are several biochemical flaws in mitochondria that have been identified. A single thing cannot be identified as having a "mitochondrial myopathy." A common outcome of mitochondrial defects involving a malfunctioning oxidative metabolism is an inclination for the muscles to produce elevated levels of lactic acid. This is a result of having to use the nonoxidative breakdown of the muscle's stored glycogen to produce energy.

10.3.8.4. Glycogenoses

In 1951, British physician Brian McArdle discovered a disorder of muscle that caused cramp-like pains yet was not associated with the normal production of lactic acid from exercise. The defect was later identified as an absence of phosphorylase, the enzyme involved in the first step in the splitting off of the glucose-1-phosphate units from glycogen. Since blood-borne glucose can still be used to make glycogen, this disorder is classified with the glycogen-storage diseases (glycogenoses).

10.3.8.5. Lipid storage myopathies

It could be confusing to refer to lipid storage myopathy because the more severe types of muscle disease (e.g., muscular dystrophy) are frequently linked to the replacement of lost muscle fibers with adipose tissue. Within the cytoplasm of the muscle fiber, triglycerides, or fat, are deposited as microscopic droplets in lipid storage myopathies. Compared to type 2 muscle fibers, normal type 1 muscle fibers contain more lipid droplets. A shuttle system component that carries free fatty acids into mitochondria for subsequent oxidation was found to be impacted by two disorders of muscle fat metabolism in the early 1970s. In the presence of the enzyme acylcarnitine transferase, this shuttle needs the fatty acid (acyl) molecule to bind to the carrier molecule carnitine. After the formed acylcarnitine passes through both the inner and outer mitochondrial membranes, it splits into carnitine and the acyl molecule, which is oxidized, in the presence of an additional form of the enzyme acyltransferase. The cytoplasm stores fat when there is a carnitine deficiency. Muscle damage occurs upon intense exertion due to acylcarnitine transferase deficiency. Since there is a chance for treatment, early detection is crucial.

10.3.8.6. Myotonic Diseases

Myotonia is the inability of a muscle to relax after contraction; this condition can show up as the inability to relax the hand following a handshake. The majority of cases of myotonia are caused by persistent electrical activity of the sarcolemma, which is the membrane of striated muscle fibers. However, slow relaxation may also result from delayed disengagement of the thick and thin filaments of myosin and actin. A single nerve action potential initiates multiple firings of the sarcolemma in this most prevalent form of myotonia, thereby perpetuating muscular contraction. Unusual ion pumps or channels in the sarcolemma are the root cause of this issue, though the precise source is unknown. The cold aggravates myotonia in many of its forms. Another symptom of the myotonic syndromes is weakness; myotonia usually becomes more noticeable after inactivity and rapidly "warms up" when exercise is initiated. The most prevalent myotonic disorder is myotonic dystrophy. It is an autosomal dominant disorder that affects not just muscle but many other body systems as well. Premature baldness, cataract development, cognitive decline, gonadal atrophy, hormone imbalances, gastrointestinal problems, and degeneration of muscle fibers are among the symptoms. Although the disease typically manifests by the time a person reaches the age of 25, some affected individuals may not experience any significant symptoms for the duration of their lives. Thomsen disease, also known as myotonia congenita, is an autosomal dominant disorder that does not exhibit dystrophic features. The condition usually starts at birth and manifests as extreme difficulty relaxing the muscle following a forced contraction, like sneezing. When startled, goats with hereditary myotonia congenita, also known as fainting goats, exhibit severe muscle stiffness. Understanding the molecular processes that underlie this reaction could provide insight on the corresponding disorder in humans. A variety of other conditions, such as periodic paralysis, can also result in myotonia. Medication that reduces the degree of myotonia, such as phenytoin, procainamide, and quinine, has varying degrees of success in treating weakness. There is presently no treatment for these illnesses.

10.3.9. The Periodic Paralyzes

People who have periodic paralysis experience recurrent episodes of muscle paralysis, which can last anywhere from 30 minutes to a full day. Attacks mostly target the muscles in the legs, with the arms and trunk receiving less attention. The muscles may become slightly swollen and tender during an attack. Attacks often happen when you're at rest following intense exercise. Periodic paralysis comes in two varieties. The blood potassium level drops during a hypokalemic periodic paralysis attack, which can also be brought on by anything that tends to lower the potassium level. Conversely, an elevated potassium level is linked to hyperkalemic periodic paralysis. Oral potassium therapy may trigger an attack. Periodic paralysis is a disorder that is inherited dominantly. Although neither is likely to cause permanent muscle weakness, there may be a significant amount of temporary incapacity. The muscle fibers become depolarized during the attack, losing their electrical potential and their ability to be excited. The illness seems to be brought on by modifications in the ions' passage through the skeletal muscle membranes. One of the ions thought to be in charge of the illness is potassium. The cause could be abnormal ion pumps or channels in the membrane. Treatment with drugs that appropriately change potassium levels, like acetazolamide, might work well.

10.3.10. Fatigue

The inability of a muscle to maintain force during an extended contraction or to regain force during repeated contractions is known as fatigue. The mechanisms that underlie fatigue and weakness are similar in that they involve electrical excitation of the muscle cell, electromechanical coupling, and the primary energy-producing processes for work, contraction, and heat production. Acetylcholine released from the presynaptic nerve terminal causes the postsynaptic membrane of the neuromuscular junction to depolarize, which in turn causes the action potential that runs the length of the muscle cell. Thus, in the chain of command for muscular contraction, the synapse may be an important control point. When curare or botulinum toxin poisoning occurs, there is a total failure of neuromuscular transmission, which leads to total paralysis. One of the characteristics of myasthenia gravis is incomplete or variable neuromuscular transmission; this condition can be diagnosed by looking for signs of fatigue in response to electrical stimulation of the muscle-supplying nerve. This behavior is a result of antibodies to the acetylcholine receptor causing immunologic damage to the postsynaptic membrane of the synapse (Figure 10.5).

Some of the mechanisms underlying muscle fatigue can be examined by electrically stimulating a muscle via its nerve at various frequencies and observing the force of the contractions that result. Myasthenia gravis causes a failure of force at high stimulation frequencies. Fatigue is also common in situations where normal muscle is either overheated or not receiving enough blood flow. There exists a connection between the onset of fatigue and the exhaustion of muscle energy reserves during exercise. Fatigue during extended exercise, like marathon running, is linked to oxidative glycolysis-induced glycogen depletion. Short, high-intensity workouts are linked to intracellular acidosis and the build-up of lactate from anaerobic (nonoxidative) glycolysis. While there is no discernible loss of adenosine triphosphate (ATP), there is a decrease in phosphocreatine in both forms of exercise. In contrast, even with low total work or power output, more noticeable alterations are observed in people with myopathies. Fatigue is not linked to the typical acidosis in people with McArdle disease, where glycogenolysis is absent. Phosphocreatine resynthesis after exercise may be sluggish in people with impaired mitochondrial metabolism, who may develop profound acidosis (Engel, 2004; Lane, 2012; Dalakas, 2015; Schapira, 2015; Merlini & Wang, 2018).

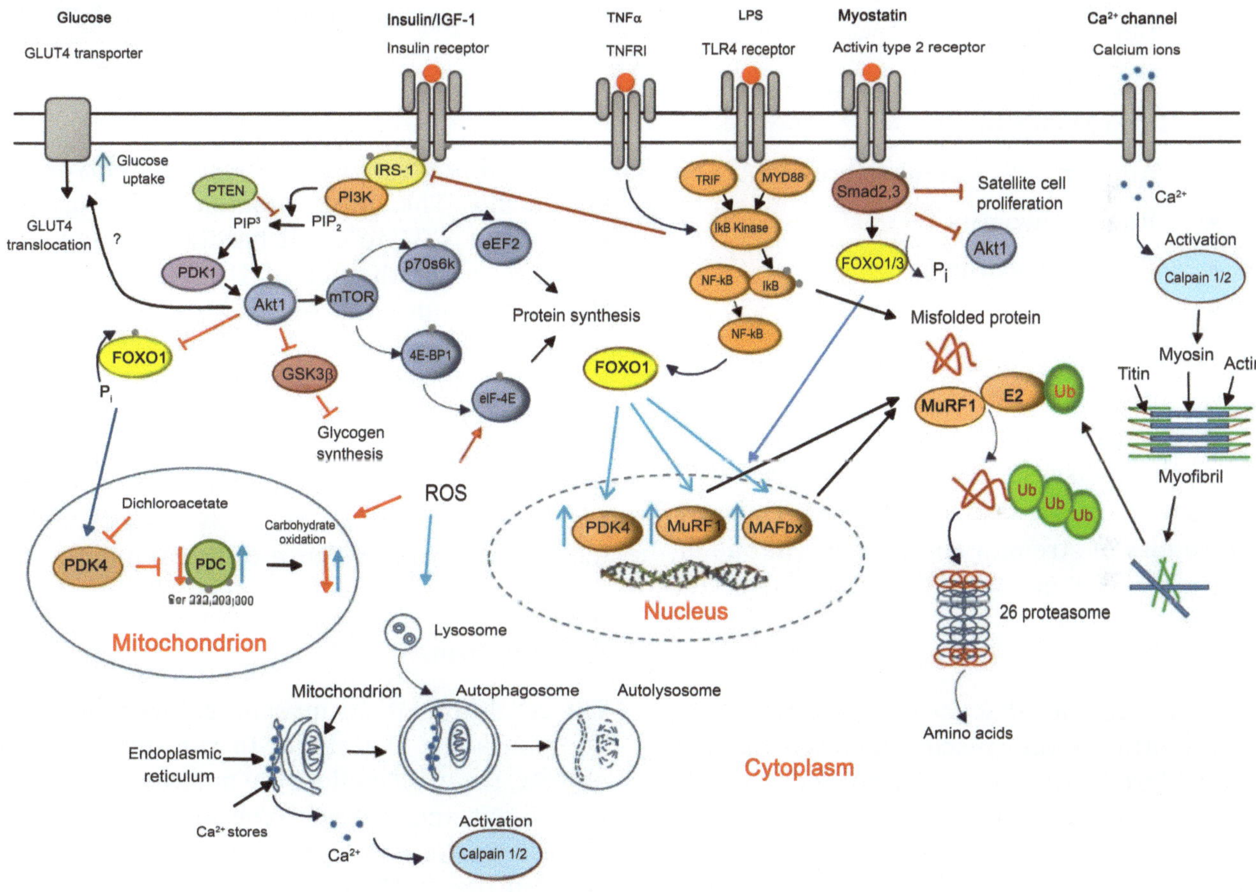

Figure 10.5. *A schematic illustration of the main molecular mechanisms underlying muscle wasting and thereby to muscle fatigue (red lines/arrows indicate downregulation, blue lines/arrows indicate upregulation).*

Source: Constantin-Teodosiu D, Constantin D. Molecular Mechanisms of Muscle Fatigue. International Journal of Molecular Sciences. 2021; 22(21):11587. https://doi.org/10.3390/ijms222111587––.

10.4. Types of Muscular System Diseases

A muscle disease is any disease that affects the human muscle system. Primary muscle diseases result from abnormalities of the muscles themselves. Secondary muscle diseases are caused by another condition that may have triggered or caused the muscle disease.

Primary muscular system diseases include:

- Polymyositis
- Dermatomyositis
- Muscular dystrophy
- Myasthenia gravis
- Amyotrophic lateral sclerosis (ALS)
- Rhabdomyolysis
- Cardiomyopathy
- Sarcopenia

Both primary and secondary muscular system diseases affect the muscles and sometimes the nerves that supply them. Because of this, these diseases may eventually result in muscle wasting or loss of muscle mass. This may involve loss of strength and function in one or more muscles. Sometimes paralysis may occur.

10.4.1. Primary Muscle Diseases

Primary muscle diseases are caused by abnormalities of the muscles. A muscle disease is considered primary if it occurs on its own, not because of any other associated diseases.

10.4.1.1. Polymyositis

Inflammation of the muscles and the tissues that surround them, including the blood vessels, is called myositis. A rare type of myositis is called polymyositis (PM). PM is more common in women over the age of twenty-five. Muscle weakness and inflammation are hallmarks of PM. An individual suffering from this ailment might have difficulties getting up after falling. Additional signs and symptoms include a persistent dry cough and/or trouble swallowing. There is no known cause for PM, and there is no cure for the illness. Fortunately, there are treatments available for the illness. Polymyositis is a condition that leads to irritated and inflamed muscles. Eventually, the muscles start to weaken and deteriorate. Every muscle in the body may be affected by the condition. This can make even seemingly simple movements challenging. Polymyositis is among the diseases classified as inflammatory myopathies.

a. Causes.

It is unknown what causes polymyositis specifically. The most common age range for it to occur is 31 to 60. It hardly ever happens to those under the age of 18. Experts believe that an autoimmune reaction or a virus may be connected to or the cause of polymyositis. When the body targets its own tissues, it is known as an autoimmune reaction. A medication may occasionally trigger an allergic reaction that damages and irritates muscles. However, medical professionals typically aren't able to identify the precise cause of the ailment.

b. Symptoms

The condition affects muscles all over the body, and can affect the ability to run, walk, or lift objects. It can also affect the muscles that allow you to eat and breathe. The muscles that are closest to the center of the body tend to be affected the most often.

The common symptoms of polymyositis include:

- Muscle pain and stiffness
- Muscle weakness, particularly in the belly (abdomen), shoulders, upper arms, and hips

- Joint pain and stiffness
- Trouble catching your breath
- Problems with swallowing
- Irregular heart rhythms, if the heart muscle becomes inflamed

Doing daily tasks can be difficult if you have polymyositis. You might experience difficulty standing up from a chair, raising your arms, or climbing stairs. Ankles, wrists, and the lower arm region may experience pain and weakness as inflammation throughout the body worsens. If eating and swallowing become difficult due to muscle weakness, weight loss and poor nutrition could become an issue.

c. Diagnosis

The process starts with a health history and a physical exam. The exam will include seeing how strong your muscles are. You may need tests such as:

- **Blood tests**. These are done to look for signs of musclc inflammation. They also check for abnormal proteins that form in autoimmune disease.
- **Electromyelogram (EMG).** This may be done to find abnormal electrical activity in affected muscles.
- **MRI**. This test uses large magnets and a computer to look for inflammation in the body.
- **Muscle biopsy**. Tiny pieces of tissue are taken to be checked with a microscope.

d. Treatment

Treatment will depend on your symptoms, your age, and your general health. It will also depend on how severe the condition is. There's no cure for polymyositis, but the symptoms can be managed. You may need more than one kind of treatment. And your treatment may need to be changed over time. In severe cases, some treatments don't work as well. Treatments include:

- *Anti-inflammatory medicines.* These are steroid medicines or corticosteroids. They ease inflammation in the body. Symptoms usually get better within 4 to 6 weeks. Your healthcare provider may lower the dose of steroids after that to ease side effects. Some people may need to take steroids ongoing to manage the disease and reduce symptoms.
- *Immunosuppressive medicines.* These are medicines that block or slow down your body's immune system.
- *Physical therapy.* This includes special exercises help to stretch and strengthen the muscles. These can help keep muscles from shrinking.
- *Heat therapy and rest.* These can help ease muscle symptoms.
- *Braces or other special devices.* These can help to support muscles and help with movement.

Talk with your healthcare providers about the risks, benefits, and possible side effects of all medicines.

10.4.1.2. Dermatomyositis

Dermatomyositis (DM) is a rare inflammatory muscle disease. It can affect people of any age or sex, though it's more often seen in women.

Common symptoms of DM include:

- A distinctive rash
- Muscle weakness
- Inflamed, painful muscles

The cause of this inflammatory myopathy is unknown, as with others. Although there isn't a cure, the illness can be controlled with medication and other treatments. A rare condition called dermatomyositis results in skin rashes and muscle inflammation. It belongs to a class of illnesses that affect the muscles and result in swelling and inflammation. It differs from other diseases of the muscles in that it also results in skin issues. The term "dermatomyositis" refers to symptoms that affect both the skin and the muscles. Although it can happen to anyone at any age, adults between the ages of 50 and 70 are the most commonly affected. The disease is twice as likely to strike women as it does men. Some patients also suffer from a connective tissue disease, like rheumatoid arthritis or lupus.

a. Causes

- The exact cause is not known, but possible causes include:
- Abnormal genes you are born with
- Cancer, especially in older people
- Autoimmune disease is a type of illness that causes the body's immune system to attack its own tissues
- An infection, medication, or another exposure in your environment that triggers the disease

b. Symptoms

The symptoms are caused by swelling and inflammation in the blood vessels that supply your skin and muscles and can include the following:

- Red or purple rash on sun-exposed areas that may be painful or itchy
- Red or purple swelling of the upper eyelids (heliotrope)
- Red or purple spots on the knuckles, elbows, knees, and toes (Gottron's papules)
- Joints that feel stuff and turn pale and painful in cold conditions and feel better when warmed (Raynaud's phenomenon)
- Scaly, rough, dry skin, which can lead to hair thinning
- Swollen, red areas around the fingernails
- Hard lumps under the skin caused by calcium deposits (calcinosis)
- Muscle weakness in the neck, hip, back, and shoulders
- Trouble swallowing and voice changes
- Tiredness, fever, and weight loss
- Muscle aches
- Trouble rising from a chair or getting out of bed due to muscle weakness

Sometimes the muscle weakness also spreads to the heart, GI tract, and lungs. This can cause breathing trouble and coughing. Adults may have a low-grade fever, along with lung inflammation and sensitivity to light.

c. Diagnosis

The process starts with a person's medical history and a physical exam. The health care provider will look for an underlying disease, such as cancer. Tests may also be done, such as:

- **Blood tests.** These are done to look for signs of muscle inflammation. They also check for abnormal proteins that form in autoimmune diseases. The most common blood tests include muscle enzyme creatine kinase and the antinuclear antibody.

- **Electromyelogram (EMG).** This may be done to find abnormal electrical activity in affected muscles.
- **MRI.** This test uses large magnets and a computer to look for inflammation in the body.
- **Skin or muscle biopsy.** Tiny pieces of tissue are taken to be checked with a microscope.

d. Treatment

Treatment will depend on your symptoms, your age, and your general health. There's no cure for the condition, but the symptoms can be managed. You may need more than one kind of treatment. And your treatment may need to be changed over time. Treatments include:

- **Physical therapy.** Special exercises help to stretch and strengthen the muscles. Orthotics or assistive devices may be used.
- **Skin treatment.** You may need to avoid sun exposure and wear sunscreen to help prevent skin rashes. Your health care provider can treat itchy skin rashes with antihistamine drugs or with anti-inflammatory steroid creams that are applied to the skin.
- **Anti-inflammatory medications**. These are steroid drugs, or corticosteroids. They ease inflammation in the body. They may be given by mouth or through an IV.
- **Immunosuppressive drugs**. These are drugs that block or slow down your body's immune system. These include the drugs azathioprine, methotrexate, cyclosporine A, cyclophosphamide, and tacrolimus.
- **Immunoglobulin.** If you have not responded to other treatments, these drugs may be given. They are donated blood products that may boost your body's immune system. They are put directly into your bloodstream through an IV.
- **Surgery**. Surgery may be done to remove the calcium deposits (calcinosis) under the skin if they become painful or infected.

Talk with your health care providers about the risks, benefits, and possible side effects of all medications.

10.4.1.3. Muscular Dystrophy

A class of inherited myopathies known as muscular dystrophy (MD) exists. Weakness and loss of muscle are the results of these conditions. Certain forms of MD manifest in early life. Some might not show up until later in life, or perhaps middle age. Symptoms differ depending on the affected muscle groups and individuals, and they are particular to the type of MD. Over time, every type of MD gets worse. Most people experience a loss of mobility. MD cannot be cured, although its symptoms can be managed. Additionally, treatment can avert complications.

Treatments include:

- Medications
- Physical therapy
- Speech therapy
- Orthopedic devices, such as canes or walkers
- Surgery

Some MD patients experience mild symptoms that develop gradually. Others experience severe, incapacitating symptoms.

A condition called muscular dystrophy (MD) causes muscles to gradually weaken. A child's muscles deteriorate with age. Fatty tissue takes their place. Movements like standing up and walking can be difficult with MD. It might even result in joint deformities. MD is an inherited illness. It is therefore inherited. Children are more likely to have the condition if there is a family history of it. Nine different types of MD exist. Certain types do not manifest until a child reaches adulthood. Some induce symptoms at a young age. Between the ages of three and six, children are typically diagnosed with the disorder. The two most prevalent kinds in children are known as Becker and Duchenne muscular dystrophies.

a. Symptoms

Children with MD often have movement problems when they are young. They may start to walk later than normal. They may have trouble getting up from a sitting or lying position. Weakness in the shoulders and pelvic muscles is an early symptom.

Children may also have these other common symptoms of the disorder:

- Clumsiness
- Problems climbing stairs
- Trouble jumping or hopping
- Frequent tripping or falling
- Walking on their toes
- Leg pain
- Weakness in the face, shoulder, and arms
- Inability to open or close the eyes
- Large calves from fat buildup

As MD progresses, a child may have heart or lung problems. He or she may also have scoliosis. Scoliosis is a condition that causes the spine to curve. A child with scoliosis may look like he or she is leaning to one side.

b. Diagnosing Muscular Dystrophy

MD may look like other health problems. To diagnose it, your child's doctor first does a physical exam. He or she may also ask about your child's medical history. A genetic blood test may help diagnose the disorder along with other blood tests.

Other tests that may confirm MD include:

- Muscle biopsy. A sample of muscle is looked at under a microscope.
- Electromyogram. This test can find out if there is the breakdown of muscle tissue.
- Electrocardiogram (ECG or EKG). This test can spot heart problems, such as an irregular heartbeat or damage to the heart muscle.

c. Treating Muscular Dystrophy

MD is a lifelong condition. There is no cure. However, managing it can prevent problems and deformities. The exact treatment depends on many things, including the child's age, overall health, and the type of MD.

A child with MD will eventually need a wheelchair because of weak leg muscles. Keeping the child as independent as possible is the main focus of treatment.Options include:

- Physical therapy
- Medicines including deflazacort
- Psychological and nutritional counseling

Braces and splints may support and protect muscles. Special devices can help a child sit, stand, or lie down. Surgery may also be needed to fix scoliosis or other related problems.

10.4.1.4. Myasthenia Gravis

An autoimmune neuromuscular disorder called myasthenia gravis (MG) affects the communication between muscles and nerves. The immune system attacks the receptors in MG patients, impairing their ability to communicate between nerve cells and muscles. Muscle weakness results from this disruption of nerve signals to the muscles. MG is the cause of the majority of chronic autoimmune neuromuscular disorders, affecting twenty out of every 100,000 individuals. The main symptom of MG is voluntary skeletal muscle weakness. While there is no known cure for MG, it is possible to manage immune system activity. The prognosis for MG varies for each individual. Some may only have mild symptoms, while others may experience disabilities. Early medical intervention can help slow the progression of the disease. Myasthenia gravis does not have hereditary or contagious forms. It typically appears later in life when the body's antibodies attack healthy muscle receptors, preventing the chemical needed for muscle contraction. When antibodies from a woman with myasthenia gravis are passed to the fetus, the fetus may develop a temporary form of the condition, which usually resolves within two to three months.

What are the symptoms of myasthenia gravis?

These are the most common symptoms of myasthenia gravis:

- Visual problems, including drooping eyelids (ptosis) and double vision (diplopia)
- Muscle weakness and fatigue may vary rapidly in intensity over days or even hours and worsen as muscles are used (early fatigue)
- Facial muscle involvement causing a mask-like appearance; a smile may appear more like a snarl
- Trouble swallowing or pronouncing words
- Weakness of the neck or limbs

The symptoms of myasthenia gravis may look like other conditions. Always see your doctor for a diagnosis.

Flare-ups and remissions (easing of symptoms) may occur now and then during the course of myasthenia gravis. Remissions, however, are only rarely permanent or complete.

1. How is myasthenia gravis diagnosed?

Your symptoms and certain tests can help your doctor diagnose myasthenia gravis. Your doctor will inquire about your symptoms and medical history during the physical examination. Assessing your response to specific medications is a common method of diagnosing myasthenia gravis. When you take an anticholinesterase medication, your muscle weakness usually significantly improves for a short while. Your response to the medication indicates that you have myasthenia gravis.

Other tests that may be done include:

- Blood tests. These tests look for antibodies that may be present in people with myasthenia gravis.
- Genetic tests. These tests are done to check for conditions that run in families.
- Nerve conduction studies. A test called repetitive nerve stimulation is used to diagnose myasthenia gravis.
- Electromyogram (EMG). A test that measures the electrical activity of a muscle. An EMG can detect abnormal electrical muscle activity due to diseases and neuromuscular conditions.

2. How is myasthenia gravis treated?

Specific treatment for myasthenia gravis will be determined by your healthcare provider based on:

- How old you are
- Your overall health and medical history
- How sick you are
- How well you can handle specific medicines, procedures, or therapies
- How long the condition is expected to last
- Your opinion or preference

Myasthenia gravis cannot be cured; however, its symptoms are frequently manageable. Myasthenia gravis is an illness that affects people forever. The secret to treating the condition is early detection. Enhancing muscle function and preventing breathing and swallowing issues are the main objectives of treatment. The majority of patients with this illness are able to strengthen their muscles and lead lives that are normal or almost normal. Assistance with breathing and eating might be required in more serious situations.

Treatment may include:

- Medicine. Anticholinesterase medicines, steroids, or medicines that suppress the immune system's response (immunosuppressive) medicines may be used.
- Thymectomy. This is the surgical removal of the thymus gland. The role of the thymus gland in myasthenia gravis is not fully understood, and the thymectomy may or may not improve symptoms. However, it reduces symptoms in more than 70% of people who do not have cancer of the thymus, possibly by altering the immune system response.
- Plasmapheresis. A procedure that removes abnormal antibodies from the blood and replaces the blood with normal antibodies from donated blood.
- Immunoglobulin. A blood product that helps decrease the immune system's attack on the nervous system. It is given intravenously (IV).

3. Complications

A myasthenic crisis is one of the most dangerous side effects of myasthenia gravis. This condition is characterized by extreme muscular weakness, especially in the diaphragm and chest muscles that support breathing. Breathing could become labored or shallow. A buildup of secretions and weakening of the throat muscles can cause blockage of the airway. Factors such as lack of medication, respiratory infection, psychological stress, surgery, or other types of stress can lead to a myasthenic crisis. In severe cases, a person might require ventilator support to assist with breathing until their muscle strength improves with therapy.

Precautions that may help prevent or reduce the occurrence of a myasthenic crisis include:

- Taking anticholinesterase medications 30 to 45 minutes before meals to lower the risk of aspiration (food entering the lungs)
- Taking anticholinesterase medications as prescribed to maintain the strength of the breathing muscles
- Avoiding crowds and contact with people with respiratory infections, such as a cold or the flu

- Taking in proper nutrition to maintain optimal weight and muscle strength
- Balancing periods of physical activity with periods of rest
- Using stress-reduction techniques and avoiding emotional extremes

Tell your healthcare providers about your condition when any medicines are being prescribed. Certain medicines may interfere either with the disease or the action of the medicines you take for myasthenia gravis.

10.4.1.5. Amyotrophic Lateral Sclerosis

Another name for amyotrophic lateral sclerosis (ALS) is Lou Gehrig's disease. This collection of rare neurological conditions affects the nerve cells in the brain and spinal cord. ALS affects the muscles involved in voluntary movement. Most cases occur in individuals aged 40 to 70 years old. Some estimates suggest that at least 16,000 Americans have this condition. Symptoms of ALS worsen over time, and there is currently no known cure. Complications can be managed, and symptoms can be controlled with treatment. However, the average life expectancy after diagnosis is only a few years.

Treatments for ALS include:

- Medication
- Speech therapy
- Physical therapy

In severe cases, patients may need nutritional and breathing support.

10.4.1.6. Rhabdomyolysis

The illness known as rhabdomyolysis results in the disintegration of skeletal muscle. Myoglobin is released into the circulation as a result of this breakdown. In the muscles, a protein called myoglobin stores oxygen. An excessive amount of myoglobin in the blood can harm the kidneys.

Causes of rhabdomyolysis include:

- Trauma
- Infection and inflammation
- Medications
- Toxins
- Genetic and metabolic disorders8

Treatment depends on the severity of symptoms and the presence of complications. Kidney damage from rhabdomyolysis may not be reversible.

10.4.1.7. Cardiomyopathy

A disease that affects the cardiac muscle is called cardiomyopathy, or heart muscle disease. The heart grows abnormally large, thick, and/or stiff when it has cardiomyopathy. The heart muscle finds it more difficult to pump blood effectively as a result. This could eventually result in heart failure. Fluids and blood can back up into the lungs and other body organs. Heart valve issues and irregular cardiac rhythms can also be brought on by cardiomyopathy.

10.4.1.8. Sarcopenia

Sarcopenia, also called geriatric muscle disease, is common in older adults. Other types of muscle diseases are less common in older adults. Sarcopenia risk in older adults ages 65 to 70 is around 14%. This risk is 53% in those over age 80.

Sarcopenia causes loss of muscle mass and strength. Risk factors include:

- Poor nutrition
- Chronic disease
- Reduced hormone levels

For some people, muscle weakness appears suddenly. For others, it comes on slowly over many years.

Sarcopenia can be diagnosed in many ways, including:

- Physical exam
- Medical history
- Blood tests to look for inflammation, genetic disease, low hormone levels, or low vitamin D levels
- Imaging, such as magnetic resonance imaging (MRI)
- Electrical activity testing
- Muscle biopsy

Physical therapy, an improved diet, and medications can improve the condition (Engel, 2004; Lane, 2012; Dalakas, 2015; Schapira, 2015; Merlini & Wang, 2018).

10.4.2. Secondary Muscle Diseases

Sometimes, muscle diseases appear as a result of other more serious health conditions. They may appear with many different diseases, including:

- Infectious diseases
- Endocrine disorders, or diseases of the glands
- Metabolic disorders, such as diabetes
- Immunological conditions such as HIV/AIDS
- Vascular diseases, conditions of the blood vessels

Primary muscle diseases that can also be secondary to another health condition include:

- Rhabdomyolysis
- Myopathy
- Myositis
- Myasthenia gravis
- Sarcopenia

Some secondary muscle diseases may even affect the respiratory muscles.

Secondary muscle diseases are diagnosed in the same way as primary conditions. Treatment involves managing the underlying cause and treating the secondary condition (Engel, 2004; Lane, 2012; Dalakas, 2015; Schapira, 2015; Merlini and Wang, 2018).

A Closer Look

Metabolic Muscle Diseases

Metabolic muscle diseases encompass a group of genetic disorders characterized by abnormalities in the biochemical pathways responsible for energy production within muscle cells. These conditions affect the way muscles utilize and store energy, leading to various symptoms ranging from muscle weakness and fatigue to more severe complications. One prominent example is mitochondrial myopathies, which result from defects in the mitochondria, the cellular organelles responsible for generating energy in the form of adenosine triphosphate (ATP). These defects can arise from mutations in genes encoding proteins essential for mitochondrial function, leading to impaired ATP production and muscle dysfunction.

Another metabolic muscle disease is Pompe disease, a lysosomal storage disorder caused by a deficiency of the enzyme acid alpha-glucosidase (GAA). This enzyme is responsible for breaking down glycogen, a complex sugar molecule, into glucose for energy. In Pompe disease, the buildup of glycogen within muscle cells impairs their function, resulting in progressive muscle weakness and respiratory difficulties. Similarly, McArdle disease, also known as glycogen storage disease type V, is caused by a deficiency of the enzyme myophosphorylase, which is involved in the breakdown of glycogen into glucose-1-phosphate. Without this enzyme, individuals with McArdle disease experience exercise intolerance, muscle cramps, and stiffness due to the inability to generate sufficient energy during physical activity.

These metabolic muscle diseases can manifest in various ways, depending on the specific biochemical pathways affected and the severity of the underlying genetic mutations. Symptoms may include muscle weakness, fatigue, exercise intolerance, cramping, stiffness, and, in severe cases, respiratory or cardiac complications. Diagnosis typically involves a combination of clinical evaluation, biochemical testing, genetic analysis, and muscle biopsy to assess enzyme activity and tissue abnormalities. Treatment options for metabolic muscle diseases are often limited and primarily focus on managing symptoms and improving quality of life. This may involve physical therapy to maintain mobility, dietary modifications to optimize energy metabolism, and, in some cases, enzyme replacement therapy or gene therapy to address underlying enzyme deficiencies.

Research into metabolic muscle diseases continues to advance our understanding of their underlying mechanisms and potential therapeutic interventions. Strategies aimed at restoring energy metabolism, reducing glycogen accumulation, or targeting specific genetic mutations hold promise for future treatments. Additionally, ongoing efforts to improve diagnostic techniques and expand access to specialized care are essential for optimizing outcomes and enhancing the quality of life for individuals affected by these challenging conditions.

Summary

- Muscle disorders are the diseases and disorders that affect the human muscle system, and their main manifestation is skeletal muscle weakness. The terms 'muscular dystrophy,' 'neuromuscular conditions,' and 'neuromuscular disorders' fall under the umbrella of the term 'muscle disorders.'
- Muscle disorders comprise a heterogeneous group of diseases that are either inherited or acquired. These can present in a wide variety of ways, but the most common symptom attributable to primary muscle disease is weakness.
- Skeletal muscle has only a limited number of responses to damage, and therefore, patients present with only a limited number of symptoms and signs. Positive symptoms include myalgias, cramps, contractures, myoglobinuria, and muscle stiffness.
- A stepwise approach to narrowing down the diagnosis of patients presenting with muscle disorders can help select the investigations that are likely to be of the highest yield. Initial investigations should screen for reversible causes of myopathy.
- Myositis-specific autoantibodies can be useful to confirm autoimmune myositis, but their main role is to subclassify and thereby assist with prognosis and choice of treatment.
- Ultrasound muscle imaging has been mainly used as a non-invasive tool in the pediatric population for the assessment of skeletal muscle disorders. Specific neuromuscular disorders can differ in the pattern of muscles involved, which is reflected in the ultrasonographic appearance of various muscles.
- Sequencing custom gene panels usually involves targeted 'capture' or amplification of a specific list of genes, for example, all genes known to cause neuromuscular disease.

References

1. Amato, A. A., & Russell, J. A. (2016). *Neuromuscular Disorders* (2nd ed.). McGraw-Hill Education.
2. Dalakas, M. C. (2015). *Inflammatory Myopathies* (3rd ed.). Springer.
3. Dubowitz, V., & Sewry, C. A. (2007). *Muscle Biopsy: A Practical Approach* (3rd ed.). Saunders Ltd.
4. Emery, A. E. (2008). *Emery's Elements of Medical Genetics* (13th ed.). Churchill Livingstone.
5. Engel, A. G., & Franzini-Armstrong, C. (2004). *Myology: Basic and Clinical* (3rd ed.). McGraw-Hill Medical.
6. Hilton-Jones, D., & Griggs, R. C. (Eds.). (2010). *Disorders of Voluntary Muscle* (8th ed.). Cambridge University Press.
7. Katirji, B., Kaminski, H. J., & Ruff, R. L. (Eds.). (2014). *Neuromuscular Disorders in Clinical Practice* (2nd ed.). Springer.
8. Lane, R. J. (2012). *Muscle Disorders in Childhood* (2nd ed.). Springer.
9. Merlini, L., & Wang, Z. (Eds.). (2018). *Myopathies: Clinical, Diagnostic and Therapeutic Aspects*. Springer.
10. Schapira, A. H. V. (Ed.). (2015). *Oxford Textbook of Neurology* (2nd ed.). Oxford University Press.

INDEX

N

O

P

R

S

T

Kolibri 360 GmbH
Ferdinand-Jühlke-Straße 7
99095 Erfurt, Deutschland
produktsicherheit@kolibri360.de